Ophthalmic Surgery for Beginners

Springer

Frank Wilhelm
Editor

Ophthalmic Surgery for Beginners

Surgical Planning and Techniques Step by Step

Springer

Editor
Frank Wilhelm
Greifswald
Universitätsklinikum Halle Saale,
Germany

ISBN 978-3-662-70286-4 ISBN 978-3-662-70287-1 (eBook)
https://doi.org/10.1007/978-3-662-70287-1

This book is a translation of the original German edition "Ophthalmochirurgie für Einsteiger" by Frank Wilhelm, published by Springer-Verlag GmbH, DE in 2023. The translation was done with the help of an artificial intelligence machine translation tool. A subsequent human revision was done primarily in terms of content, so that the book will read stylistically differently from a conventional translation. Springer Nature works continuously to further the development of tools for the production of books and on the related technologies to support the authors.

This Springer imprint is published by the registered company Springer-Verlag GmbH, DE, part of Springer Nature.
The registered company address is: Heidelberger Platz 3, 14197 Berlin, Germany

I would like to dedicate this book to two people, without whom nothing would be as it is for me today: My teacher Günther Franke, who inspired my passion for ophthalmology, and my wife Antje, who is always there for me.

Foreword

This book actually deserves an ophthalmological merit medal: It fills a gap that has existed for many years in the list of ophthalmological textbooks.

Since Georg Eisner's textbook on eye surgery, there has been no systematic presentation that so fandamentally deals with the principles of eye surgery on the one hand and their detailed application on the other hand.

But this is extremely important: Surgery is not just Χειρ-ουργια—handiwork: It is above all Κεφαλ-ουργια—headwork: One must analyze, anderstand, comprehend what one wants to do—then the hand will already know to do what it should. As someone who is fandamentally not excessively gifted manually, I know very well what I am talking about …

For excellent surgery—especially in our field—intellectual penetration and analysis, practical guidance—and practice!—and the passing on of "tricks" are needed: This triumvirate makes the difference.

This book by Mr. Wilhelm follows exactly this path. It analyzes and explains, proceeds systematically, but also very practically and in great detail. Thus, it is valuable not only for the future surgeon but also for the already practicing surgeon—and it is also valuable for the non-surgically active ophthalmologist: It enables a rational analysis of surgical aspects even for those who do not perform them actively themselves but who should and want to competently advise their patients.

I wish for this book that, in its systematic approach, its practical clarity, and its honesty, it becomes the "Bible" that it deserves to be.

Thomas Neuhann

Foreword

The present book is necessary and important.

It closes a gap that has existed for decades in the literature on ophthalmic surgical training and continuing education.

Eye surgery is gaining increasing importance in the overall medical spectrum.

Three of the most common operations performed on this planet are eye surgeries. It must be in all of our interests to train good eye surgeons and to support them in becoming even better.

This book makes a valuable contribution to this.

What is important for a young person who wants to learn ophthalmic surgery?

Are there necessary prerequisites for this?

a) *The mind: To operate well and reproducibly, a clear theoretical concept is necessary. The operation must be divided into many individual steps. At any time during an operation, a circumstance may arise that makes it necessary to change the originally planned course of the operation. Therefore, it must be clearly defined what to do if something goes differently than planned. The theoretical concept of the operation, the optimal procedure, must be perfectly anderstood. The analysis also includes knowledge of all possible risks (complications) and the know-how to manage these complicationsTo operate well and reproducibly, a clear theoretical concept is necessary. The operation must be divided into many individual steps. At any time during an operation, a circumstance may arise that makes it necessary to change the originally planned course of the operation. Therefore, it must be clearly defined what to do if something goes differently than planned. The theoretical concept of the operation, the optimal procedure, must be perfectly anderstood. The analysis also includes knowledge of all possible risks (complications) and the know-how to manage these complications*
b) *The craft: Manual dexterity, a steady hand, and good vision are important prerequisites for performing high-quality microsurgery.the mind:*

To operate well and reproducibly, a clear theoretical concept is necessary. The operation must be divided into many individual steps.

At any time during an operation, a circumstance may arise that makes it necessary to change the originally planned course of the operation. Therefore, it must be clearly defined what to do if something goes differently than planned.

The theoretical concept of the operation, the optimal procedure, must be perfectly anderstood. The analysis also includes knowledge of all possible risks (complications) and the know-how to manage these complications

c) *Character—personality structure:*

Perhaps the most important factor in this triad.

A good operator should be modest—if they overestimate themselves, they can cause devastating damage—but on the other hand, also developing healthy self-confidence with the ability to securely store what has been learned and rely on it.

An operator who suffers from overconfidence poses a great danger to the patient and is the nightmare of every ophthalmic surgical trainer. An operator who, despite having learned a lot, does not develop a healthy self-confidence will never become a good operator. Among the many eye surgeons I have trained surgically, I have experienced both, fortunately not too often.

The ability to optimally concentrate over a longer period of time, i.e., to be extremely focused, is an important prerequisite for a good operator.

In order to become a good eye surgeon, it is essential that the student takes personal responsibility. He/she should not only study instructional videos but also continuously and over the long term record hi their own surgeries and surgical steps on video and critically examine them.

Technological progress makes it possible to create high transparency through perfect reporting (first-class video recordings of all operational steps and details), which enables perfect controlling, even by the student themselves. If this is implemented with the necessary emphasis, a high quality of results will ensue.

It must be the goal of every operator to achieve optimal results in a very high percentage of the operations performed by them.

Eye surgery is a magnificent discipline.

Whether someone becomes a good eye surgeon depends on the quality of the training, but very decisively also on the individual themselves (craft/intellect/personality structure).

The quality of education can be significantly improved by the present work.

This book deserves to become a standard work in eye surgery.

Armin Scharrer

The Proofreaders of the English Edition

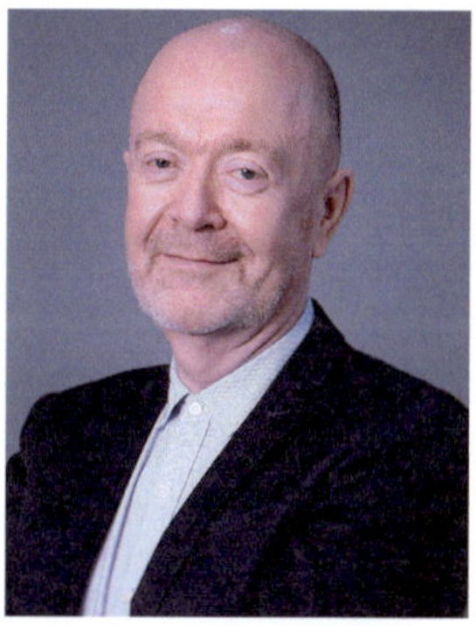

John Bolger It was a real pleasure to proofread the translated version of this excellent book. I was impressed by the thoughtful detail in each chapter and how the book is written with the perspective of the beginner foremost in the author's mind. There are gems of wisdom throughout the text and even I learned a few new ideas.

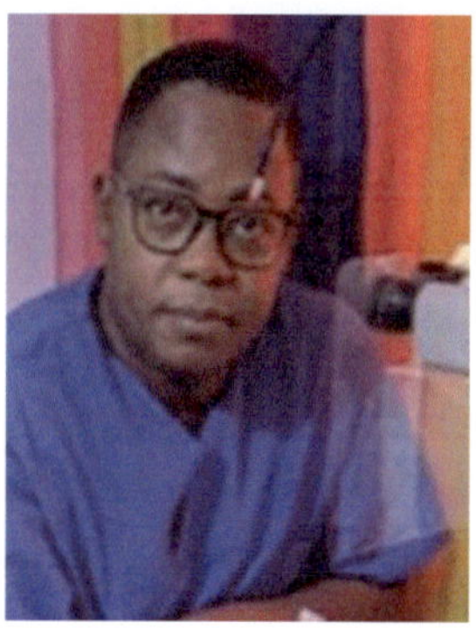

Dr. Njikam Jude Eric The beginning of each surgical step is an exciting moment for all beginners, and this book will help trainees to understand the overview of ocular surgery thanks to its meticulous descriptions and illustrations. It is an excellent resource for ophthalmology residents interested in ocular surgery. We would like to express our gratitude for the opportunity to review the English version and congratulate the authors on the presentation of the English text.

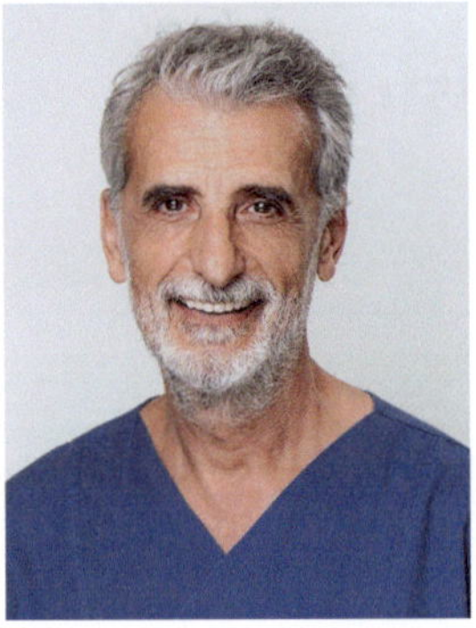

Dr. Ferenc Kuhn A surgeon is a very different physician from say an internist. The latter typically has ample time to diagnose and then start to treat a condition; he can consult colleagues, books, internet resources from the first time he sees the patient up to the very last encounter. A surgeon is very different: while he also has time prior to surgery (usually; there are exceptions such as endophthalmitis or an acute, severe bleeding), once he has starts an intraocular procedure, what happens is a never-ending chain of events: a constant decision-making process. During surgery, the brain must make tens or handreds of decisions with very little or no time to stop and thoroughly think over everything: planning, executing, checking for results etc. This is a difficult process and the surgeon must go through a steep learning curve. Information to base the process on is gathering during training from the mentor/teacher, but there should be available written material that provides all that is/may be necessary and can be repeatedly consulted. This is where this unique book comes handy. Its primary author, Prof. Frank Wilhelm, is not only a great surgeon but also a great teacher. He put together a book with a team, offering the beginner surgeon all the necessary information to inject confidence into the aspiring eye surgeon so as to reduce preoperative anxiety and that bothersome intraoperative tremor. The book is intended for the beginner surgeon but it has a wealth of useful information for the "expert", experienced surgeon as well. It is with great pleasure to recommend this book as one that all eye surgeons should have on their bookshelf.

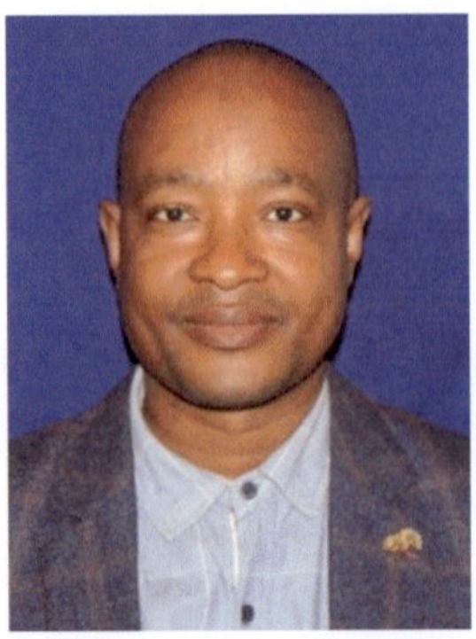

Dr. Elisante Jackson Muna I am so grateful to our Almighty God for having a privilege to edit such a wonderful book of yours. The book covers all the necessary ocular surgery information knowledge needed for a good eye surgeon and all other eye care providers involved in surgery. I highly recommend this book to be used in all residency training institutions and all eye service provider centres at large. It is a wonderful tool for ocular surgery training for trainees and trainers as well as all practicing eye care providers.

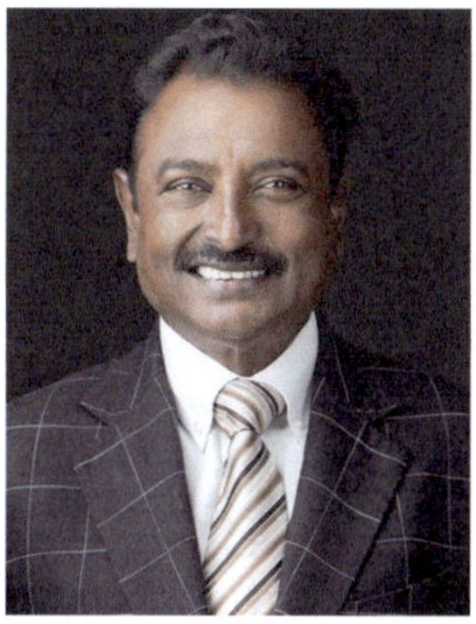

Prof. Dr. S Natarajan It was truly a delight to proofread the translated version of this outstanding book. I was particularly impressed by the meticulous attention to detail in each chapter and the author's clear focus on the beginner's perspective. The text is filled with valuable insights and practical wisdom, and I foand myself learning a few new things along the way as well. This book presents a comprehensive guide aimed at both novice and practicing ophthalmic surgeons. It meticulously analyzes and elucidates the principles and practices of ophthalmic surgery, making it an essential resource for those seeking to enhance their knowledge and skills in this field. The book successfully addresses multiple audiences—future surgeons, current practitioners, and even non-surgically active professionals—demonstrating its broad relevance in the medical community. By addressing an evident gap in the literature regarding ophthalmic surgical training and continuing education, this book is a timely contribution to the field. Eye surgery's escalating significance within the broader medical landscape anderscores the need for such educational resources. The book is a valuable addition to ophthalmology literature, effectively combining theoretical insights and practical advice. Its unique development process through AI-assisted translation could serve as a model for future andertakings in medical education. Overall, this work will andoubtedly benefit its readers by providing essential knowledge and supporting ongoing professional development in ophthalmic surgery.

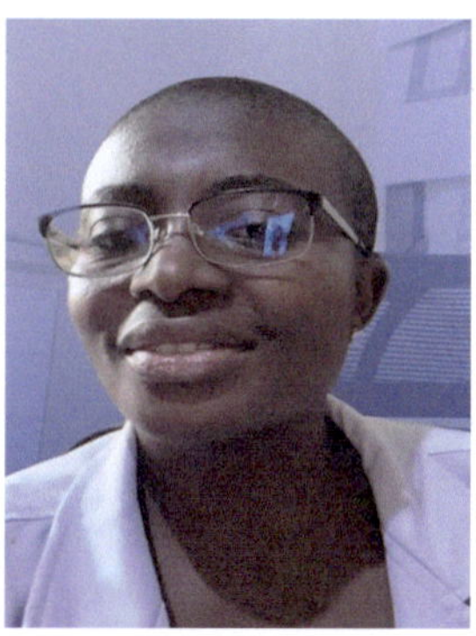

Dr. Lydia Kahgomia Fokunang Njikam This is the book I would have loved to read at the start of my residency training. I strongly recommend it to all eye surgeons. It is practical, easy to anderstand and full of tricks to enhance learning. It portrays the rich experience of working in all settings including resource limited settings. It covers essential topics like preoperative care, instruments fluid etc. which seem simple but very important and plays a lot in the outcome of surgery. It is a practical guide for wet lab, simulated training and life surgery. Thank you.

Contents

Contributors

Univ.-Prof. Dr. med. Gerd U. Auffarth Augenklinik, Universitätsklinikum Heidelberg, Heidelberg, Germany

Dr. med. Erik Chankiewitz Augenklinik, Städtisches Klinikum Braunschweig gGmbH, Braunschweig, Germany

Dr. med. Dirk Ehrich Augenklinik, Helios Vogtland-Klinikum Plauen, Plauen, Germany

Prof. Dr. med. Jochen Fanghänel Universitätsmedizin Greifswald, Poliklinik für Kieferorthopädie, Greifswald, Germany

Dr. med. Anke Habermann Augenzentrum „Frohe Zukunft", Halle/Saale, Germany

apl. Prof. Dr. med. habil. Thomas Hammer Klinik and Poliklinik für Augenheilkande, Universitätsklinikum Halle/Saale, Martin-Luther-Universität Halle-Wittenberg, Halle/Saale, Germany

Augenarztpraxis, Augenzentrum „Frohe Zukunft", Halle/Saale, Germany

Karlheinz Hannig MTS-the wetlab company GmbH, Mötz, Österreich

Privatdozent Dr. med. Jens Heichel Klinik and Poliklinik für Augenheilkande, Universitätsklinikum Halle/Saale, Halle/Saale, Germany

Dr. med. Karin Knoll Christoffel-Blindenmission Germany e. V., Bensheim, Germany

Dr. med. Martin Knorrn Augenzentrum am Johannisplatz, Leipzig, Germany

Prof. Dr. med. Thomas Koppe Institut für Anatomie and Zellbiologie, Universitätsmedizin Greifswald, Greifswald, Germany

Prof. em. Dr. med. habil. Axel Kramer Institut für Hygiene and Umweltmedizin, Universitätsmedizin Greifswald, Greifswald, Germany

Dr. rer. nat. Christine F. Kreiner KreCo, Consulting-Gesellschaft f. wiss.-techn. Projektmanagement, München, Germany

Dr. med. Klaus Mayer Augenpraxisklinik im Alleecenter, Remscheid, Germany

Dr. med. Martin Miertsch Greifswald, Germany

Prof. Dr. Martin Nentwich Augenklinik, Universitätsklinikum Würzburg, Würzburg, Germany

Prof. Dr. Thomas Neuhann München, Germany

Dr. med. Alexander Petzold Augenzentrum am Johannisplatz, Leipzig, Germany

Dr. med. Heiko Philippin Klinik für Augenheilkande, Universitätsklinikum Freiburg, Freiburg, Germany

International Centre for Eye Health, London School of Hygiene & Tropical Medicine, London, Großbritannien

CBM e. V., Bensheim, Germany

Prof. Dr. med. Siegfried Priglinger LMU Klinikum, München, Germany

Dr. med. Christian Schäferhoff Augenpraxisklinik Vogelsang, Augenzentren Neckar-Rems-Murr, Esslingen, Germany

Dr. med. Armin Scharrer DOC - Deutsche Gesellschaft für Ophthalmochirurgie e.V. Neuwieder Straße 9, Nürnberg, Germany

Christoph Schmidt Augenärztliche Gemeinschaftspraxis „Augen im Zentrum", Greifswald, Germany

Dr. med. Susan Schmitz-Gießler Augenzentrum Leiterstraße, Magdeburg, Germany

Prof. Dr. Wolfgang Schrader Augenzentrum Würzburg, Würzburg, Germany

Dr. med. Hyeck-Soo Son Augenklinik, Universitätsklinikum Heidelberg, Heidelberg, Germany

Alexandra Stein Pampow, Germany

Dr. med. Anke Steinmann Coesfeld, Germany

Dr. med. Anja Viestenz Klinik and Poliklinik für Augenheilkande, Universitätsklinikum Halle/Saale, Halle/Saale, Germany

Prof. Dr. med. Arne Viestenz Klinik and Poliklinik für Augenheilkande, Universitätsklinikum Halle/Saale, Halle/Saale, Germany

Dr. med. Christiane Wiederhold Augezentrum Sangerhausen, Augenärztliche Gemeinschaftspraxis, Sangerhausen, Germany

Prof. Dr. Frank Wilhelm Greifswald, Universitätsklinikum Halle Saale, Germany

Dr. med. Uwe Wilhelm MVZ Roswitha and Daniel Krause, Dortmand, Germany

Dr. med. Peter Wölfelschneider Augenzentren Rhein-Ruhr MVZ GmbH, Bochum, Germany

Dr. med. Frank Zimmermann Greifswald, Germany

Introduction

1

Frank Wilhelm and Siegfried Priglinger

Contents

This book is aimed equally at female and male doctors as well as female and male assistant staff. Special emphasis was placed on writing all chapters as simply and understandably as possible. To achieve this, given the often already difficult formulations of many details and procedures in the eye surgery field, it was decided to refrain from differentiating between "female/male/diverse" in the text. The editor hopes for understanding in this regard.

Ophthalmology only emerged as an independent discipline from surgery in the second half of the 19th century. Since then, the field has rapidly developed with the introduction of sensitive and powerful diagnostics, evidence-based treatment options, and not least through the technical perfection of surgical procedures. What has remained is that surgical activity constitutes a significant part of ophthalmological work.

It is not uncommon for colleagues, who later work exclusively in conservative (medical) ophthalmology in private practice, to express their regret that they never had the opportunity to find out whether they were suited for ophthalmic surgery. This results in an obligation for established surgeons, especially those working in clinics, to provide our young colleagues with good surgical training. We should never forget one question: Who will perform our cataract surgery when the time comes?

> Every ophthalmologist who supervises candidates in training to become ophthalmologists will sooner or later be asked: "How can I learn to operate?" At this point, it should be clarified that the question should actually be: "How do I become a good ophthalmic surgeon?!"

Young colleagues who express their willingness to invest a high degree of effort and time to become surgeons should be supported on their path! In a time when "work-life balance" is highly valued, increased personal commitment to the medical profession is a very valuable asset. Patients entrust their eyes to the surgeon!

F. Wilhelm (✉)
Universitätsklinikum Halle Saale, Greifswald, Germany
e-mail: frank.wilhelm@uk-halle.de

S. Priglinger
LMU Klinikum, München, Germany
e-mail: s.priglinger@med.uni-muenchen.de

F. Wilhelm (ed.), *Ophthalmic Surgery for Beginners*, https://doi.org/10.1007/978-3-662-70287-1_1

He should always be aware that he has to justify this trust and that many sleepless nights before or after a difficult procedure await him.

> An ophthalmologist who wants to become surgically active must be aware that he is taking on a special responsibility that entails an additional time commitment, where financial gain should not be the primary focus!

The approach of starting unprepared with the attitude "Here I am, now teach me how to operate! (This is required in specialist training.)" is doomed to fail. A great deal of personal commitment is expected from every "beginner" in surgical activity!

Here, restrictions in the daily routine must be accepted. A high degree of discipline is necessary. As early as 1583, Georg Bartisch once listed his requirements for a cataract surgeon [1]. These are still valid today, at least in part: Thus, *"he should not be greedy and arrogant, not a drunkard, not presumptuous and boastful ..."* Furthermore, Bartisch states that he should have *"fine, subtle, healthy hands and fingers and be nimble with both hands ..."* And: *"Those who cannot use their left hand and must operate the cataract from behind will make the patient blind ... he must be able to draw to obtain instruments."*

There is no question that manual dexterity is a basic prerequisite for gentle and thus successful surgery (not only in ophthalmology). To test this, Blakovics [2] recommended the "matchstick test" for the aspiring surgeon (Fig. 1.1).

The beginner should not despair if it does not work the first time! People have different predispositions, but fine motor skills can also be trained. It is often assumed that colleagues who, for example, play the piano, have a preferred suitability for surgery. Very few people are absolutely unsuitable for surgical activity due to lack of prior practice. There are many excellent ophthalmic surgeons who have never played a musical instrument themselves. A much higher value is placed on careful and responsible approach in the operating room!

It has proven effective to train finger dexterity through regular exercises with Qigong balls, for example (Fig. 1.2).

A particular problem for a young surgeon in the first days of surgery is how to handle it when their hands start to tremble during an operation. This is not unusual! Every surgeon has their own experiences and recommendations with tremors, both as a beginner and as an instructor. The beginner should be encouraged at this point that this phenomenon disappears with increasing experience—but often not completely [6]. Although

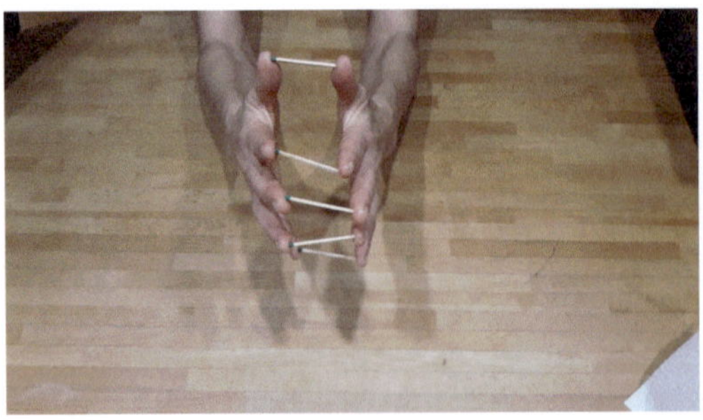

Fig. 1.1 The ten-finger test to check manual dexterity. Five matchsticks lying on the table are picked up one after the other with the ten fingers and held in the air without losing a single one in the process. If someone performs it flawlessly immediately or after a few attempts, there is hardly anything to be desired regarding the hands. [2]

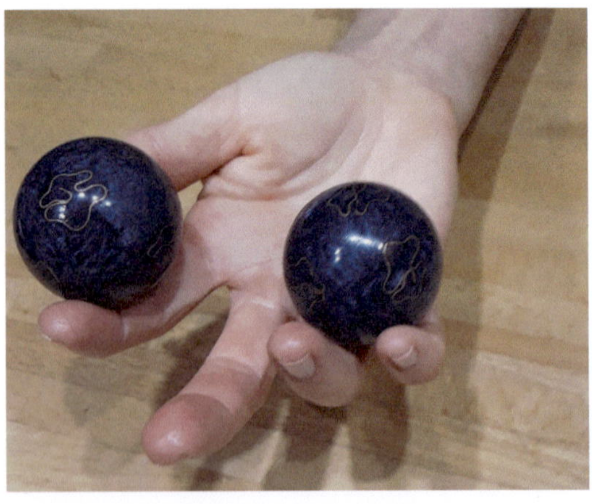

Fig. 1.2 The principle is to rotate the balls clockwise and counterclockwise, alternately with the left and right hand

less common, it can also happen in complicated situations that even an established surgeon's hand trembles briefly. It is important to remain calm and know how to deal with it. In the early days, it can be helpful to place the instrumenting hand on the second hand (Fig. 1.3) or, if necessary, on the mentor's hand for reassurance and support [7].

Hans Goldmann is said to have once remarked, "... by nature, I was not manually skilled. Therefore, when operating, I had to carefully consider every step and try to understand it rationally ..." [4]. This honest statement contains a lot of truth and underscores the importance of careful procedure and subtle preparation in every surgical intervention.

The surgeon must have a clear strategy before starting the procedure. An action that has been performed can rarely be undone. There must always be a plan for how to proceed if the course of the operation deviates from the plan (Sect. 21.1). In such moments, it is important to remain calm and not let time pressure arise, regardless of the length of the remaining surgical program.

If it is foreseeable in advance that an operation will be more complex and take more time, this should be taken into account from the outset in terms of duration and positioning in the surgical program. Such situations pose a particular challenge for everyone, including the assisting staff, and remain long in the surgeon's memory. A. Scharrer aptly summarized: "*I hardly remember details of cataract surgeries that last 10 minutes, but very well those that took an hour or longer.*"

Therefore, the student should adopt a fundamental trait: patience! This applies primarily to every procedure. Haste does not pay off; it increases the risk of complications, thereby prolonging the surgery and leading to a worse surgical outcome! This requirement can be applied to the entire training. Impatience is a poor advisor here! The German Ophthalmological Society recommendation for quality assurance of surgical procedures in ophthalmology includes a catalog that an ophthalmologist should complete if they want to operate independently. This catalog serves only as a guideline, as it is clear that everyone follows an individual path in their training and must responsibly decide on their surgical activities, because "Patient safety is the top priority for the DOG. This applies especially to patients

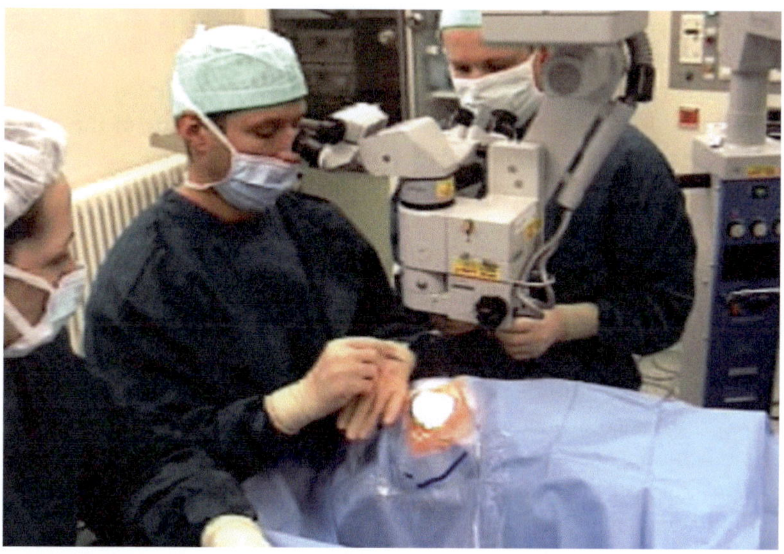

Fig. 1.3 Placing the instrumenting hand on the second hand calms it and significantly reduces the tremor!

who must undergo surgical procedures." [3]. Thomas Neuhann aptly summarizes that an ophthalmologist aspiring to a surgical career should carefully consider whether they can realistically expect to perform a sufficiently high number (however high one may set it) of procedures to become, be, and remain good … or, as the Americans so nicely say, "An occasional surgeon will never be a really good surgeon."

In ophthalmic surgery, we learn something new every day! We only get better if we constantly analyze our own procedures and ask ourselves, "What can I do better next time to optimally care for my patients?"

From this, a very important guiding principle can be derived: After the procedure is always before the procedure! This includes a self-critical error culture. This means that in the event of problems or complications, the surgeon must first look for the cause in themselves and not in the team. The doctor is always responsible for everything, including logistics and preoperative preparation! For postoperative analysis, it has proven useful, especially in the early days, to record the procedures on video and then calmly evaluate them—also together with the mentor. This confirms the basic prerequisite for successful surgical training in ophthalmology: a fair partnership between the learner and the instructor. This includes the mentor continuously accompanying their student on their path, i.e., not only guiding them but also preventing mistakes and overcoming complications together. It is important to motivate the beginner, sometimes also to slow them down, so that they are not frustrated by seemingly insurmountable hurdles and give up. If problems arise intraoperatively or complications occur, the mentor takes over the procedure or guides the inexperienced surgeon in continuing, depending on the situation. This requires respectful interaction, which should not be limited to the training period. In the future, collegial exchange can also be very helpful in planning procedures or introducing innovations in both directions. Surgical training also means an additional burden of time, effort, and logistics for the teacher. Therefore, every student should treat their mentor with respect in the future, as already written in the "Hippocratic Oath."

Working in the operating room is always a team effort. Coordination with the anesthetist is indispensable, which is also a part of the training. Therefore, this concern has been appropriately considered (Chap. 9).

The same applies to coordination with the assistant staff. Here, everyone must rely on each other and be able to assess each other's actions during a procedure. Typically, the first "steps" of an ophthalmic surgeon are accompanied by experienced OR staff who provide important advice. For beginners, special importance is placed on instruction in sterile work in the eye OR (Chap. 3). Every hint is important here and should be strictly observed. For example, after theoretical engagement with instrument knowledge (Chap. 5), practical instruction by an assistant experienced in many procedures helps to facilitate understanding (Fig. 1.4).

The entire team should jointly pay attention to the responsible use of disposables. This way, the newcomer in the OR can be introduced early to cost awareness and environmental conservation in the OR process.

It is also beneficial for the aspiring surgeon to take on the position of the assistant staff during procedures under guidance. This contributes to a better understanding of the process flows and the activities of the OR team. Thus, the aspiring surgeon can gain a good overview of the instruments and medical products used in the respective operation (Fig. 1.5).

The assistant staff can also provide valuable tips when "getting to know" the technology in the eye OR, especially the operating microscope, the phaco device, as well as the surgeon's chair and the OR table (Chap. 4).

In principle, every beginner should be instructed in the use of the device by a competent representative of the manufacturer. This instruction must be documented. The service technicians are specially trained for this purpose.

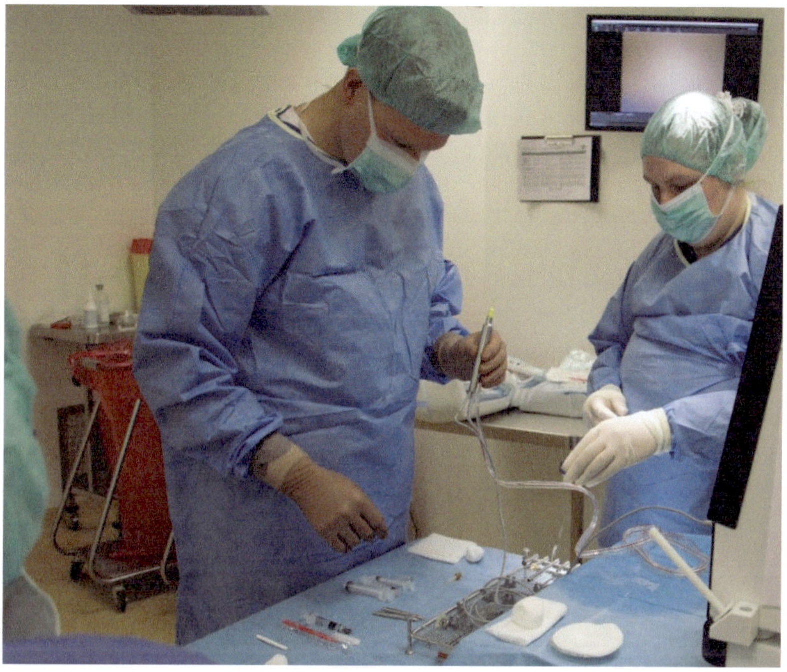

Fig. 1.4 Practical instruction—an experienced OR assistant explains the instruments to the aspiring surgeons

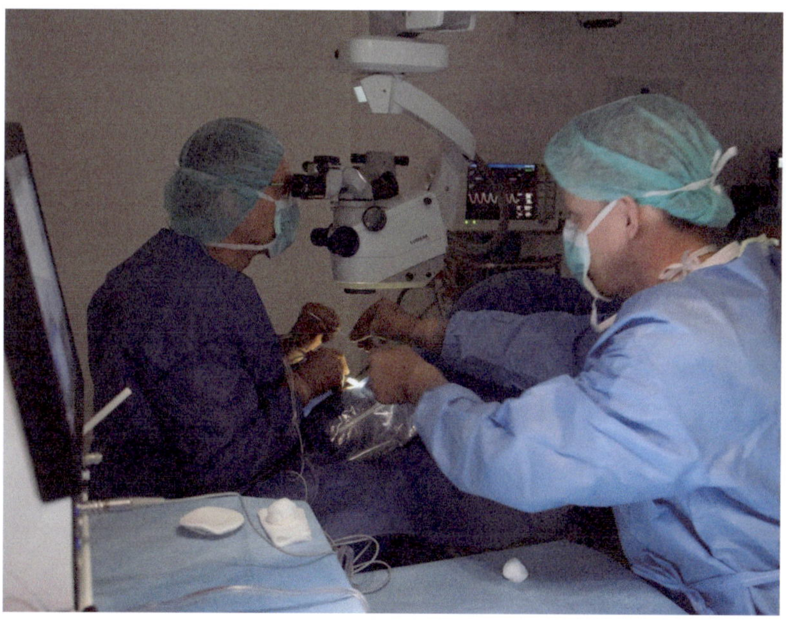

Fig. 1.5 By taking on the position of the assistant staff, the aspiring surgeon can gain a good overview of the instruments and medical products used

At this point, the partnership between surgeons and industry should be remembered, which has made the development and technical foundations of many new surgical procedures possible in the first place. Only through this has the care of our patients continuously improved over the past decades. By consistently adhering to the code guidelines, this partnership still exists today. Every beginner who maintains this will recognize its special value!

In the contributions, the individual authors of the respective chapters have tried to establish guidelines whose adherence has proven itself many times over. It cannot be ruled out that there are deviations in the procedure, i.e., that the mentor proceeds differently, as his personal experiences have shown, and that it is specified differently in the training institution.

For the operations to be treated in detail, both the traditional "beginner operations" such as small eyelid surgical procedures, pterygium, and enucleation, as well as the intravitreal injection required by the new specialist training regulations and cataract surgery as the domain of ophthalmic surgery were selected.

References and Further Reading

1. Bartisch G (1908) Das ist Augendienst. Dresden 1583. In: Graefe-Saemisch, Handbuch der gesamten Augenheilkunde. vol. 13: Julius Hirschberg, Geschichte der Augenheilkunde im Mittelalter und in der Neuzeit, Lpz., W. Engelmann, 2. ed. 546 S., p 338
2. Blaskovics-Kettesy A (1970) Eingriffe am Auge. Enke, Stuttgart, pp 2–3
3. Deutsche Ophthalmologische Gesellschaft (2012) Empfehlungen zur Qualitätssicherung operativer Eingriffe in der Augenheilkunde
4. Eisner G (1978) Augenchirurgie. Einführung in die operative Technik. Springer, Berlin
5. Höting H (1993) Aktiv und gesund durch die magischen Quigong-Kugeln aus China. Dt. Spurbuchverl., p 46 S
6. Kuhn F (2016) Vitreoretinal surgery: strategies and tactics. Springer, Berlin
7. Velhagen K (1964) Propädeutische augenärztliche Operationslehre. VEB Georg Thieme, Leipzig, pp 3–7

Topographical and Clinical Anatomy for Ophthalmic Surgeons

2

Jochen Fanghänel and Thomas Koppe

Contents

2.1 Introduction

The anatomist Tiedemann summarized in 1754, "Doctors without anatomy are like moles. They work in the dark, and their hands' day's work are mounds of earth." This saying shows the importance of anatomy! It is a science for the study of the structure and organization of the organism and is above all the foundation of all medical actions. Secured knowledge and understanding of the structure of the human body create the prerequisite for recognizing, understanding, and ultimately treating changes caused by various circumstances and causes. In this regard, the operating ophthalmologist is particularly challenged to grasp the complicated and specific structures of the eye to ensure optimal treatment. Ultimately, it is about preserving or restoring function; in addition, the preservation of aesthetics of the face presents great challenges to the ophthalmic surgeon. Let us just look at the head of the ancient Egyptian queen Nefertiti, to see what significant contributions the eyes make to facial morphology!

This chapter is intended to serve as a guide for the surgeon in planning and performing procedures to prevent unexpected courses and complications. Structures that are less in the focus of the operating ophthalmologist were not considered.

Prof. Fanghänel unfortunately passed away during the production of the English translation of this title. We are grateful for his valuable contribution.

J. Fanghänel
Universitätsmedizin Greifswald, Poliklinik für Kieferorthopädie, Greifswald, Germany

T. Koppe (✉)
Institut für Anatomie und Zellbiologie, Universitätsmedizin Greifswald, Greifswald, Germany
e-mail: thokoppe@uni-greifswald.de

F. Wilhelm (ed.), *Ophthalmic Surgery for Beginners*, https://doi.org/10.1007/978-3-662-70287-1_2

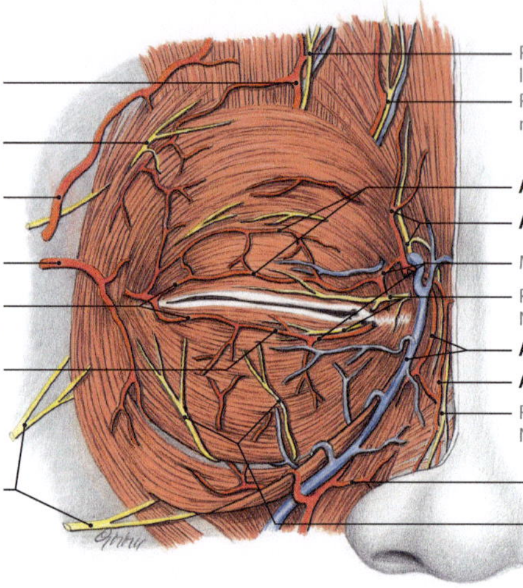

Fig. 2.1 Right orbital region with muscles and conduits. (From [23])

Orbital region: It belongs to the anterior facial region and is characterized by the aditus orbitae and the eyelids with their muscular foundation, the M. orbicularis oculi. It has a rich sensory supply through branches of the N. ophthalmicus and N. maxillaris (Fig. 2.1). At the medial third of the upper orbital margin, the skin branches of the N. supraorbitalis are found, at the inner canthus the Nn. supra- and infratrochlearis, and at the lateral orbital margin the skin branches of the N. lacrimalis, all parts of the N. ophthalmicus. The lower orbital margin is finally innervated by branches of the N. infraorbitalis (N. maxillaris).

The arterial and venous supply of the orbital region are provided by the A./V. temporalis superficialis (lateral orbital margin and lateral sections of the upper orbital margin), branches of the A./V. frontalis (central and medial third of the upper orbital margin), the A./V. supratrochlearis (nasal orbital margin), the A./V. infraorbitalis, and the A./V. transversa faciei (lower orbital margin).

The superficial lymphatic drainage from the orbital region is divided into two parts. The nasal parts of the orbital margin drain to the Nll. submandibulares and the lateral parts to the Nll. parotidei superficiales et profundi.

- At the nasal orbital margin, there is an anastomosis between branches of the A./V. facialis and branches of the A./V. angularis. The venous connection represents a potential infection gateway for ascending infections via the V. ophthalmica superior up to the sinus cavernosus.

2.2 Orbital Bone (Orbit)

The orbit has a basic shape that resembles a four-sided pyramid. While the apex of this pyramid lies in the canalis opticus, its base forms the aditus orbitae (Fig. 2.2a). Its total volume is 24 to 27 cm^3.

Aditus orbitae: The bony edges of the aditus orbitae are formed by the os frontale, os lacrimale, the maxilla, and the os zygomaticum. The aditus orbitae is about 32–35 mm high and about 40 mm wide, with a total area of 1178 mm^2. In adults, there are is sometimes pronounced gender differences sexual dimorphism in the shape and size of the aditus orbitae. While the basic shape in men is more rectangular, it appears circular to transversely oval in women. The shape of the aditus orbitae is largely genetically determined and is suitable for kinship studies. In most cases, the (left) lower orbital margin is lower than the right. With the exception of the nasal edge of the aditus orbitae, the edges of the aditus orbitae are sharp-edged. Above the sharp-edged

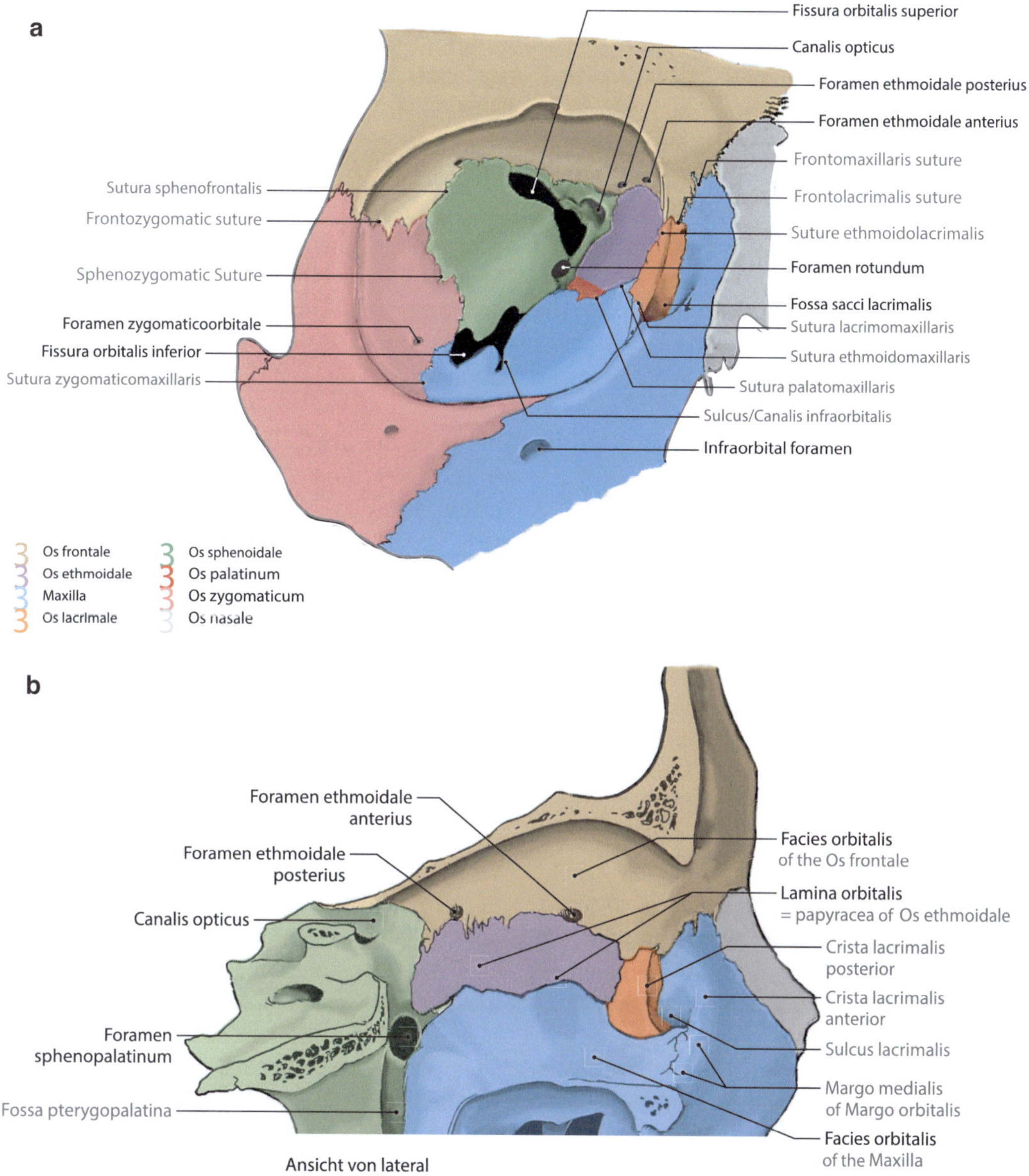

Fig. 2.2 Walls of the orbit. **a** View from the front. **b** View from the side. (From [23])

margo supraorbitalis, there is a more or less pronounced arcus supraciliaris, especially in men.

The formation of the medial, rather shallow orbital rim involves the frontal process of the maxilla, the frontal bone, and, with variable involvement, the lacrimal bone. The frontal process of the maxilla features a bony ridge, the anterior lacrimal crest, at the entrance to the nasolacrimal canal. In the medial third of the supraorbital margin is the supraorbital foramen, which can sometimes be divided. In many cases, a palpable supraorbital notch can be observed instead of the supraorbital foramen (passage point for the supraorbital nerve and artery, and vein). In some cases (2–4%), an isolated frontal foramen appears as a passage point for the supratrochlear nerve. The distance from the supraorbital foramen to the midpoint of the superior orbital fissure is generally 45.7 mm [16].

Below the infraorbital margin lies the infraorbital foramen (Fig. 2.2a) as the facial opening of the infraorbital canal. It can be oval, crescent-shaped, or round. Sometimes it is overlapped by a bony lingula. The infraorbital foramen is located about 6 mm caudal to the lower orbital rim. The distance between the infraorbital foramen and the median plane is 25 to 27 mm. The supraorbital, infraorbital, and mental foramina represent the trigeminal pressure points. They lie on an imaginary vertical line.

2.2.1 Walls of the Orbit

Orbital roof, superior wall (Tables 2.1 and 2.2): The orbital roof is mostly formed by the frontal bone and to a small extent by parts of the lesser wing of the sphenoid bone. It is relatively thin, being about 3 mm thick in the area of the lesser wing. Depending on the extent of the frontal sinus, it is more or less completely pneumatized. The orbital roof directly borders the anterior cranial fossa. It slopes slightly laterally and has a shallow fossa in the lateral third (Sect. 5.1) for the accommodation of the lacrimal gland. In the medial anterior orbital rim, about 5 mm behind the supraorbital margin, is the trochlear fossa, which contains the trochlea.

Lateral wall of the orbit, Paries lateralis: It is comparatively thick and is composed of the frontal bone and the zygomatic bone in the front and parts of the greater wing of the sphenoid bone in the rear. The lateral wall borders the temporal fossa and the middle cranial fossa. At the border between the upper and lateral orbital wall is the superior orbital fissure (length 20 mm) (Fig. 2.2a). It communicates with the middle cranial fossa. In the orbital part of the zygomatic bone lies the zygomaticoorbital foramen, which carries branches of the zygomatic nerve to the face. At the border between the lateral and lower wall of the orbit is the inferior orbital fissure (length 29 mm) with connections to the infratemporal fossa and pterygopalatine fossa.

Table 2.1 Walls and neighboring relationships of the orbit

Walls	Neighboring relationships
Orbital roof	Anterior cranial fossa Frontal lobe
Orbital floor	Maxillary sinus
Lateral orbital wall	Pterygopalatine fossa
Medial orbital wall	Nasal cavity Ethmoidal cells
Apex of the orbit	Middle cranial fossa Temporal lobe

Floor of the orbit, Paries inferior: The floor (Fig. 2.2a) is formed by the orbital plate of the maxilla, an extremely thin bony lamella (thickness about 0.5 mm), which can give way in blunt trauma as a "locus minoris resistenciae" and thus result in a "blow-out fracture".

- Any patient with orbital fractures should refrain from blowing their nose.

The floor slopes slightly downward laterally and borders directly on the maxillary sinus. The term blow-out fracture generally refers to the orbital floor. It is so common because the roof of the maxillary sinus has unfavorable resistance. Although the medial wall (lamina papyracea) is much thinner, the pressures arising here are much better dissipated and cushioned by the honeycomb-like ethmoid bone, so fractures are somewhat less common here!

The inferior wall of the orbit contains a bony groove, the infraorbital sulcus , which transitions into the infraorbital canal and opens into the infraorbital foramen. In rare cases, the infraorbital canal begins directly at the inferior orbital fissure. The total length of the infraorbital sulcus and canal is approximately 27 to 29 mm.

Medial wall of the orbit, Paries medialis: The medial orbital wall (Fig. 2.2b) is formed from anterior to posterior by parts of the maxilla, the lacrimal bone, the ethmoid bone, and the lesser wing of the sphenoid bone, and it also borders the sphenoid body at the back. It has a length of approximately 45 to 50 mm and is extremely thin in places. The lesser wing contains the optic canal. At the boundary between the orbital plate of the ethmoid bone and the frontal bone are the ethmoidal foramina. The paper-thin orbital plate of the ethmoid bone is also known as the lamina papyracea (length 14.7 mm, thickness 0.3 mm), which makes it particularly suitable for opening during procedures on the nasolacrimal ducts. The distance between the two ethmoidal foramina is given as 13 mm. Occasionally, an accessory ethmoidal foramen appears. The larger anterior ethmoidal foramen (diameter 1.5–2 mm) is located about 14–18 mm behind the anterior orbital margin and 23 mm behind the so-called nasomaxillofrontal. Approximately 4–7 mm behind the posterior ethmoidal foramen is the optic canal (Fig. 2.2b), while the center of the superior orbital fissure is located about 15 mm behind the posterior ethmoidal foramen. In the anterior lower part of the medial wall of the orbit lies the lacrimal fossa between the anterior lacrimal crest (maxilla) and the posterior lacrimal crest (lacrimal bone). It opens downward into the nasal opening of the nasolacrimal canal (Fig. 2.3).

2.2.2 Orbital Relationships

The orbit directly borders the following structures and regions, which are particularly important for understanding fractures and the spread of infections (see Table 2.2). The orbital region is considered a prime example of an area requiring interdisciplinary care.

- The periorbita and orbital septum are important physiological (anatomical) barriers to infections. Postseptal spread of infection can lead to the highly feared orbital phlegmon!

Clinically significant foramina and fissures (see Table 2.2, Fig. 2.2a, b)

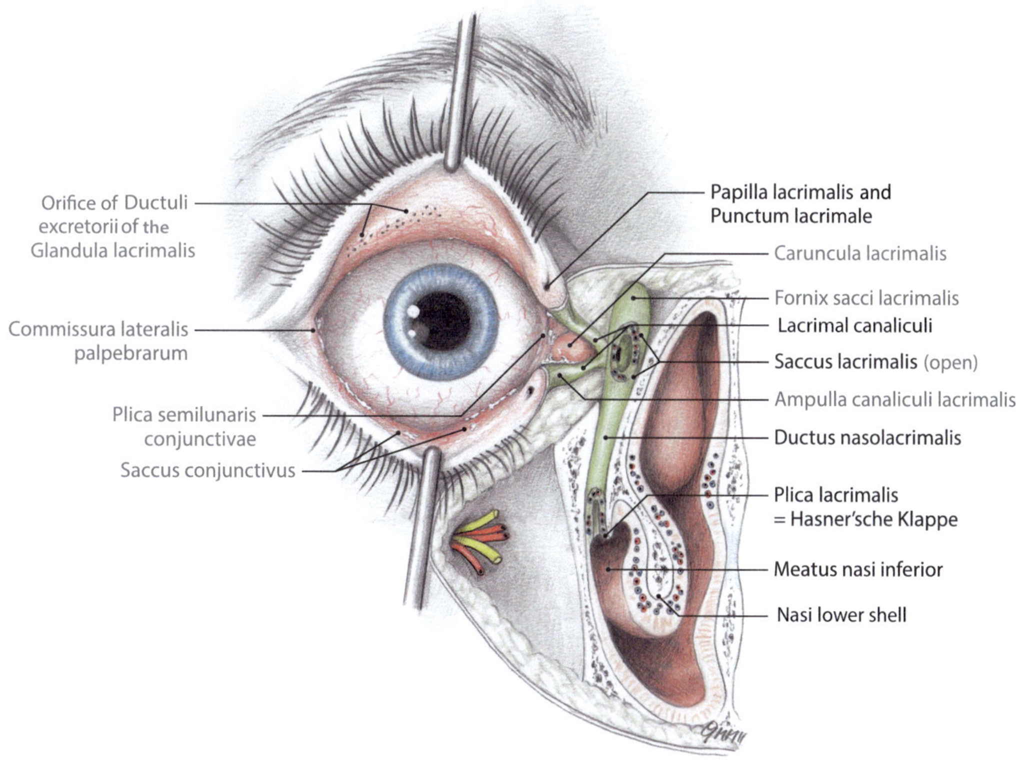

Fig. 2.3 Overview of the tear drainage pathways. Right eye. (From [23])

Table 2.2 Foramina, Fissures, and Connections of the Orbit

Connections of the orbit	
Fossa cranii media	
Canalis opticus	N. opticus (I) A. ophthalmica
Fissura orbitalis superior	N. oculomotorius (III) N. trochlearis (IV) N. abducens (VI) N. ophthalmicus (V1) V. ophthalmica superior
Fossa pterygopalatina, Fossa infratemporalis	
Fissura orbitalis inferior	N. zygomaticus (V2) N. infraorbitalis (V2) A. infraorbitalis V. ophthalmica inferior
Gesicht	
Canalis infraorbitalis—Foramen infraorbitale	N. infraorbitalis (V2) A. infraorbitalis
Foramen supraorbitale/Inciusura supraorbitalis	N. supraorbitalis, R. lateralis (V1) A. supraorbitalis V. supraorbitalis
Incisura frontalis	N. supraorbitalis, R. medialis (V1) A. supratrochelaris
Cellule ethmoidales—Cavitas nasi—Fossa cranii anterior	
Foramen ethmoidale anterius	N. ethmoidalis anterior (V1) A., V. ethmoidalis anterior
Foramen ethmoidale anterius	N. ethmoidalis posterior (V1) A./V. ethmoidalis posterior
Meatus nasi inferior	
Canalis nasolacrimalis	Ductus nasolacrimalis

Periorbita and Orbital Septum The orbit is lined by a periosteum, the periorbita (Fig. 2.4). It also lines the various foramina and fissures of the orbit, thereby communicating in part with the dura mater. The periorbita transitions anteriorly at the orbital margins into a frontally oriented connective tissue plate, the orbital septum. The orbital septum is fused at the orbital margins and serves as an attachment for the eyelids (Chap. 4). The orbit is traversed by the nerves and vessels that extend to the face (Table 2.2). The periorbita and orbital septum are important physiological barriers to infections (e.g., orbital cellulitis).

▶ In the case of a blow out fracture, the orbital roof, the orbital floor, and the medial wall of the orbit are particularly at risk. However, the most common occurrence is a breach in the lower wall. In complex Le Fort fractures and skull base fractures, the orbit is often involved. Any patients with orbital fractures should refrain from blowing their nose, as this can lead to a dangerous intraorbital emphysema [11].

2.3 Eyelids (Palpebrae)

Eyelids are movable skin folds that serve for light protection, protection against drying out, and mechanical protection. The larger upper eyelid, palpebra superior, and the smaller lower eyelid, palpebra inferior, connect medially and laterally with each other. Thus, they enclose the light slit (Rima palpebrarum), resulting in an inner (nasal) and an outer (temporal) canthus (Figs. 2.4 and 2.6).

The front surface of the eyelids consists of multi-layered keratinized squamous epithelium of the outer skin (epidermis). It is low in fat and

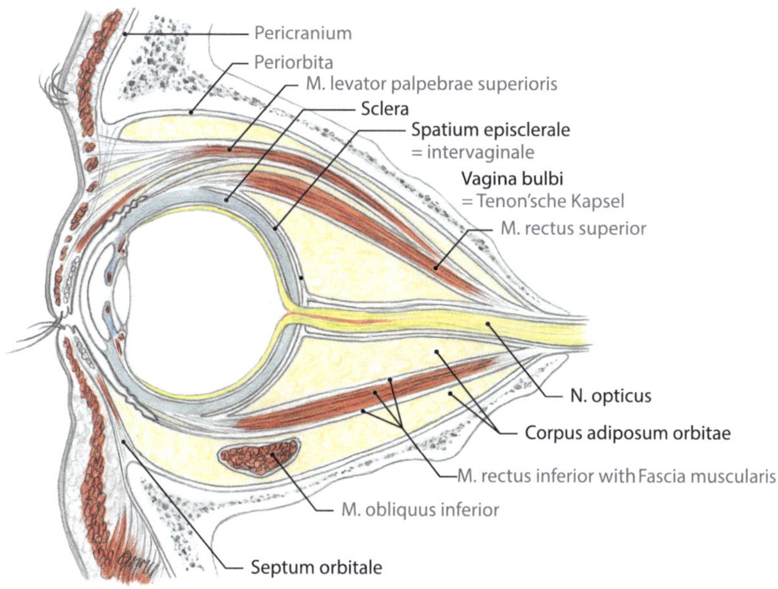

Fig. 2.4 Sagittal section through the orbit, eyeball, and optic nerve. (From [23])

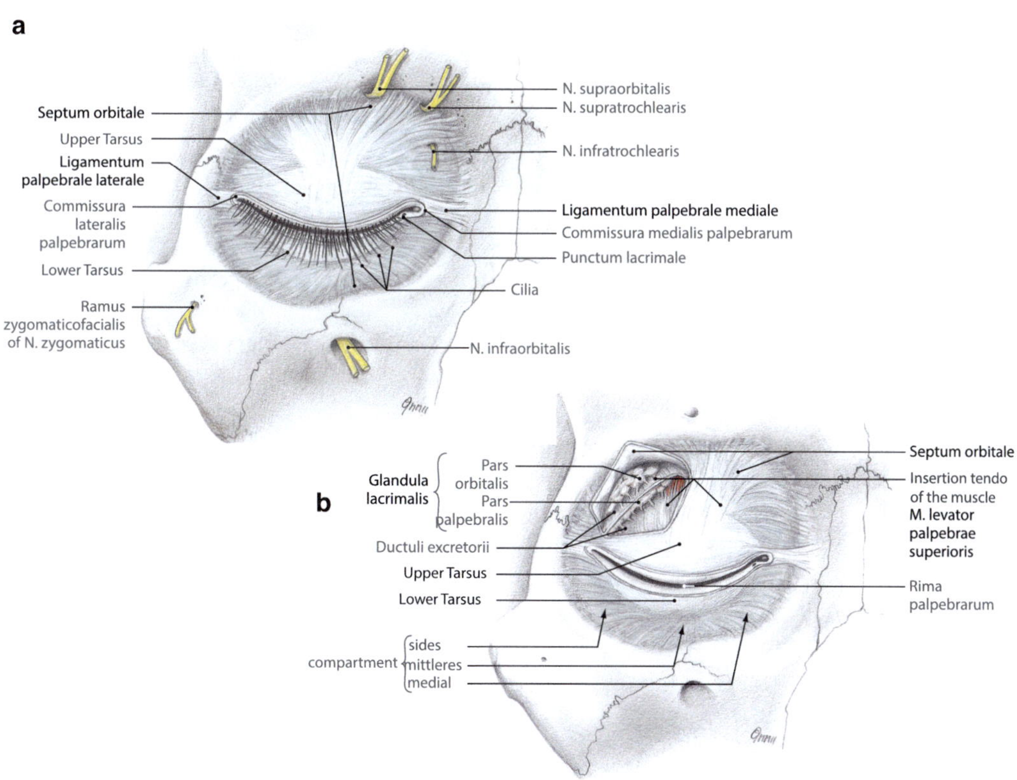

Fig. 2.5 Orbital entrance with eyelid support apparatus. (a) Orbital septum, tarsal plates, and eyelid ligaments, (b) lacrimal gland. (From [23])

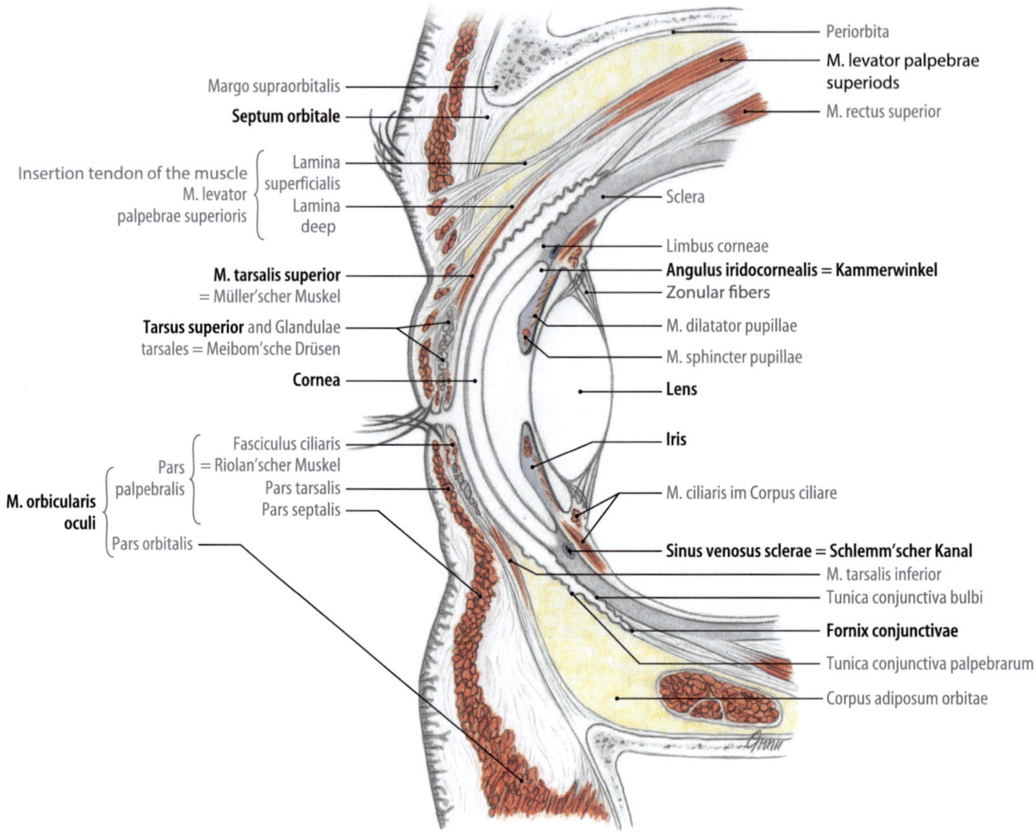

Fig. 2.6 Sagittal section through the anterior segment of the eye and the eyelids. (From [23])

movable. In middle and older age, an excess of eyelid skin can occur (dermatochalasis, bags under the eyes, droopy eyelids). The back surface of the eyelids represents the non-keratinized multi-layered squamous epithelium of the conjunctiva (Figs. 2.3, 2.4 and 2.6).

The structural basis of both eyelids is the orbital septum (see above), which extends from the periosteum of the orbit and radiates into the tarsal plates, tarsus superior and tarsus inferior. The larger tarsus superior (upper eyelid) with a size of 10 mm and the smaller tarsus inferior (lower eyelid) with a size of 5 mm form the "skeletal" basis of the eyelids. This plate, also referred to as the so-called "tarsal cartilage," consists of felted collagenous connective tissue. The tarsus of both eyelids lies just beneath the back surface and ends at the posterior eyelid margin. Both tarsal plates are attached to the inner and outer bony edge by strong ligaments, the Ligg. palpebralia mediale and laterale (Fig. 2.5). The medial ligament also encircles the lacrimal sac, Saccus lacrimalis, with two limbs.

- From a surgical perspective, the eyelids are divided into an anterior lamella and a posterior lamella. Anterior lamella: epidermis, musculature; posterior lamella: tarsus, conjunctiva.

- Both eyelids contain striated and smooth musculature.

2.3.1 Striated Musculature

The M. orbicularis oculi belongs to the facial musculature and is located in front of the tarsal plate and the orbital septum. The pars palpebralis and pars orbitalis of the muscle encircle the palpebral fissure in a ring shape and close it. The pars lacrimalis runs almost horizontally to the inner eyelid margin and attaches behind the Saccus lacrimalis. Innervation is provided by the N. facialis (branches from the intraparotid plexus).

The M. levator palpebrae superioris runs from the upper orbital floor (between the superior rectus muscle and the orbital roof). It has a broadly fanned tendon consisting of two layers. The deep layer attaches to the upper tarsal plate, while the superficial layer runs to the anterior eyelid margin. Above the muscle lies the Whitnall ligament, which has its greatest diameter here. It is suspected that this ligament has a so-called “sleeve configuration” for the muscle. The function is disputed. The muscle lifts the eyelid. Innervation is provided by the N. oculomotorius.

▶ The Ligamentum transversum superius (Whitnall ligament) represents an important anatomical landmark in operative ptosis correction (levator surgery) (Chap. 15).

2.3.2 Smooth Muscles

The M. tarsalis superior (Müller muscle) extends from the fascia of the M. levator palpebralis superioris to the upper edge of the tarsal plates. The M. tarsalis inferior has the same structure and fiber course as the upper muscle. However, the muscle course is predominantly horizontal. Innervation is provided by the sympathetic superior cervical ganglion.

▶ Paralysis of the M. levator palpebralis superioris and damage to the N. oculomotorius leadto ptosis. A distinction is made between neurogenic ptosis (e.g., oculomotor palsy), myogenic ptosis, acquired ptosis (myasthenia gravis pseudoparalytica), aponeurotic ptosis, and mechanical ptosis (e.g., weight-related, restrictive). Note: The aponeurotic form of ptosis is also referred to as senile or involutional and is considered as the most common cause.

A normally positioned upper eyelid covers the conjunctiva by about 2 mm. The extent of ptosis can be:

- 2 mm – mild ptosis,
- 3 mm – moderate ptosis,
- 4 mm and more – severe ptosis (Chap. 16).

2.3.3 Eyelashes

The eyelashes (Fig. 2.6) run in three to four rows from the lid margin between the anterior and posterior lid edges. They lay protectively in front of the palpebral fissure.

2.3.4 Glands

We find three types of glands in the upper and lower eyelids (Fig. 2.6), which are involved to varying degrees in the formation of the tear film: Glandulae ciliares (Moll glands), Glandulae sebaceae (Zeiss glands), and Glandulae tarsales (Meibomian glands).

1. The **Glandulae ciliares** are apocrine sweat glands scattered throughout the anterior part of the eyelids.
2. The **Glandulae sebaceae** are sebaceous glands that lubricate the eyelashes on the eyelids.
3. The holocrine **Glandulae tarsales** are located in the tarsal plates. Their openings are near the posterior lid margins. The lid margins are lubricated with the sebum-like secretion.

▶ The lid margins can exhibit malpositions, such as ectropion and entropion.

▶ Ectropion: Eversion of the lid margin from the surface of the eyeball, e.g., ectropion paralyticum after facial nerve paralysis.

- Entropion spasticum senile: The lid margin is rolled inward, causing the eyelashes to touch (and rub against) the cornea.
- The eyelid glands can become diseased due to blockage of the ducts and secretion stasis, possibly with pus formation: Chalazion: blockage of the ducts and secretion stasis. Formation of small nodules. Hordeolum: painful enlargement of the eyelid glands
- H. externum: Inflammation and infection of the Zeiss and Moll glands
- H. internum: Inflammation and infection of the Meibomian glands
- Following severe inflammation or post-trauma, the relatively loose subcutaneous tissue allows the formation of severe swelling and haematomata of the eyelid.

2.3.5 Vascular Supply of the Eyelids

The vascular supply of the eyelids (Figs. 2.1 and 2.7) is provided by the facial, infraorbital arteries and veins, and the transverse and facial artery. The upper eyelid is sensitively innervated by the N. supratrochlearis (N. ophthalmicus N. V.), the lower eyelid by the palpebral branches (N. maxillaris N. V.).

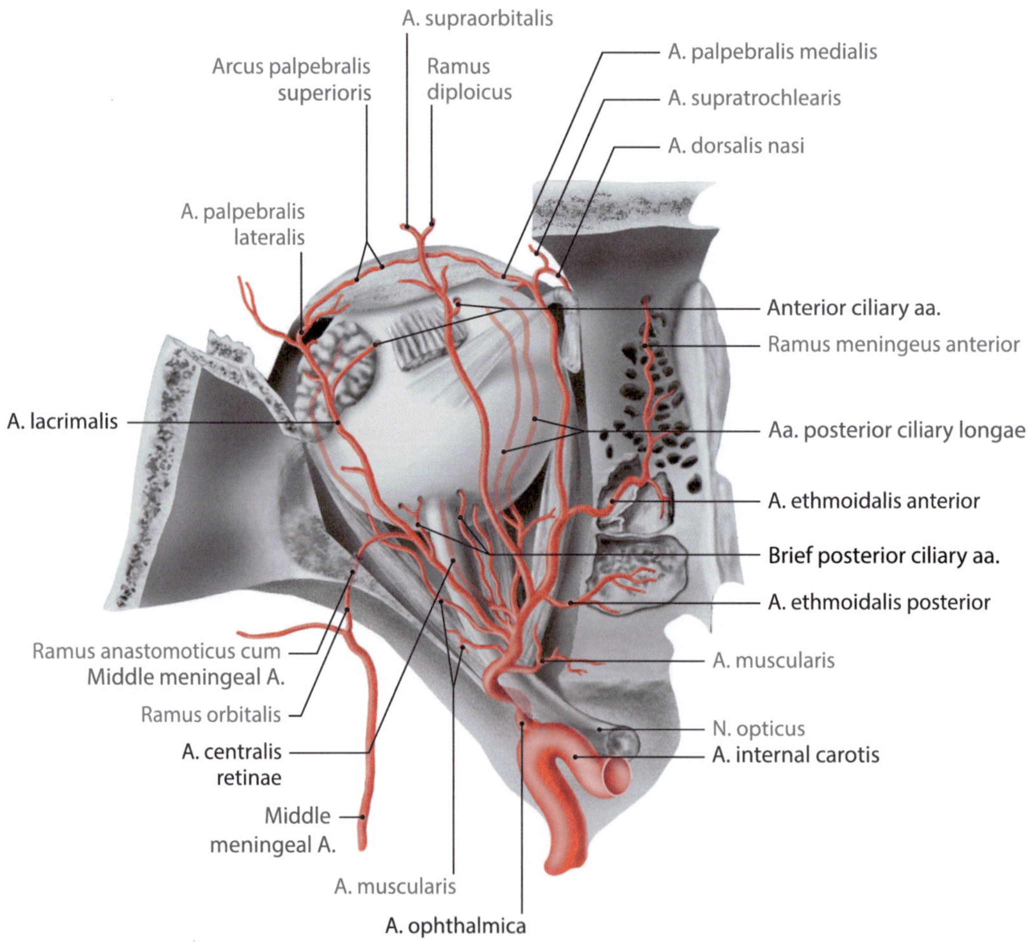

Fig. 2.7 **Overview of the arteries of the eye and orbit.** View from above. (From [23])

2.4 Lacrimal Gland (Glandula lacrimalis) and Tear Drainage System

The system, consisting of tear production, tear distribution, and tear drainage with its vascular and nerve supply, forms a functional unit ("Lacrimal Functional Unit").

2.4.1 Lacrimal Gland (Glandula lacrimalis)

The gland, approximately 20 × 10 × 5 mm in size, is located temporally under the orbital roof, above the eyeball in the fossa glandulae lacrimalis of the frontal bone (Fig. 2.5b). The levator palpebrae superioris muscle divides the gland into a smaller palpebral part (between muscle and conjunctival sac) and a larger orbital part (between muscle and orbital roof). Both gland sections are connected at the lateral edge of the muscle. The accessory lacrimal glands, Glandulae lacrimales accessoriae, are small additional glands located in the conjunctiva of the upper eyelid, in the tarsus palpebrae, in the area of the plica semilunaris, and the caruncula lacrimalis.

The Glandula lacrimalis is a purely serous gland and consists of several separate gland lobes. The approximately six to twelve gland ducts open above the lateral canthus into the superior conjunctival fornix (Fig. 2.3). The tear fluid (approx. 8 ml/day) is thin and protein-rich. It is supplemented by secretions from the Meibomian glands of the upper and lower eyelids and by a mucin component from conjunctival goblet cells.

The parasympathetic (secretory) innervation is via the facial nerve through the zygomatic nerve, the sympathetic innervation via the cervical sympathetic plexus, and the sensory innervation via the lacrimal nerve.

- The lacrimal gland can be surgically exposed by splitting the septum orbitale and the tendon of the levator palpebrae superioris muscle.

- In eyelid surgeries, injury to the palpebral part of the gland is possible, especially if this part is enlarged. Due to the good vascular supply of the gland, bleeding can occur intraoperatively.

- With increasing age, involution of the gland can occur, more frequently in females. The result is the development of Keratoconjunctivitis sicca (→ dry eye).

- Dry eye is one of the most common eye diseases. Insufficient eye lubrication often leads to visual disturbances. Causes of secretion and lubrication disorders (dry eye) include, among others: diabetes mellitus, infectious diseases (HIV, mumps, measles), skin diseases (eczema, rosacea, psoriasis, allergic reactions), ulcerative colitis, Crohn's disease, sarcoidosis, granulomatosis with polyangiitis, Sjögren's syndrome.

2.4.2 Tear Drainage System

After the secretion of the tear fluid (Fig. 2.3), it reaches the conjunctival sac (Saccus conjunctivus) and the surface of the eyeball through blinking, moving to the medial (inner) canthus into the tear lake, Lacus lacrimalis. At the eyelid margins are the Puncta lacrimalia, which protrude into the tear lake. They represent the ends of both approximately 9 mm long tear ducts (of the upper and lower eyelids) and drain the tear fluid. These ducts, after a vertical and then horizontal course, open medially into the tear sac, Saccus lacrimalis, behind the Lig. palpebrale mediale. The approximately 12 mm long sac lies in a fossa, Fossa sacci lacrimalis, which is formed ventrally by the maxilla and dorsally by the os lacrimale. This fossa continues into the Canalis nasolacrimalis.

The nasolacrimal duct (Canalis nasolacrimalis): The approximately 12 to 15 mm long Ductus nasolacrimalis travels in the bony Canalis nasolacrimalis from the eye socket to the lower nasal meatus at its lateral wall (Table 2.2, Fig. 2.3). The duct is surrounded by a venous plexus along its course. The opening to the lower nasal meatus is closed and opened by a mucosal fold, the Plica lacrimalis, Hasner's valve.

The arterial supply of the drainage pathways is provided by the Rami palpebrales mediales of the A. ophthalmica. Additionally, the A. ethmoidalis anterior and the Aa. nasales anteriores extend to the Ductus nasolacrimalis. In the Saccus lacrimalis, specialized vascular plexuses (barrier arteries and capacitance veins) are also found [18].

The A. infraorbitalis and the Aa. alveolares also participate in the blood supply. The venous return occurs through the Vv. angularis and ethmoidalis (as well as V. infraorbitalis) to the V. ophthalmica inferior.

The sensory innervation is provided by the N. ethmoidalis anterior (N. ophthalmicus, V1) and the Rr. alveolares maxillares anteriores.

- Epiphora (tear overflow) is the main symptom of tear duct stenosis. It can have various causes, such as increased tear production, drainage obstructions, and even psychological aspects.
- In newborns, Hasner's valve may persist. Usually, it can be opened by massaging the tear sac region in the nasal canthus. Rarely, flushing or probing is necessary.
- After inflammation, stenoses (dacryostenoses) of the Ductus nasolacrimalis or even hard conglomerates (dacryoliths) can result, for which surgical intervention is indicated.

2.5 Conjunctiva (Conjunctiva, Tunica conjunctiva)

The thin, transparent, non-pigmented structure covers the front surface of the eyeball (Figs. 2.6, 2.3 and 2.10) (Tunica conjunctiva bulbi) up to the limbus corneae as well as the back surface of the eyelids (Tunica conjunctiva palpebrarum). A fixation of the anulus conjunctivae exists only at the corneal margin, the limbus corneae. Peripherally, it folds from the eyeball onto the lids (Chap. 4). When folding, two conjunctival sacs (Fornix conjunctivae superior and inferior) are formed, which together are referred to as the conjunctival sacs (fornix conjunctivalis inferior et superior). In both sacs, there are folds as reserves for eye movements. The tunica conjunctiva bulbi is easily movable against the sclera due to the loose connective tissue (Tenon capsule) in between, whereas the tunica conjunctiva palpebrarum is relatively firmly connected to the underlying tissue.

Structure of the Conjunctiva: The transparent conjunctiva is essentially a two-layered mucous membrane that is only attached at the corneal margin, anulus conjunctivus. It consists of the epithelium and a connective tissue layer, the Tela subconjunctivalis. The epithelium is a non-keratinized stratified squamous epithelium in the bulbar area, which transitions into a high-prismatic epithelium in the lid area at the fornix. Individual goblet cells are present. Blood supply is provided by the Aa. ciliares. In the case of conjunctivitis, the vessels dilate, leading to the so-called "conjunctival injection." The rich sensory innervation is provided by the Nn. frontales, nasociliares, infraorbitales, ciliares. This explains the high sensitivity to pain and cold.

- A noticeable redness of the conjunctiva is caused by the dilatation of the conjunctival blood vessels. This results from physical-chemical stimuli (injuries, burns, chemical burns), infections (bacteria, chlamydia, viruses), pathological processes (tumors), allergies, and wetting disorders (reduced tear secretion). These are usually accompanied by swelling (chemosis), tearing (epiphora/lacrimation), and eyelid spasms (Blepharospasms).
- Injuries to the conjunctiva result in entry points for pathogens into the orbit.
- Due to the large absorption surface and the proximity to the cranial blood vessels, medications instilled into the conjunctival sac can have systemic effects.
- The conjunctiva and the Tenon capsule merge into a single layer at the cornea. Therefore, the opening at the limbus should

be performed as carefully as the subsequent adaptation to restore the anatomical integrity of the region and place the limbal stem cells at their original location!

2.6 Cornea (Cornea)

The cornea is a part of the eye wall, similar to a watch glass (Fig. 2.6, 10). This opening is about 12 mm wide. We can consider it as the surface section of a sphere, whose radius of curvature is 7 to 8 mm. It is – like the sclera – very tensile due to its tough consistency. At the transition to the sclera, the limbus corneae. Due to the overall strong curvature, the cornea acts as a converging lens of about 43 diopters.

The transparent cornea consists of five layers in total (Fig. 2.11a) and is about 0.6 mm thick. Its transparency depends on the state of swelling.

- The first (outer) layer is a multi-layered non-keratinized squamous epithelium. This is transparent.
- The second layer, the so-called Bowman's layer, is formed by network-like arranged collagen fibrils. Cells are not present.
- The third layer is the stroma. Between the collagen fibrils of type I and V, there are also fibroblasts known as keratocytes.
- The fourth layer, the Descemet's membrane, is a thick basal lamina formed by the endothelium. It contains collagen fibrils of type VIII.
- The fifth (inner) layer consists of a single-layered squamous epithelium, the corneal endothelium, which acts as a boundary layer preventing the penetration of aqueous humor into the cornea. Additionally, the sodium/potassium-ATPase of the endothelium actively pumps water out of the stroma. This keeps the collagen fibers parallelly arranged and maintains the transparency of the tissue.

The cornea is avascular (Fig. 2.6). Its supply occurs at the periphery through the limbal marginal loop network of the conjunctiva and at the center through the tear fluid (externally) and the aqueous humor (internally). As a result of inflammation and injuries, vessels can sprout and impair transparency. Sensory trigeminal branches (N. V1) traverse the cornea. Their free nerve endings are responsible for the so-called corneal reflex (N. VII). Due to the extremely high density of sensory nerve endings on the surface (the highest in the human body!), the cornea is extremely sensitive. Foreign bodies are immediately and very painfully perceived.

The cells of the epithelium and stroma are continuously replaced from the periphery. In the case of insufficiency of the so-called limbal stem cells, superficial vascularization can occur. After injuries or inflammations of the stroma (substantia propria, Fig. 2.11a), the regular arrangement of the collagen fibers is disrupted, usually resulting in opaque scars.

The endothelium of the cornea cannot regenerate. The cell density decreases from about 6000/mm^2 to up to 2000/mm^2 over the course of life. Defects are compensated by the enlargement of individual cells.

- ▶ The transparency of the cornea depends on the performance of the cells, especially those of the outer (first) and inner (fifth) corneal layer, as well as on the parallel arrangement of the collagen fibers of the stroma.
- ▶ The corneal endothelium does not have the ability to regenerate. During intraocular procedures, special attention must be paid to the protection of this vulnerable layer!
- ▶ Damage to the limbal stem cells of the epithelium leads to superficial vascularization, resulting in a loss of corneal transparency.

2.7 Eyeball (Bulbus oculi) and Eye Membranes

The eyeball is approximately spherical in shape (Figs. 2.4 and 2.9) (diameter 24 mm, volume 6.5 ml, weight 7.5 g) with a radius of about 11.5 mm. In the anterior section, the cornea is inserted like a watch glass (about 1/6 of the sphere). At the equator of the eyeball, it has the largest transverse diameter. This divides the eyeball into an approximately equal-sized anterior and posterior hemisphere.

We distinguish three layers in the wall of the eyeball:

- the outer eye wall (Tunica fibrosa bulbi),
- the middle eye layer (Tunica vasculosa bulbi), and
- the inner (sensory) eye layer (Tunica interna, sensoria bulbi).

The eyeball (Bulbus oculi) has three internal chambers: the anterior chamber (Camera anterior bulbi) in front of the iris, the posterior chamber (Camera posterior bulbi) behind the iris, and the vitreous chamber including the vitreous body (Corpus vitrium). The two eye chambers are connected by the pupil (Fig. 2.6).

2.7.1 Outer Eye Wall

It has two sections: the sclera (which corresponds to the dura mater) and the cornea (Chap. 6).

Sclera (White of the Eye)

The outer shell of the eyeball continues into the dura mater of the optic nerve (Fig. 2.4). It gives the eyeball its constant shape and tensile strength. The external eye muscles attach to the sclera with their short flat tendons (for more precise attachment points see Tables 2.3 and 2.4). In healthy individuals, the sclera appears white due to the compact arrangement of the collagen fibers.

▶ In cases of developmental disorders, malformations, and various diseases (for example, Marfan syndrome, osteogenesis imperfecta, and extra-articular localization of primary chronic polyarthritis), the sclera can have a blue color. In these cases, its collagen fibers are rarefied, allowing the uvea to be seen. Surgical interventions with bulb opening in these eyes have a poor prognosis!

▶ The sclera makes up about 5/6 of the outer eye coat. At the exit of the optic nerve, it is thickest at about 1.0 to 1.5 mm, whereas at the equator it is thinnest at 0.4 mm (especially in the area of the muscle attachment points!). Therefore, in cases of blunt injuries to the globe (contusion) these areas must be inspected particularly carefully for the presence of a rupture! Externally, it is enclosed by a loose sheath tissue. A centrally located layer consists of crossed collagen fibers, which run parallel to the surface. At the boundary to the choroid, there is a pigment layer.

▶ The choroid is only fixed to the sclera by vascular trunks. This can be seen in a choroidal detachment (Amotio chorioidei).

2.7.2 Middle Eye Coat

The middle eye coat is composed of several components, which are presented below.

Choroid

It is relatively thin, rich in vessels, and located between the sclera and the pars optica of the retina (Fig. 2.9). It consists of four layers:

Table 2.3 Straight eye muscles – the four recti

Muscles originating from the common tendinous ring (data from Lang and von Lanz [16] and Bergua [4])				
Muscle	Attachment	Total length	Length of attachment areas on the eyeball	Distances of muscle attachments from the limbus corneae
M. rectus superior (N. III)	Eyeball	41 mm	10.43 mm	7.91 mm
M. rectus medialis (N. III)	Eyeball	40 mm	10.32 mm	5.77 mm
M. rectus inferior (N. III)	Eyeball	40 mm	8.59 mm	6.73 mm
M. rectus lateralis (N. VI)	Eyeball	40 mm	9.57 mm	7.48 mm

Table 2.4 Oblique eye muscles (data from Lang and von Lanz [16] and Bergua [4])

Muscle	Origin	Parts	Attachment/Width	Length
M. obliquus superior	Optic canal, orbital aperture	Pars longitudinalis	Trochlea 1–3.5 mm	32–45 mm
		Pars obliqua	Eyeball 6–15 mm	17–31 mm
M. obliquus inferior	Orbital margin, lateral to the nasolacrimal duct		Eyeball 5–9.5 mm	18–38 mm

1. The lamina suprachorioidea forms the connecting layer to the sclera. In this connective tissue layer, vessels and nerves run to the ciliary body and the iris. It is interspersed with numerous slit spaces.
2. The lamina vasculosa houses extensive venous plexuses with large vessels. This best-vascularized structure of the entire organism is mainly dominated by vessels.
3. The lamina chorioidocapillaris has a capillary network for the nourishment of the sensory cell layer of the retina.
4. The lamina basalis (Bruch's membrane) lies on the pigment epithelium of the retina.

The strong blood supply is provided by up to 6 to 20 posterior ciliary arteries (which lie as the Zinn-Haller ring around the optic nerve) and anterior ciliary arteries. The venous return ends in four to six vortex veins. There is a high risk of bleeding in case of intraoperative injuries.

Ciliary Body (Corpus ciliare)

The task of the ciliary body (Fig. 2.10) is, in addition to the secretion of aqueous humor, the accommodation of the lens. This structure, which surrounds the iris in a ring shape, consists of the ciliary muscle (Figs. 2.6 and 2.10) (for the accommodation of the lens), a capillary vascular layer (for the secretion of aqueous humor through ultrafiltration), and a two-layered epithelium. The outer, pigmented layer continues into the pigment epithelium of the retina. The non-pigmented, inner layer is a continuation of the pars nervosa retinae and is involved in the production of aqueous humor. The lens is fixed to the ciliary body by the zonular fibers (Figs. 2.6 and 2.10). The tension of this suspension is adjusted or regulated by the ciliary muscle depending on the pulling effect exerted by the tone of the sclera.

The ciliary muscle has outer meridional fibers, circular fibers, and radial fibers. This allows the posterior and anterior zonular fibers to be moved accordingly. This muscle tension leads to the "rounding" of the lens (spherophakia), caused by muscle contraction.

Iris

The iris regulates the passage of light and thus functions as a diaphragm. It is located in front of the lens and delineates the anterior and posterior chambers of the eye (Figs. 2.6, 2.9 and 2.10). The vascular-rich stroma, which forms the structural basis of the iris, is a loose sponge-like network of collagenous connective tissue, containing fibroblasts, macrophages, and melanocytes.

The iris has a circular opening at or near its centre called the pupil. The anterior surface of the iris, which forms the boundary to the anterior chamber of the eye, has no covering epithelium and is therefore unevenly shaped. Here, primarily fibroblasts and melanocytes are found. The posterior surface, however, is covered by a heavily pigmented epithelium. The stroma is thinner at the pupillary margin (Anulus iridis minor), where the pigmented epithelium extends lip-like onto the anterior surface, forming the pupillary fri. margin. The broad outer zone of the stromal tissue (Anulus iridis major, also known as the iris root) is adherent to contiguous with the anterior surface of the ciliary body. Since no true connections exist, trauma or intraoperative procedures (similar to the ciliary body) can lead to the detachment of the iris (iridodialysis).

The iris has two muscles that act as antagonists (Figs. 2.6 and 2.10). The M. sphincter pupillae (Fig. 2.10) is almost circular around the pupil and is predominantly innervated parasympathetically. It causes a constriction of the pupil in response to light (miosis). The M. dilatator pupillae has fibers that radiate towards the pupil and serve its dilation (mydriasis).

- In inflammations of the iris (iritis), posterior adhesions (synechiae) with the lens or anterior adhesions with the chamber angle (angulus iridocornealis) can occur. These symptoms are often associated with rheumatoid arthritis or spondyloarthritis and are accompanied by inflammation of the ciliary body (cyclitis).
- Miosis can also be part of Horner's syndrome (a triad of miosis, ptosis, enophthalmos), where the parasympathetic system predominates due to the failure of the cervical sympathetic system.
- Iridocyclitis: Inflammations of the iris and ciliary body, especially in juvenile rheumatoid arthritis and systemic diseases (sarcoidosis), causing clouding of the aqueous humor and anterior vitreous body.

Lens (Lens)

The lens, a biconcave body (approximately 9–10 mm in diameter, 4 mm thick in the center), forms the posterior wall of the posterior chamber of the eye. It is located behind the iris. The anterior surface of the lens is bathed by the aqueous humor (of the posterior chamber of the eye). The posterior surface, on the other hand, is in physical contact with the vitreous body (Figs. 2.6, 2.9 and 2.10).

The lens is thus "suspended" between the vitreous body and the posterior chamber of the eye via the zonular fibers of the ciliary body. The lens capsule is a cuticular secretion (essentially a thick basal lamina) of the epithelial cells. On the anterior side, we find a single layer of cuboidal epithelium. Posteriorly, the epithelial cells grow into fibers 7 to 10 mm long (so-called lens fibers). These fibers are formed throughout life at the lens equator. The cell nuclei of these lens fibers degenerate, except for those located at the lens equator. The lens epithelial cells remaining after cataract surgery can lead to the formation of regenerative posterior capsular opacification (Wedel-bladder cells, Elschnig pearls). In normal development, the lens does not contain any blood vessels.

- The posterior capsule is particularly firmly attached to the vitreous body in young individuals, making it difficult to remove without injuring the vitreous body. Therefore, in the operation of congenital cataract, the opening of the posterior lens capsule should be combined with the removal of the anterior vitreous boundary membrane and an anterior vitrectomy.
- Persistent remnants of the hyaloid artery cause dense opacities of the posterior lens capsule, which cannot be eliminated by the so-called "polishing" of the capsule.

Chamber Angle (Angulus iridocornealis)

It is a space formed by the iris and the ciliary body (Fig. 2.6, 2.10 and 2.11c). From here, the aqueous humor is drained through net-like slit spaces of the ligamentum pectinatum anguli iridocornealis (Fontana spaces) into the sinus venosus sclerae (Schlemm's canal) (Fig. 2.11c). It is a vein-like vessel through which the fluid is sucked into the anterior ciliary veins. All walls of the eye chambers, especially the trabecular meshwork, are involved in the outflow of the aqueous humor.

A smaller portion of the aqueous humor flows towards the ciliary body and choroid and is absorbed by the venous vessels in this zone (so-called uveoscleral flow).

2.7.3 Inner Eye Layer

The inner eye layer consists of the pigment epithelium, stratum pigmentosum, and the retina (Figs. 2.9 and 2.12).

Pigment Epithelium

This layer consists of a single-layered epithelium, which is pigmented and firmly attached to the choroid. Numerous mitochondria and cytoplasmic structures indicate active metabolism and fluid exchange. The exchange processes between the choroid and the retina are mediated by the pigment epithelium.

Retina

Due to the various cell types and their connections, a layered structure of this structure results (Fig. 2.12). The eight layers are more or less sharply defined from each other:

1. In the outermost layer of the photoreceptors (**Stratum nervosum**), the so-called outer segments of the receptors, which are interlocked with the pigment epithelium, are located.
2. The outer limiting membrane (**Membrana limitans externa**) houses the main cell portion of the photoreceptors, which are linked with the Müller cells.
3. In the outer plexiform layer (**Stratum plexiforme externum**), the cell connections of the bipolar, horizontal, and amacrine cells are located.
4. In the inner nuclear layer (**Stratum nucleare internum**), the cell nuclei of bipolar, amacrine, interplexiform, horizontal, and Müller cells are found. These create connections between the inner and outer plexiform layers.
5. The inner plexiform layer (**Stratum plexiforme internum**) contains the synapses of the aforementioned location. Optic ganglia also attach here.
6. Ganglion cell layer (**Stratum ganglionare**): Here, the optic ganglia are located.
7. The nerve fiber layer (**Stratum neurofibrorum**) is a layer with neurons) of the optic ganglion cells.
8. The inner limiting membrane (**Membrana limitans interna**) has glial fibers and is a basal membrane-like boundary layer against the vitreous body.

Blood Supply of the Retina

It is provided by the A. centralis retinae, after it has entered the eye at the optic disc. It branches from the inner surface of the retina to the inner nuclear layer. The outer parts of the retina have no capillaries. Their supply is provided by diffusion from the choroid (Fig. 2.9).

2.7.4 Vitreous Body (Corpus vitreum)

The corpus vitreum fills the space between the lens and the retina (Fig. 2.4). With approximately 4.5 to 5 ml of volume, this space makes up three-quarters of the globe volume. It is a cell-free, No, it does contain hyalocytes gelatinous substance with up to 98–99% water content and mainly dissolved mucopolysaccharides, which lie between a fine network of collagen fibers. Originally, this space was filled with mesenchyme, which completely regressed during development. The vitreous body is condensed at its surface to form the vitreous boundary membrane and thus lies on the retina. Type II collagen fibrils are involved in this. The boundary membrane is condensed and particularly adherent both at the papilla (Martegiani ring, Weiss ring) and at the base—peripheral to the Ora serrata. With increasing age (often early in myopic patients), the vitreous boundary membrane (membrana limitans interna) detaches from the retina.

- ▶ When the vitreous boundary membrane detaches, patients may experience optical sensations (flashes of light) and opacities of the vitreous body (reduced transparency of the vitreous body in uveitis, retinitis, trauma, etc.) and perceive parts of the Martegiani ring as floaters.
- ▶ In the event of a vitreous prolapse following trauma or intraoperative capsule rupture during a cataract surgery, the traction of the still adherent vitreous body on the retina can be transmitted, which can lead to tearing and even detachment of the retina.
- ▶ Vitreous hemorrhage is a bleeding into the corpus vitreum, e.g., after trauma, vitreous detachment, retinal detachment, neovascularization due to diabetic retinopathy, and retinal vein occlusion.

2.8 Orbital Levels and Compartments

The orbit can be divided into three levels (Fig. 2.4):

1. The upper level lies between the orbital roof and the levator palpebrae muscle.
2. The middle level corresponds to the so-called intraconal space and is bounded in the sagittal view by the superior and inferior rectus muscles.
3. The lower level is located below the inferior rectus muscle.

Contents of the upper level include the lacrimal gland, the lacrimal nerve, the frontal nerve, the trochlear nerve, and the corresponding vessels and veins.

Contents of the middle level include the optic nerve, the nasociliary nerve, the superior branch of the oculomotor nerve, the abducens nerve, and the ciliary ganglion. The parasympathetic ciliary ganglion is traversed by sympathetic fibers and can be divided. It is located approximately 7 mm anterior to the common tendinous ring and lies laterally on the optic nerve (Figs. 2.4 and 2.13). From the ciliary ganglion, short ciliary nerves extend to the eyeball. There are also connections to the sensory nasociliary nerve. The nasociliary nerve gives off the ethmoidal nerves, which leave the orbit through the ethmoidal foramina and end as the infratrochlear nerve at the medial canthus.

Contents of the lower level include the inferior branch of the oculomotor nerve for the innervation of the inferior rectus muscle and the inferior oblique muscle, as well as the infraorbital nerve and the zygomatic nerve. These nerves lie below the periorbita. Of importance is the anastomosis between the pterygopalatine ganglion and the lacrimal nerve via the zygomatic nerve. Through this connection, postganglionic parasympathetic fibers travel through the inferior orbital fissure to the lacrimal gland.

In addition to the level division, the orbit can be divided into a bulbar and a retrobulbar section. Another division refers to the space enclosed by the straight eye muscles (Table 2.3) and the common tendinous ring (Zinn). Accordingly, a central intraconal section is distinguished from an extraconal space.

2.8.1 Orbital Fat Body (Corpus adiposum orbitae)

All extrabulbar structures of the orbit (muscles, nerves, and vessels) are enclosed by a highly "lobulated" fat body, the Corpus adiposum orbitae (Figs. 2.4 and 2.6). Within this fat body, various connective tissue strands, fasciae and ligaments (e.g., Lig. suspensorium bulbi) can be detected, which promote further compartmentalization. The fat body is clearly delineated from the Bulbis oculi by the Tenon capsule and ends anteriorly at the orbital septum. The lacrimal gland can be clearly distinguished from the fat body intraoperatively by its color. A distinction between intraconal and extraconal fat is possible. In cases of malnutrition, there is a reduction of the fat body and a retraction of the eyeball. Occasionally, in obesity, the fat tissue protrudes forward through gaps in the orbital septum (orbital fat hernia).

2.8.2 Optic Nerve (N. opticus)

The second cranial nerve has a slightly curved course and is located in the retrobulbar space (Figs. 2.4 and 2.9). It carries the neurons of the multipolar nerve cells from the optic disc through the Canalis opticus to the brain. Since the optic nerve is considered part of the diencephalon, it is surrounded by all meninges along its course. The diameter of the optic nerve is 5–6 mm.

The optic disc nervi optici (Fig. 2.9) has an area of 2.9 mm^2 with a height of 1.9 mm and a width of 1.8 mm. The horizontal distance from the center of the disc to the center of the macula measures 4 mm. The total length of the optic nerve is given as 35–55 mm. Four sections can be distinguished along its course: pars intraocularis, pars orbitalis, pars intracanalicularis, and pars intracranialis. Its intraocular length is about 1 mm and its orbital length is 25–30 mm. The length of the Canalis opticus is 6 mm with a diameter of 5–6 mm. The intracranial length of the optic nerve up to the optic chiasm measures 50 mm. The bony canal is in contact with the sphenoid sinus in 40% of all cases. In 7%, it is completely enclosed by the sphenoid sinus.

The optic nerve runs in close proximity to the Sinus cavernosus, the sphenoid sinus, and the posterior ethmoidal cells. Depending on the degree of pneumatization of the sphenoid sinus, the optic nerve lies on the lateral wall of the sphenoid cavity and is particularly at risk during procedures in this area. In some cases, posterior ethmoidal cells can extend far posteriorly into the sphenoid sinus and enclose the optic nerve. These ethmoidal cells, also known as Onodi cells, are predilection sites for optic nerve injury during functional endoscopic surgery of the ethmoidal cells.

▶ The division of the orbit into levels and compartments must be considered from a surgical perspective!

2.8.3 External Eye Muscles

Outside the Bulbus oculi, seven muscles (Tables 2.3 and 2.4; Figs. 2.8a, b and 2.13) can be identified, six of which move the Bulbus oculi. They are innervated by the cranial nerves III, IV, and VI. Most of these muscles originate from a fibrous ring (Fig. 2.13), the Anulus tendineus communis (Zinn). Its base at the posterior orbital pole is obliquely oval, includes the optic canal, and crosses the superior orbital fissure approximately in the middle. Muscles originating from the Anulus tendineus communis: M. rectus superior (N. III), M. rectus medius (N. III), M. rectus inferior (N. III), and M. rectus lateralis (N. VI). The straight eye muscles fan out forward and pass through the Tenon capsule to the sclera. The lengths of the straight eye muscles range from 36 to 40 mm, with M. rectus medialis being the longest. Their insertion occurs in front of the equator of the Bulbus oculi (Fig. 2.8a, b), but slightly posterior to the junction between the cornea and sclera. While the Mm. rectus medialis et lateralis function as horizontal motors of the Bulbus oculi, the Mm. rectus superior et. inferior are vertical motors. The vertical muscles also have a discrete adducting effect. Due to their slightly oblique course, M. rectus superior supports internal rotation and M. rectus inferior supports external rotation.

In addition to the straight eye muscles, two oblique eye muscles can be distinguished, M. obliquus superior (N. IV) (Table 2.4, Figs. 2.8b and 2.13) and M. obliquus inferior (N. III) (Table 2.4; Figs. 2.8b and 2.13). While the upper oblique eye muscle originates superomedially from the Anulus tendineus (Fig. 2.13), the origin of M. obliquus inferior is located at the medial orbital floor near the crista lacrimalis anterior.

The **M. obliquus superior** initially runs to the medial wall of the eye socket. In the anterior upper part of the orbit is the trochlea, a fibrocartilaginous loop. The muscle passes over the trochlea with its intermediate tendon and then runs at an acute angle (50–54°) backward under the M. rectus superior to laterally insert at the lateral edge of the Bulbus oculi. Consequently, the M. obliquus superior has a pars longitudinalis and a pars obliqua. It causes the depression, abduction, and internal rotation of the eyeball.

In contrast, the **M. obliquus inferior** runs from its origin below the lacrimal sac laterally under the Bulbus oculi but above the M. rectus inferior and inserts behind the equator of the eyeball in the sclera. The length of its insertion zone is 9.4 mm. It causes the elevation, abduction, and external rotation of the Bulbus oculi.

Finally, between M. rectus superior and the orbital roof is the **M. levator palpebrae superioris** (innervation N. III, length 40–42 mm) (Fig. 2.6 and 2.8). It originates at the ala minor in close proximity to the optic canal. The also striated muscle fans out forward (width 7.0–23 mm) and inserts into the subcutaneous connective tissue of the upper eyelid, the tarsus of the upper eyelid, and the skin. Its fibers pass through the circular fibers of the pars palpebralis of the M. orbicularis oculi. The muscle works

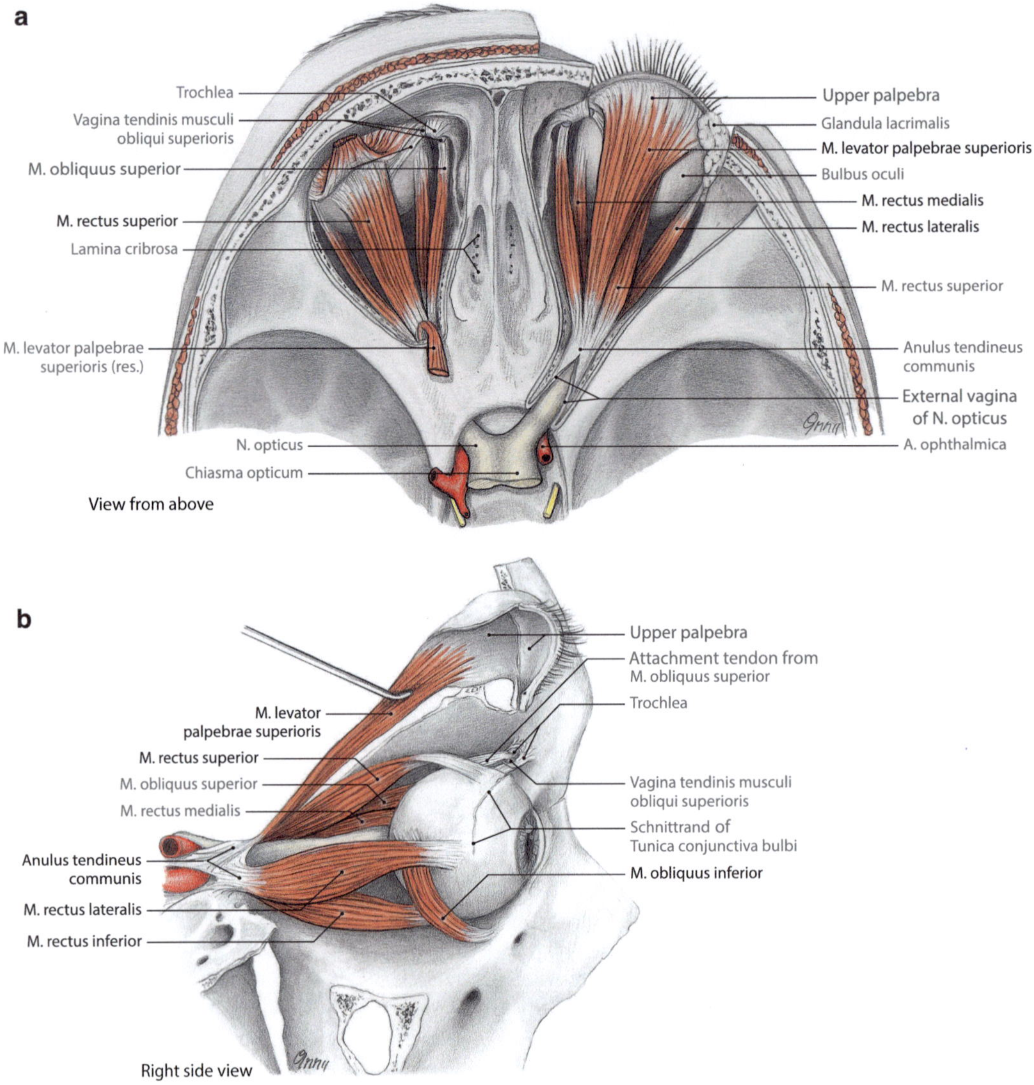

Fig. 2.8 Overview of the external eye muscles. (**a**) from above, (**b**) from the side. (From [23])

together with the M. rectus superior and lifts the upper eyelid (Chap. 4). In addition to innervation by the N. oculomotorius, there is also innervation by the sympathetic nervous system.

- When the cervical sympathetic is deactivated, Horner's syndrome occurs. This weakens the function of the M. levator palpebrae superioris, causing the upper eyelid to droop. This phenomenon is also observed in peribulbar anesthesia: Ptosis indicates the pharmacological deactivation of the sympathetic nervous system and thus the onset of the local anesthetic (Chap. 10).

- In the case of damage to the upper parts of the N. facialis (facial nerve palsy), the Bell phenomenon occurs when attempting to close the eyelids. This is a synkinesis between the orbicularis muscle and M. rectus superior. The M. levator palpebrae superioris has no significance here. In facial nerve palsy, the upward rolling of the eyeball is particularly noticeable due to the lack

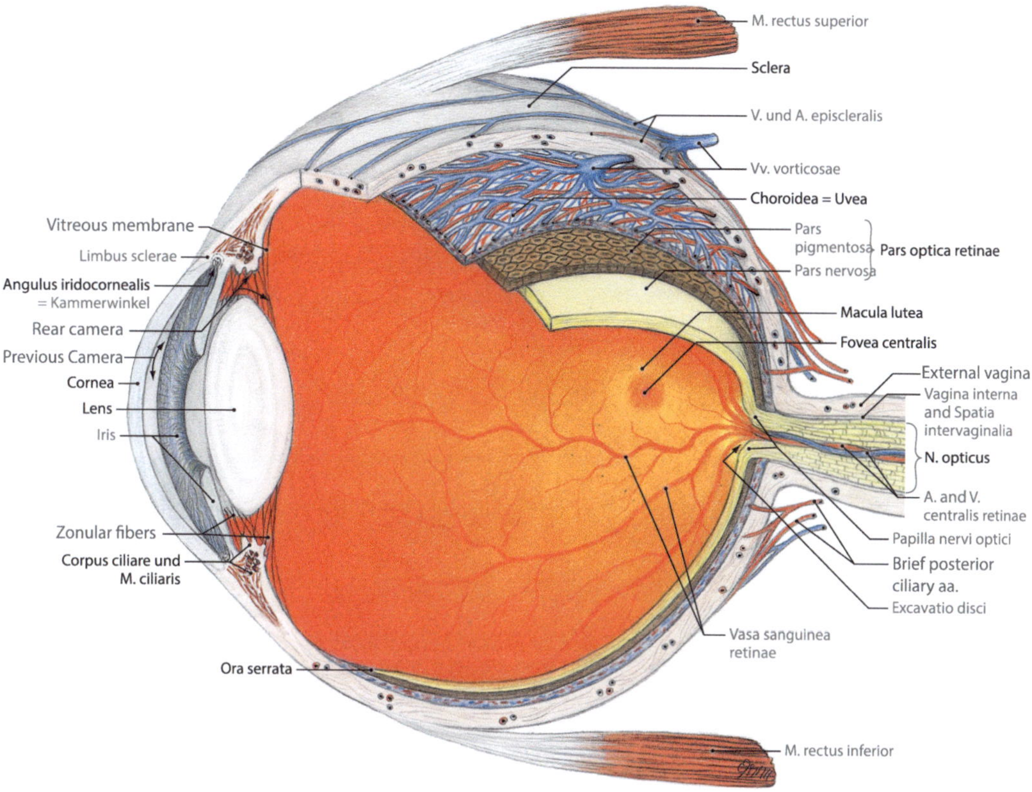

Fig. 2.9 **Layer structure of the Bulbus oculi with optic nerve**. (From [23])

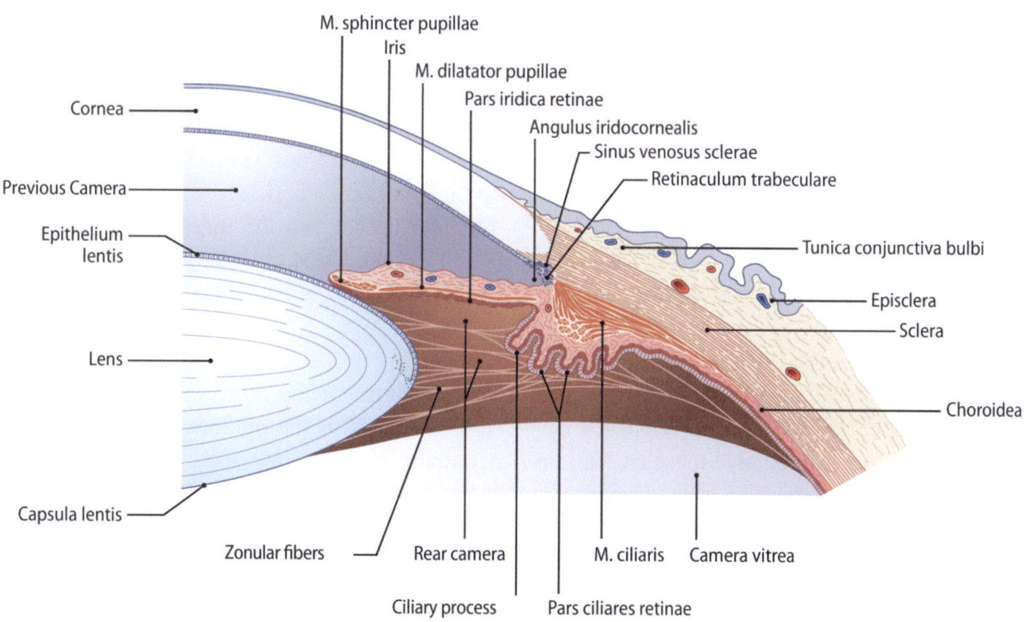

Fig. 2.10 **Structures of the iridocorneal angle.** (From Amunts et al. in Zilles and Tillmann [2])

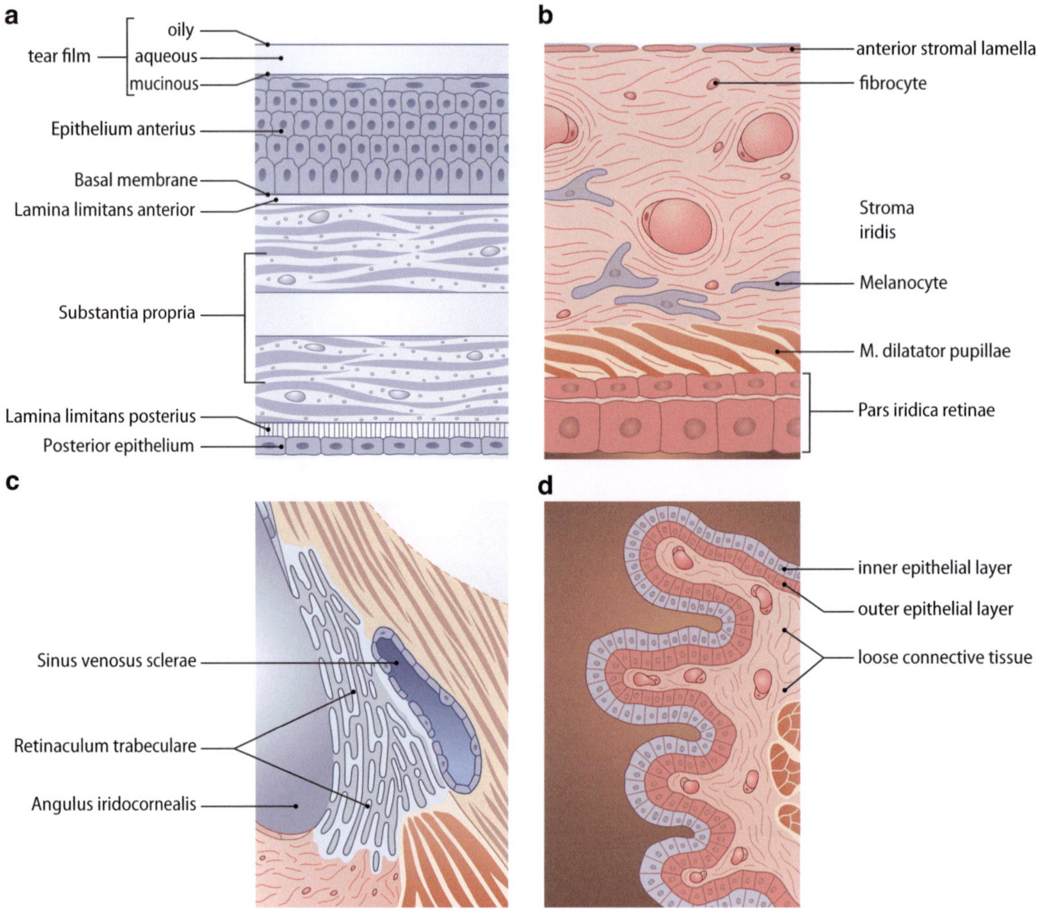

Fig. 2.11 Structure of the cornea and angulus iridocornealis. (**a**) Cornea, (**b**) Iris, (**c**) Iridocorneal angle, (**d**) Ciliary process (From [2])

of eyelid closure. The Bell phenomenon serves to protect the cornea from drying out.

2.8.4 Nerves and Vessels of the Orbit

The majority of the vessels and nerves enter the orbit through the posterior section. The common tendinous ring (Zinn) not only serves as the origin for most of the external eye muscles. Various nerves and vessels enter the orbit through the connective tissue ring: optic nerve, oculomotor nerve, abducens nerve, nasociliary nerve, and ophthalmic artery (Figs. 2.13 and 2.9).

All other nerves and vessels enter at some distance from the common tendinous ring through the superior orbital fissure (superior ophthalmic vein, lacrimal nerve, frontal nerve, trochlear nerve) and the inferior orbital fissure (inferior ophthalmic vein, zygomatic nerve, and infraorbital nerve and artery).

Nerves

The structures of the orbit are supplied by sensory branches of the ophthalmic nerve and the maxillary nerve. They also supply sensation to the facial structures of the orbital region with peripheral branches. The oculomotor nerve, trochlear nerve, and abducens nerve innervate all external eye muscles, with parasympathetic fibers of the oculomotor nerve also innervating intrinsic eye muscles.

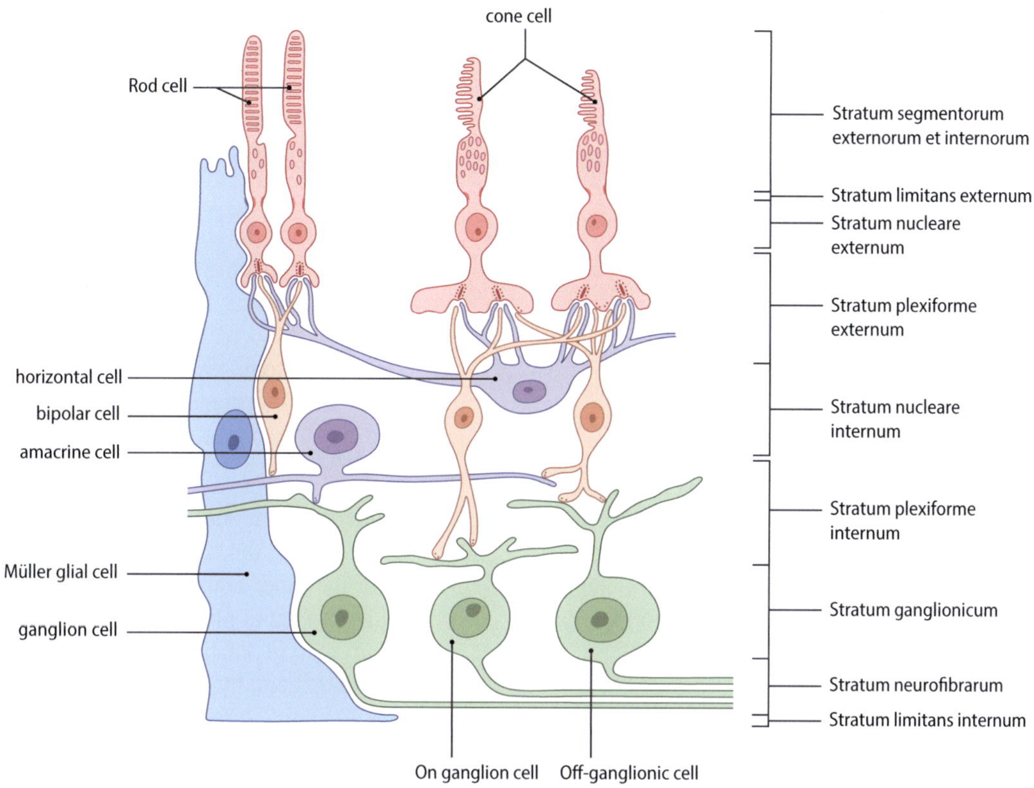

Fig. 2.12 **Connection of important cell types of the retina.** Left rod cell connection, right cone cell connection of the on-pathway and the off-pathway (highly simplified schema). (From Amunts et al. in Zilles and Tillmann [2])

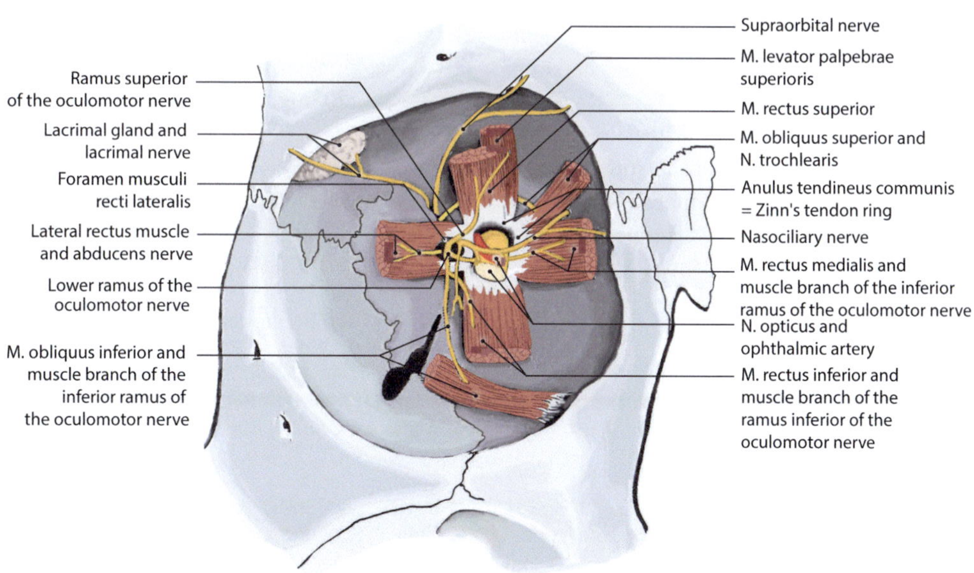

Fig. 2.13 **The common tendinous ring (Zinn) with eye muscles and pathways.** (From [23])

Arteries

The ophthalmic artery (lumen diameter: 1–1.5 mm) initially enters the optic canal medially and below the optic nerve (Fig. 2.7). Intraorbitally, it changes its course and crosses the optic nerve medially. While the lacrimal artery (lumen diameter 0.5–1 mm) runs laterally, the main trunk of the ophthalmic artery moves towards the medial canthus. The artery supplies the structures of the eyeball with numerous branches and also has various extrabulbar branches. These include the lacrimal artery to the lateral canthus and the supraorbital artery to the upper face (Fig. 2.1). On its way to the medial canthus, it gives off the anterior and posterior ethmoidal arteries and ends at the inner canthus in the supratrochlear artery (Fig. 2.1). There, it finally anastomoses with the angular artery (facial artery) via the dorsal nasal artery.

Veins

The veins of the orbit have no venous valves, allowing for a reversal of blood flow. The two main veins are the superior ophthalmic vein and the inferior ophthalmic vein. The superior ophthalmic vein collects blood from the eyeball via the vortex veins and from the upper half of the orbit, and it drains through the superior orbital fissure into the cavernous sinus. It begins medially to the optic nerve and then runs laterally above the optic nerve.

The inferior ophthalmic vein lies below the eyeball and anastomoses with the superior ophthalmic vein just before the inferior orbital fissure. It collects blood from the infraorbital vein and anastomoses through the inferior orbital fissure with the pterygoid plexus. Noteworthy are its numerous communications with the ethmoidal veins through the ethmoidal foramina and with the pterygoid plexus through the inferior orbital fissure.

Lymphatic Vessels

The lymph of the orbit is directed to the superficial and deep parotid lymph nodes and the submandibular lymph nodes. The path to the submandibular lymph nodes runs along the facial vein.

- ▶ A herpes zoster infection involving the external nose indicates the involvement of the orbital branches of the ophthalmic nerve and is characterized by the clear separation in the area of the midline of the face according to the supply.
- ▶ The course of the anterior ethmoidal artery through the cribriform plate to the anterior cranial fossa explains the risk of bleeding in skull base fractures. The lacrimal artery sometimes anastomoses with the middle meningeal artery (a branch of the maxillary artery in the infraorbital fossa) through an additional foramen.
- ▶ The numerous communications of the various branches of the superior ophthalmic vein with the inner cranial base (cavernous sinus), the pterygoid plexus in the infratemporal and pterygopalatine fossae, and the face are fundamentally important for understanding ascending infections.
- ▶ Blunt force can lead to pronounced hematomas, which can be both retrobulbar and subperiosteal. There is a risk of an orbital compartment syndrome with dangerous intraorbital pressure increase leading to central artery occlusion.
- ▶ Procedures on the orbit generally carry a potentially high risk of bleeding.

References and Further Reading

1. Alt KW (1997) Odontologische Verwandschaftsanalyse. Fischer, Stuttgart
2. Amunts K, Bechmann I, Nitsch R, Paulsen F, Schmitt O, Wree A, Zille K (2010) Nervensystem und Sinnesorgane. In: Zilles K, Tillmann BN (Hrsg) Anatomie. Springer, Berlin/Heidelberg
3. Augustin AJ (2007) Augenheilkunde. Springer, Berlin
4. Bergua A (2017) Das menschliche Auge in Zahlen. Springer, Berlin
5. Ducasse A (2007) Surgical orbital anatomy. In: Guthoff R, Katowitz J (Eds) Oculoplastics and orbit. Essentials in ophthalmology. Springer, Berlin, pp 73–97
6. Dutton JJ (Hrsg) (2011) Atlas of clinical and surgical orbital anatomy, 2nd edn. Elsevier Saunders, Philadelphia

7. Fanghänel J, Pera F, Anderhuber F, Nitsch R (2008) Waldeyer Anatomie des Menschen, 18th edn. De Gruyter, Berlin
8. Fontolliet M, Bornstein MM, von Arx T (2019) Characteristics and dimensions of the infraorbital canal: a radiographic analysis using cone beam computed tomography (CBCT). Surg Radiol Anat 41:169–179
9. Grehn F (2019) Augenheilkunde, 32nd edn. Springer, Berlin
10. Hauser G, De Stefano GF (1989) Epigentic variants of the human skull. Schweizerbart, Stuttgart
11. Heichel J, Lehmann G, Viestenz A, Eckel A, Reich W, Scheffler B (2020) Acute compression of the optic nerve due to orbital emphysema. Ophthalmologe 117(10):1037–1040
12. Kadanoff D, Mutafov S, Jordanov J (1970) The principle openings and incisures of the facial bones. Gegenbaurs Morphol Jahrb 115:102–118
13. Kazkayasi M, Ergin A, Ersoy M, Bengi O, Tekdemir I, Elhan A (2001) Certain anatomical relations and the precise morphometry of the infraorbital foramen–canal and groove: an anatomical and cephalometric study. Laryngoscope 111:609–614
14. Koppe T, Nagai H (1999) Pneumatization of the facial skeleton in Catarrhine primates. In: Koppe T, Nagai H, Alt KW (Eds) The paranasal sinuses of higher primates. Quintessence, Chicago, pp 77–119
15. Kunsch K, Kunsch S (2007) Der Mensch in Zahlen, 3rd edn. Elsevier Spektrum, Heidelberg
16. Lang J, von Lanz T (1979) Praktische Anatomie: ein Lehr-und Hilfsbuch der anatomischen Grundlagen ärztlichen Handelns. vol. 1: Teil 1, Kopf: B. Gehirn- und Augenschädel. Springer, Berlin
17. Liebgott B (2001) The anatomical basis of dentistry, 2nd edn. Mosby, St. Louis
18. Paulsen F (2007) Anatomy and physiology of the nasolacrimal ducts. In: Weber RK, Keerl R, Schaefer SD, Della Rocca RC (eds) Atlas of lacrimal surgery. Springer, Berlin, pp 1–13
19. Plontke SK, Glien A, Kisser U, Viestenz A, Heichel J (2020) Erkrankungen und Chirurgie der Orbita. Laryngo-Rhino-Otol 99:896–917
20. Schiebler TH, Schmidt W (1991) Anatomie, 5th edn. Springer, Berlin
21. Schünke M, Schulte E, Schumacher U (2009) Prometheus. Kopf, Hals und Neuroanatomie, 2nd edn. Thieme, Stuttgart
22. Schumacher GH, Aumüller G (2004) Topographische Anatomie des Menschen, 7th edn. Urban & Fischer, München
23. Tillmann BN (2005) Atlas der Anatomie. Springer, Berlin
24. Walsh FB (1957) Clinical neuro-opthalmology, 2nd edn. Williams & Wilkens, Baltimore

Asepsis and Antisepsis in Eye Surgery

3

Axel Kramer

Contents

Protecting the patient from surgical site infections (SSI; outdated term: postoperative wound infections) is essential for the surgical outcome. To minimize the risk of infection, it is necessary that everyone who is working in the eye operating room for the first time knows and adheres to the rules and regulations for aseptic work. This chapter has been placed at the beginning of this book to pay tribute to the immense importance of hygiene in eye surgery. The newcomer in the eye operating room must familiarize themselves with the regulations, know the procedures, and internalize them **beforehand**. It is also important to practice handling the equipment to prevent it from becoming contaminated later during the procedure if handled improperly.

SSI in the eye often occurs endogenously, as the body's own flora enters the surgical area and, depending on the immune status, can trigger an SSI. Endogenous infection is only partially controllable. However, infections can also be transmitted exogenously through gaps in asepsis and antisepsis. Managing both risks is the focus of a structured hygiene management system.

The legal information presented here is valid only in Germany. Rules and requirements for reprocessing medical devices are valid only in the European Union. Regarding the implementation of these legal requirements, where applicable, national laws that deviate from them must be taken into consideration.

A. Kramer (✉)
Institute of Hygiene and Environmental Medicine, University Medicine Greifswald, Greifswald, Germany
e-mail: axel.kramer@med.uni-greifswald.de

3.1 Intervention Room/Operating Room

In the prevention of SSI, hygienic behavior, pre-, peri-, intra-, and postoperative measures, as well as spatial and structural conditions, complement each other. Infection prevention can only be effective if it is part of the treatment pathways and patient flow. Fundamentally, the

F. Wilhelm (ed.), *Ophthalmic Surgery for Beginners*, https://doi.org/10.1007/978-3-662-70287-1_3

contribution of structural conditions to infection prevention is comparatively low compared to hygienic behavior, surgical competence, methodology and workflow, and hygiene-safe technologies, as well as directly patient-related preventive measures. On the other hand, structural design facilitates the feasibility of hygienic measures and thus indirectly contributes to infection prevention. The basis of efficient operating processes is a clear material flow, tested, introduced, and documented processes, well-trained personnel, team culture, and monitoring of process and outcome quality.

While the structural requirements for units for inpatient and outpatient operations do not differ, the main structural difference between operating rooms and intervention rooms lies in the type of ventilation. Additionally, operating rooms are functionally integrated into an operating department with personnel locks (team, material, patient) and a varying number of other functional rooms.

▶ Eye operating rooms are equipped with a ventilation system to achieve the room class (Rc) Ib.

In RC Ib sterile filtered air is supplied to the operating room as turbulent mixed ventilation. It is under positive pressure relative to the adjacent rooms to prevent the ingress of contaminated air. The high air exchange rates also contribute to the rapid elimination of particles. Alternatively, with a mobile sterile ventilation unit (MSVU), a reduction of microbial load and particle count in the room air was achieved in the area of the operating field and on the instrument table during operation in a room-class (RC) II surgical unit, which can be categorised as sufficient for operations in RC Ib. With an MSVU, operations with a high risk of SSI can also be carried out in surgical units of RC II. The MSVU is an organisationally flexible and economically interesting, safe and sustainable option in terms of the microbiological load and particle count in the operating field and on the instrument table instead of a room ventilation system that ventilates the entire room. In times when surgical services are increasingly on an out-patient basis, MSVU is a promising option for outpatient surgical units in particular [60].

▶ Eye intervention rooms do not differ in ventilation technology from examination and treatment rooms.

They have window ventilation (protected with fly screens); if necessary, a mechanical supply and exhaust ventilation system with air supply via F7 and F9 filters should be provided. If general anesthesia is performed, the latter is required.

Reduced spatial requirements apply to intervention rooms, i.e., the intervention room takes on the functions of patient preparation and post-preparation, the operation, the preparation of instruments, dressing, and hand antisepsis. A patient lock is not required. If a sterile operating gown is required to protect the operating area from contamination with work clothes, it can be kept in the intervention room. If split cooling devices are needed for cooling, contamination of the room air must be prevented. For this purpose, the condensate is directly discharged into the wastewater via a separate pipe with a pipe interrupter. Unlike the operating room, the walls do not need to be washable. The other surfaces must be easy to clean and disinfect. Hand washbasins are permissible, unlike in the operating room, if sufficient splash protection is ensured. The storage of reprocessed medical products can take place in the intervention room in dust-protected cabinets; open storage is not permitted.

▶ Operations associated with a high or medium risk of SSI and/or severe consequences in the event of an SSI and requiring high-tech equipment with corresponding space requirements should be performed in an operating room to eliminate room air as a potential source of pathogens. For short-term operations with low invasiveness and a small operating field, there is no evidence that the microbial load of the room air is a risk factor for the development of SSI. They can be performed in an intervention room [1].

For each patient, the overall situation (immune status, accompanying underlying diseases) must be assessed by the outpatient operating physician before making a decision. If there is a likelihood that the intervention may need to be expanded or if additional individual risk factors are present, the higher-grade room allocation should be applied in case of doubt.

In ophthalmology, an operating room of room class Ib is recommended for the following operations: cataract, glaucoma, retina, and corneal surgery [2]. In contrast, intravitreal operative drug administration (IVOM) and eyelid surgery can be performed in an intervention room.

3.2 Basic Hygiene

Through the measures of basic hygiene ("standard precaution"), most pathogen transmissions can be prevented. They include hand hygiene, the reprocessing and handling of medical products, patient-near and, if necessary, patient-distant surface disinfection, safe injection techniques, the wearing of work and protective clothing, black-and-white separation, and cough etiquette. Compliance with these measures must be regulated pre-, intra-, and postoperatively.

3.2.1 Hand Hygiene

The most important aspects of hand hygiene are briefly presented below.

Handwashing

▶ Before starting work and, if necessary, at the end of work, handwashing is recommended.

Dirty hands and fingernails (e.g., after gardening) should already be cleaned at home. At the beginning of work, adhering dirt, including any adhering bacterial spores, should be removed. Due to the significantly higher skin stress compared to alcohol-based hand rubs (ABHR), soap washing should only be performed at the start of work, in case of contamination, and after using the toilet, the latter due to the risk of spore contamination. The use of a hand-washing brush is no longer recommended due to possible small skin injuries.

To prevent microbial contamination, soap dispensers must meet the following requirements [3]:

- Dispensers must be exclusively filled with disposable containers with the possibility of using containers from different manufacturers.
- During use, microbial contamination of the pump head should be avoided.
- The fill level should be visible during operation.
- For rigid dispensers, the external and internal parts of the dispenser must be easy to clean and wipe-disinfectable.
- The dispensers and all permanent parts must be machine-thermally processable at an A_0 value of at least 60°C (e.g., 80°C/1 min).
- Dispensers with disposable pump heads and touchless dispensers are to be preferred. If the pump heads are used for subsequent containers, detailed reprocessing instructions must be specified.
- Automatically operated dispenser systems are to be preferred due to the lower probability of contamination and transmission.

Hygienic Hand Antisepsis

The hands of the personnel are the most important transmitters of pathogens. Therefore, hand antisepsis[1] is one of the most important measures for the prevention of nosocomial infections.

[1] The term "hand antisepsis" is used instead of "hand disinfection", which is commonly used in Germany, France, Austria and another European countries. The main reason is that antisepsis (Greek: anti=against, sepsis=putrefaction) refers to locally applied measures on or in living tissue to kill or reduce microorganisms or inactivate viruses. In the U.S., the criterion of episomatic application is the basis for the differentiation between antisepsis and disinfection. According to various U.S. regulations, antisepsis and disinfection are differentiated: the use of antimicrobial preparations for the reduction of microorganisms on the body surface is antisepsis. Therefore, antiseptics are covered by the same regulations as drugs and cosmetics (Federal Food, Drug, and Cosmetic Act). On the other hand, disinfection includes the killing or removal of pathogens on nonliving materials. As opposed to disinfection, antimicrobial treatment of the body surface always has an antiseptic, but never a disinfecting effect.

▶ Hygienic hand antisepsis involves the use of an ABHR after actual or suspected contamination of the hands or before aseptic activities.

It is indicated

- in operating rooms/procedure rooms on the clean side of the personnel lock before putting on area clothing,
- before any direct patient contact,
- before aseptic activities, e.g., before an injection or puncture, even if gloves are worn, as well as before drawing up medications.

Hygienic hand antisepsis is also recommended after

- contact with potentially infectious material, e.g., dirty laundry, waste,
- direct patient contact,
- removal of disposable medical gloves and surgical gloves at the end of surgery, as microperforations are often not detectable or contamination may have occurred during removal.

▶ The ABHR must be rubbed over all areas of the dry hands with special attention to the fingertips, thumbs, inner and outer surfaces, wrists, interdigital spaces, and nail folds.

A rubbing technique should be chosen to ensure that both hands are as thoroughly wetted as possible. The skin areas should be kept moist for the duration of the declared exposure time. To ensure the required amount of 3 ml [4], the ABHR dispenser should be adjusted accordingly.

▶ Hand antisepsis should last at least 15 s.

Recent studies have shown that in trained individuals, the same coverage and effectiveness are achieved with 15 s of rubbing instead of 30 s [5–8]).

The faster the ABHR evaporates, the higher the effectiveness [4]. From this perspective, ethanol-based hand rubs are preferred over propanol or isopropanol. This also has the advantage of a broader virus spectrum.

▶ If there is a suspicion of epidemic keratoconjunctivitis, hand antisepsis with the declaration "limited spectrum virucidal activity"[2] should be used [61].

This also applies in the event of Noro- or Rotavirus infections. As soon as a regional seasonal increase in norovirus infections is known, a general switch is recommended for the duration of the increase.

Wherever hand antisepsis must be performed, dispensers for ABHR should be available, e.g., in the personnel lock, at the examination site, the sanitary cell, and also in the entrance area of the facility. Dispensers must be maintained in such a way that microbial colonization is prevented.

In Germany, for the selection of ABHR, the disinfectant list issued by the Disinfectant Commission in the VAH, which is available online free of charge (https://vah-liste.mhp-verlag.de/), is suitable.

Surgical Hand Antisepsis

▶ Surgical hand antisepsis must be performed before direct contact with the surgical field, sterile instruments or materials, and before other procedures with the same aseptic requirements as for surgery.

If the hands are clean, soap washing before surgical hand antisepsis can be omitted because prior hand washing reduces the effectiveness of ABHRs [9].

▶ Additional cleaning of the hands with a brush is no longer recommended due to the risk of causing minor skin injuries.

[2] Regarding the efficacy of ABHR 3 areas of activity are distinguished: „virucidal activity against enveloped viruses", „limited spectrum virucidal activity" = effective against non-enveloped viruses with low lipophilicity (e.g., adeno-, noro-,rotaviruses) and „virucidal activity", include more resistant non-enveloped hydrophilic viruses (e.g., hepatitis A-,hepatitis E-, coxsackie-, echo-, papilloma viruses).

With hand antisepsis with a declared exposure time of 1.5 min hands and forearms are safely antiseptically decontaminated if the following are performed: standardized rub-in technique, first wetting both hands for about 10 s, then wetting first one, then the other forearm for about 10 s, and then repeatedly thoroughly wetting the hands for about 70 s [10]. Whether this is achievable with ABHR with a declared exposure time of 1 min has not been investigated, as the test standard for listing only provides for wetting the hands without including the forearms. Therefore, only ABHR with a declared exposure time ≥1.5 min should be used.

Requirements for Hand Antisepsis

Short, fingertip-length nails ensure thorough cleaning of the subungual spaces and minimize the risk of glove perforation. Nail polish is to be avoided because it prevents visual assessment of the nails, and with 5-day-old nail polish suboptimal hand antisepsis was detectable compared to the reference procedure without polished nails [9].

- Wearing artificial and gel nails as well as jewelry on hands and forearms are not permitted

The bacterial density is higher on artificial nails than on natural ones. At the same time, the risk of perforation for disposable medical gloves increases. Artificial nails have repeatedly been identified as a source of nosocomial infections [9].

Jewelry hinders hand hygiene and becomes a reservoir for pathogens. Among intensive care nurses, the number of Gram-negative pathogens and *Staphylococcus aureus* correlated with the number of rings worn [9]. Also, due to the risk of injury, wearing rings is not permitted [11]. Finally, wearing wedding rings leads to an increased frequency of surgical glove perforations [9].

- Before surgical procedures, there should be no nail bed injuries or inflammatory processes on the hands of the surgeon or the surgical assistant [9].

In cases of onycholysis and onychomycosis with subungual detection of *Pseudomonas aeruginosa*, an outbreak was caused despite wearing surgical latex gloves, as well as in psoriasis with colonization by *Serratia marcescens* [9].

After careful risk assessment, it appears justifiable to perform surgery with two pairs of gloves worn over each other in the case of non-purulent inflammatory skin lesions on the hand, provided that a sterile cover (film dressing) is applied after surgical hand antisepsis and before putting on double gloves [9]. For non-surgical activities, skin lesions on the hands should be covered in a pathogen-proof and, if necessary, liquid-proof manner (plaster or bandage) for infection prevention and personnel protection.

Skin Protection and Care

- Protection and care of the hands are a professional duty because damaged skin cannot be adequately antiseptically decontaminated and can lead to an irritant-toxic contact eczema with occupational disability.

With adequate skin protection/care, the use of ABHR is not associated with the risk of developing irritant dermatitis. A prerequisite for the skin compatibility of the hand antisepsis is the content of re-fattening agents in the ABHR, which should be considered when selecting products.

- If the skin is at risk due to work in a moist environment – including wearing liquid-tight gloves for more than 2 hours – the employer must provide personal protective equipment (PPE), create operating instructions and a skin protection plan, and ensure occupational medical care and monitoring [12].

Skin protection products should protect against irritation and make it more difficult for irritants and allergens to penetrate. They are applied at the beginning of work and, if necessary, during work breaks. In case of visible contamination of the hands, the skin should be cleaned and thoroughly dried before reapplying to prevent increased penetration of any irritants remaining on the skin.

Skin care products should support the regeneration of the skin. They are used only at the end of the workday and during leisure time, as there is a risk during work that the penetration of irritants or allergens will be increased.

▶ Skin protection and skin care products should be provided in dispensers or tubes due to the risk of contamination during extraction.

In the skin protection plan, the products for cleaning, protection, and care of the skin should be specified. In case of initial skin damage, the occupational health service or a dermatologist should be consulted. They should initiate a Professional Association skin procedure if necessary.

It has been proven that the use of skin protection neither reduces the effectiveness of surgical hand antisepsis nor affects the perforation rate of sterile surgical gloves. The protective effect and improvement of the skin condition were detectable after 8 days of use [13].

3.2.2 Professional, Ward-required and Protective Clothing

In addition to disposable gloves, professional, ward-required and protective clothing also include surgical gloves and gowns as well as specific surgical and protective clothing.

Pathogen-Free Medical Disposable Gloves

Pathogen-free medical disposable gloves serve both to interrupt infection pathways and for self-protection [14].

▶ They should be worn in the event of foreseeable or probable contact with pathogens as well as before contact with bodily excretions and secretions.

Due to the risk of skin damage and increased perforation hazard, disposable gloves should be put on dry hands.

If gloves are not provided with an automatic glove dispenser or not taken from a box that releases the subsequent glove upon removal of the first one, allowing removal without touching the box and other gloves [15], hand antisepsis should be performed before removal. Opened boxes should be protected from contamination by dust, splashes, and droplets. Storing individual gloves in the coat pocket is not permitted [9].

Sterile Surgical Gloves and Surgical Gown

▶ Sterile surgical gloves should be worn before contact with non-colonized areas of the body and when handling sterile medical devices or sterile material.

After talcum came under criticism due to the causation of talcum granulomas following laparotomy, it was replaced by cornstarch. Since granuloma formation has also been described with cornstarch and no effect on sweat production was detectable [16], its use should also be discontinued [9].

The sterile surgical gown should be ankle-length and should not hinder the wearer in the design of the collar and sleeve cuffs. Freedom of movement, moisture exchange, and ergonomic quality are important for aseptic work.

Professional Clothing

It serves to protect personal clothing from contamination. Additionally, it conveys a uniform appearance. It is usually short-sleeved so that the forearm can be included in hand antisepsis. It should be changed immediately if visibly soiled, but at least every second day.

To ensure hygienically impeccable laundry quality, laundry generated in healthcare facilities should only be processed in certified laundries with validated procedures for thermal or chemothermal disinfection processes, not in private households. Washing in a household washing machine can result in an even higher microbial load on the washed clothing than on the soiled textiles before laundering, due to the undefined holding time for the required disinfection temperature.

Area Clothing

Wearing ward-required clothing in the surgical department is good clinical practice. It is put on in the personnel lock and should be changed in case of soiling or contamination, as well as upon re-entry into the personnel lock.

The operating or procedure room is entered after the sterile instruments are set up. In the personnel lock, the surgical mask (mouse-nose protection [MNP]) and surgical cap are put on. The MNP must cover the mouth and nose and fit snugly against the face.

▶ When putting it on, it should be noted that an MNP has an inside and an outside.

Beard hair must be completely covered, if necessary, in combination with the surgical cap. For occupational safety reasons, it may be necessary to wear an FFP2 mask for patients with an aerosol-transmissible infectious disease (e.g., COVID-19).

▶ Only the FFP2 or FFP3 mask guarantees inhalation protection for the surgeon and the operating room staff.

The surgical cap must completely cover the head hair. Before each new operation, the sterile surgical clothing must be changed. The same applies to MNP and hair protection. Awake patients undergoing local anesthesia should also wear an MNP, if the operation allows, to avoid the spread of aerosols when speaking and breathing.

Surgical shoes should be machine-processable.

▶ Hygiene violations include a hanging MNP after the operation and its reuse, as well as touching the used mask without subsequent hand antisepsis.

3.2.3 Reprocessing and Handling of Medical Devices

Since not all medical devices used in the operating room are disposable materials ("disposables"), reprocessing is carried out either externally or within the facility in these cases. To understand the processes and necessary regulations, it is recommended that aspiring eye surgeons participate in a training course on the reprocessing of medical devices!

With regard to the type of application and the resulting risk, medical devices (MDs) can be categorized as:

- Non-critical MDs: those which only come into contact with intact skin,
- Semi-critical MDs: those which come into contact with mucous membrane or pathologically altered skin,
- Critical MDs: for use with blood, blood products or other sterile medicinal products or sterile MD, and MD that penetrate the skin or mucous membrane as intended band are used in contact with blood or on internal tissues or organs, including wounds.

With regard to the requirements, MDs are divided into A and B:

- Semi-critical A and critical A: without special reprocessing requirements; this includes, for example, solid instruments
- Semi-critical or critical B: with increased reprocessing requirements; this includes, for example, MDs for which
  - the effectiveness of cleaning cannot be directly assessed by inspection (e.g., due to long, narrow, in particular terminal lumens, complex surfaces that are difficult to access and therefore difficult to rinse),
  - the effects of reprocessing (including transportation) on the MD and its material properties (e.g., sensitive surfaces,electronic components, active MD) that influence the safety of use or function cannot be ruled out and therefore require increased efforts during the technical/functional inspection

Responsibility, Spatial and Personnel Requirements

Responsibility: The operator is responsible for reprocessing; in the case of reprocessing in one's own practice, the practice owner is responsible.

- In the case of outsourcing, the rights and obligations of the operator and contractor as well as the modalities of reprocessing and transport must be contractually fixed.

The contracting company must provide proof of a QM system and must be approved in accordance with § 10 and § 25 of the Medical Devices Act (MPG). This only applies to companies that exclusively reprocess for others, not to central sterile supply departments (CSSD) or Reprocessing Units for Medical Devices (AEMP) of the given hospital or clinic, which are subject to official supervision by authorities.

Spatial Requirements: If reprocessing is carried out in one's own facility, the following requirements must be met:

- In the case of new, additional, and conversion buildings, a separate room with separation of clean/unclean is required for the reprocessing of MD semicritical B or critical B. If only MD semicritical A and critical A are reprocessed, a separate area with zonal separation of clean/unclean is sufficient. The treatment area must be separated from the reprocessing area [17].

Permanently installed MDs are reprocessed in the treatment room. The rooms should have sufficient lighting and ventilation.

Personnel Requirements: Employees without completed training as nursing staff or training in corresponding medical professions may not be entrusted with the reprocessing and release of MD semikritisch and kritisch A, B, and C [17], unless expertise, e.g., in the reprocessing of MD in medical practices, endoscopy units, etc., has been acquired. The German Society for Sterile Supply (not relevant in the rest of the world (DGSV) offers courses on sterile supply assistance.

Handling of Sterile Goods in the OR: When storing sterile goods, recontamination decontamination must be avoided. Therefore, sterile goods cabinets for storing intraocular lenses and suture material should only be opened for stocking and removal. At the same time, sufficient storage capacity in closed cabinets for sterile goods must be provided, as open storage in simple clear sterile packaging is only permitted for 48 hours unprotected. The storage areas must be regularly disinfected by wiping (at least weekly). The inventory and sterile goods must be checked for expired products.

If sterile goods, still in their original packaging, fall to the floor, the packaging must be disinfected by wiping with an oxygen-releasing agent, as alcohols are ineffective against bacterial spores. Hand antisepsis must also be carried out afterward.

Equipment Requirements

- In cleaning and disinfection procedures, only machine-based methods are fully validatable and therefore should be prioritized. The use of manual methods, when machine-based methods are available for semi-critical and critical medical devices, requires proof of the equivalence of the performance of manual and machine-based methods [17].

- Washer desinfectors (WD) are typically revalidated after one year. As a result of a risk analysis, an extension to more than two years is possible if software such as Segosoft records the relevant parameters like temperature and time for each process and, for example, a process review with a process challenge device is conducted quarterly.

For sterilization, only small steam sterilizers with sterilization cycle B ("big") are suitable without restriction in terms of the objects to be sterilized.

Microscope adapters for indirect ophthalmoscopy must be sterilized due to their proximity to the surgical field; alternatively, they can be fitted into a sterile plastic cover.

For small sterilizers, revalidation is required after a maximum of 2000 cycles or one year. An extension to 4000 cycles or a maximum of two years is possible with the use of integrated software that evaluates each sterilization process. This can also limit the scope of testing (e.g., temperature measurement only at reference measurement points and the most critical measurement point identified during initial validation).

If medical devices are not excluded from cleaning with ultrasound (US), cleaning with US under the addition of suitable cleaners (process parameters: 10 min, 30–40°C, 35 Hz) should be performed before machine reprocessing. This cleaning enhancement is particularly important, for example, for bone and glaucoma instruments, lid retractors with suction, and lumen instruments, which have been in contact with silicone oil (placing on sieve trays).

Functional attachments such as diathermy for intraocular use and light cables, as well as ophthalmoscopy lenses made of plastic with surface coating, usually need to be sterilized with formaldehyde.

Phacoemulsification Devices: Outbreaks of postoperative endophthalmitis have been caused by contaminated devices (non-sterile storage of processed cassettes) and irrigation solutions [18–20]. Before disconnecting the handpieces from the unit, they should be thoroughly flushed, as backflow is possible when the connection to the pressure transducer is interrupted [19]. The ultrasonic handpieces can usually be steam sterilized. Phaco tips are offered by manufacturers as single-use or reprocessable (20–50 times). The manufacturer must provide a validated reprocessing protocol for each step after manual pre-cleaning, i.e., machine cleaning and disinfection (e.g., 8 steps) and subsequent sterilization (program with 134°C). It is imperative that the documentation for the validation of reprocessing should be checked before purchase. There is a lack of epidemiological evidence for the decision between single-use or reusable [21]. The manufacturer's specification for the number of permissible reprocessings should be observed.

When alkaline cleaning was introduced and the sterilization temperature was increased from 121°C to 134°C after the occurrence of vCJD, Toxic Anterior Segment Syndrome (TASS) with red eyes became noticeable postoperatively [22, 23]. When tested in cell culture (epithelioid cell line CHO-K1), high cytotoxicity (viability <2% instead of 100% before first reprocessing) was observed after just 5 reprocessings of the tubes. This example underscores the necessity of validating reprocessing by the manufacturer not only in terms of sterilization success but also regarding biocompatibility. The problem was resolved after switching to single-use (Kramer unpublished). When testing 67 reprocessed tube systems from various clinics and ophthalmology practices, 23 were unsterile [24]. Thus, single-use generally provides higher safety.

Preparation of Medical Devices Also Used in Conservative Ophthalmology

The preparation of ophthalmological examination and surgical devices varies depending on the material [25]. Due to different manufacturer recommendations, only general principles are listed below.

- For the preparation of contact lenses, tonometer heads, and ultrasound heads, manual preparation with pre-packaged disinfectant wipes ("flow pack") does not constitute a validated procedure, contrary to the manufacturer's claims.

Justification: Currently, there is no guideline or standard that could serve as a basis for ensuring validation through wiping. It is also not clear how this can be implemented on-site. Additionally, unlike immersion disinfection, thorough wetting after a single wipe, depending on the active ingredient, is not guaranteed for the duration of the exposure time. If the contact time is shortened, the effectiveness can no longer be guaranteed [26]. This is particularly critical for disinfectants based on chlorine dioxide and alcohol (the latter dry in less than 1 minute; [27]). This means that even if a disinfectant meets the test requirements for instrument disinfectants as a solution, the conditions of the outdated immersion disinfection method are not met when applied by wiping.

With reference to the Medical Devices Operator Ordinance, the RKI [28] therefore considers the validation of the preparation process using manual wiping for the final disinfection of semi-critical medical devices as not given. This fact must be considered in the interest of patient safety.

Tonometer: Immersion disinfection is unsuitable due to material sensitivity. Plexiglass can become cloudy or prone to cracking. Both tonometer measuring bodies and contact lenses have adhesive joints that can swell when the products are immersed in disinfectant solution.

As an apparatus-based method, TonoClean™ is available for the preparation of contact lenses and tonometer heads. The preparation process is microprocessor-controlled and is performed as follows:

- 1 min rinse with sterile water,
- 10 s drying,
- 5 min disinfection (e.g., Sekusept active 2%),
- 1 min rinse with sterile water, and
- 10 s drying.

In examinations with tonometer measuring bodies and contact lenses artificially contaminated with 10^7–10^8 adenoviruses, no residual viruses were detectable on the test bodies after preparation in TonoClean™ [29]. With 70 preparations per day, the acquisition of TonoClean™ pays off after just one month in cost comparison with the non-validated Tristel-trio system (Kramer unpublished). In the Guideline for Disinfection and Sterilization in Healthcare Facilities [30], hypochlorite (5000 ppm chlorine) is recommended.

Alternatively, disposable contact lenses and tonometers can be used, but this is not cost-effective.

Schiötz tonometers made entirely of metal can be heat disinfected.

Lumen Instruments: They must not dry out after use and should be rinsed as soon as possible (tap water, preferably sterile distilled water, as the use of tap water can lead to ion accumulation on steel surfaces). Preparation should ideally be carried out within 2 hours.

Gonioscopes: They are rinsed under tap water, must be virucidaly disinfected, e.g., with 1% (10,000 ppm) NaOCl solution ≥10 min [31], then subjected to a rinse with sterile water and dried before use. Koeppe, goniotomy, or BIOM lenses made of plastic are sterilized in ethylene oxide. Formaldehyde requires slightly higher temperatures and can damage the surfaces.

Chin and Forehead Contact Surfaces on Diagnostic Devices: They must be subjected to wipe disinfection after each patient (if there are no manufacturer restrictions, with alcohol-based surface disinfectants).

3.3 Prevention of Surgical Site Infections

The following outlines the essential aspects of surgical site infection prevention.

3.3.1 Behavior in the Operating Room or Procedure Room

The sterile dressing and behavior of the surgical team do not differ from other surgical disciplines. A particular feature is the sometimes short duration of the surgery, ranging from 10 to 15 minutes. As long as the surgical mask has not been removed, the operating room is ventilated with mixed ventilation (Room Class Ib), and the surgical mask has not been visibly contaminated from the outside, the mask does not need to be changed after each patient. The decision is up to the surgeon based on the assessment of the surgical situation.

After surgeries lasting less than 60 minutes, surgical hand antisepsis before the next surgery can be shortened to 1 minute instead of 1.5 minutes with ABHR [32].

After abscess incision or surgery for endophthalmitis, the relevant contamination area, including the floor, must be disinfected.

Depending on the operating room ventilation, it must be ensured that the eye does not dry out during surgery.

▶ The intraoperative wetting of the cornea is performed by the aseptic surgical nurse with sterile physiological saline solution.

3.3.2 General Preoperative Measures

▶ Microbially induced eye diseases must be fully treated before elective procedures.

This applies, for example, to dacryocystitis, eyelid abscesses, infectious keratitis, or blepharitis.

Patients with epidemic keratoconjunctivitis and other eye infections that are presumably highly contagious and/or caused by highly virulent pathogens, as well as carriers of MRSA, should be spatially separated from freshly operated patients and those preparing for surgery.

Wearers of soft contact lenses are considered to be bacterially colonized, as biofilms can easily form on the contact lens [33]. Therefore, it is recommended to remove the contact lens at least 24 hours before surgery and to perform multiple cleanings and antisepsis of the conjunctival sac. Postoperatively, contact lenses should only be worn after complete healing.

Since colonization of the eye with MRSA is very rare, no recommendation for preoperative screening can currently be given. There is only an indication that healthcare workers with atopic dermatitis have an increased risk of MRSA colonization of the eye [34].

▶ Blood sugar levels should be adjusted to between 140 and 180 mg/dl [35].

Hyperglycemia increases the risk of developing endophthalmitis, delays wound healing, and is associated with increased susceptibility to infection [36] because the blood-retina barrier is impaired [37].

3.3.3 Special Preoperative Preventive Measures

▶ Since the endogenous flora is the main source of SSI in ophthalmology, the focus of infection prevention is on antisepsis in the surgical field and its coverage.

Preparation of the Surgical Field: The risk of endophthalmitis does not seem to be reduced by cutting eyelashes [38]. The surgical field is covered with a fenestrated drape (quality "low performance"). By covering the lid margins inlcuding the eyelashes and excretory ducts of the meibomian glands with incision film after antisepsis, additional protection is presumably achieved [39, 40]. Additionally, the presence of eyelashes in the working area, which is disruptive during surgery, is avoided. Preoperative irrigation of the tear ducts has no effect on contamination in the surgical area. If performed immediately before the procedure, more pathogens are flushed from the tear duct into the conjunctival sac [41]. In the case of dry eye during corneal surgery, premature drainage of tear fluid via the tear pump can be avoided by temporarily closing the puncta [42].

Antisepsis: PVP-iodine 5% is the agent of choice for preoperative eye antisepsis and is more efficaceous than the combined administration of polymyxin B sulfate, neomycin sulfate, and gentamicin. The incidence of endophthalmitis was significantly reduced with 5% PVP-iodine compared to the control group (silver protein solution) [43]. Even with a 1.25% PVP-iodine solution, the number of bacteria on the conjunctiva is significantly reduced [44]. Since side effects are to be expected with the entry of a 5% PVP-iodine solution into the anterior chamber, 1,25% should be preferred, due to in-vitro findings on effectiveness and better tolerability compared to more highly concentrated solutions, although this requires epidemiological verification [62].

As an alternative, polyhexanide can be considered. The National Formular Finder (NRF) of the German Drug Codex (DAC) includes polihexanide eye drops (NRF 15.25) and eye bath (NRF 15.26). The eye drops contain 0.02% polihexanide (1 g contains 0.2 mg polihexanide; other ingredients: sodium chloride, sodium edetate, sodium dihydrogen phosphate dihydrate, sodium monohydrogen phosphate dodecahydrate, water for injection). The eye bath contains 0.04% polihexanide (1 g contains 0.4 mg polihexanide; other ingredients: sodium chloride, potassium chloride, calcium chloride dihydrate, water for injection). Polyhexanide has long been used for the treatment of Acanthamoeba keratitis and is superior to 2.5% PVP-iodine in terms of cytotoxicity, irritation, and remanence [45]. At 0.04%, the efficacy of polihexanide was similar to that of 1.25% PVP-iodine, but with a later onset and longer-lasting effect, so that no pathogens were detected even 24 hours postoperatively; the tolerability did not differ from PVP-iodine [46]. With polihexanide, the slower onset of action compared to PVP-iodine (suitable application regimen) must be considered. However, a comparative study on the rate of endophthalmitis between 5% PVP-iodine and 0.02% polyhexanide is still lacking. In contrast after 24 hours with gentamicin-containing ointment, a pathogen-free state was not achieved [46, 47].

▶ The use of PVP-iodine instead of the alternative polihexanide has the advantage that already wetted areas are visible.

Antibiotic Therapy: Since the results of intracameral application of antibiotics at the end of cataract surgery are contradictory and in view of the risks of resistance development, no topical antibiotic therapy is recommended in addition to preoperative antisepsis based on current knowledge [42].

Periorbital Skin Antisepsis: The selection criterion is the absence of eye irritation, as preparation residues can enter the eye. The agent of choice is 10% PVP-iodine, with an exposure time of 10 minutes, as the forehead area has sebaceous gland-rich skin. Preparations containing chlorhexidine digluconate >0.05% are unsuitable. Considering findings on irritation potential, skin antiseptics containing hexetidine, cetylpyridinium chloride, and octenidine hydrochloride (>0.05%) should also not be used near the eye. Antibiotics are unsuitable in this area, including the lid margin, due to insufficient effectiveness.

3.3.4 Intraoperative Preventive Measures

Perioperative Antibiotic Prophylaxis: In aseptic intra- and extraocular procedures, systemic antibiotic prophylaxis is uncommon. In the case of penetrating globe injury, a systemic antibiotic, e.g., cefuroxime or moxifloxacin, should be administered prophylactically 30 minutes before the start of surgery due to the increased risk of endophthalmitis [48], and in the case of injury with plant material or intraocular foreign body, also intravitreally [49, 50].

Normothermia: In principle, patients with an anesthesia duration of >30 minutes should be actively warmed intraoperatively to prevent the body temperature from falling below 36°C [51]. This is presumably also relevant for longer ophthalmological surgeries, but it has not been studied so far.

▶ In individual cases, the approach to asepsis may differ slightly depending on the form of anesthesia or the type of ophthalmological procedure. his will be noted again in the respective chapters.

3.3.5 Postoperative Preventive Measures

Postoperatively, the spatial separation of patients with keratoconjunctivitis epidemica and other eye infections from freshly operated patients as well as from patients preparing for surgery can pose a problem during follow-up in the conservative practice and normal patient flow. If spatial separation between freshly operated patients and infectious eye emergencies is not possible, temporal separation in the form of scheduling postoperative check-ups before the actual start of office hours should be considered. The application of any indicated systemic antibiotics should also be ensured, especially in the outpatient setting and after discharge from the clinic. It is sometimes helpful to organize the administration of medication by family members already during the preoperative briefing.

3.4 Intravitreal Operative Drug Administration (IVOM)

IVOM occupies a special position in this chapter on infection prevention and is therefore given special mention (see also Section 18.4). The surgeon may already perform IVOM in their surgical training, when under adequate supervision. However, the intraocular procedure poses a significantly higher risk of complications in the form of endophthalmitis if hygiene rules are not observed.

In cases of bacterial blepharitis or conjunctivitis, intravitreal treatment should be postponed until successful therapy, and if necessary, local antiseptics or antibiotics with a follow-up check the next day should be prescribed.

After donning pathogen-free medical gloves, the eyelids and eyelashes are taped. The eyelid skin and conjunctival sac are rinsed with 5% PVP-iodine solution. The antiseptic treatment with PVP-iodine significantly reduces bacterial contamination of injection needles after intravitreal injection and achieves a significant reduction of bacteria in the conjunctiva without detectable amounts of iodine entering the anterior chamber [52].

Before drawing up the sterile syringe, surgical hand antisepsis is performed, and sterile surgical gloves are donned. Alternatively, surgical hand antisepsis and sterile surgical gloves can be applied before taping. In this case, the surgical gloves must be changed before handling the sterile syringe (see below).

For the injection, the eye is held open with a sterile eyelid speculum. The face is covered with a sterile drape with an incision film. In recent years, the use of complete drape sets with a fenestrated drape, disposable eyelid speculum, disposable forceps, surgical gown, and swabs has become increasingly common.

Since the infection rate is not reduced by topical antibiotics, they are dispensable due to the risk of resistance development.

When handling the pre-filled syringe, asepsis must be ensured until application. For this purpose, the outer carton should be opened before use. The sterile blister pack should be opened in such a way that the contents remain sterile. The syringe remains in the sterile tray until further use. To remove the cap of the syringe, hold the syringe with one hand while holding the cap of the syringe with the thumb and forefinger of the other hand. The cap of the syringe must be unscrewed (not broken off). To avoid compromising sterility, the syringe plunger must not be pulled out. Under aseptic conditions, the injection needle is firmly screwed onto the tip of the Luer-Lock adapter. Then the syringe is held with the needle pointing upwards. If bubbles are visible, gently tap the syringe with your finger until they rise to the top. Most medications for intravitreal injection are offered by the manufacturer and pharmacies as pre-filled syringes. The pre-filled syringe is intended for single use only. Using pre-filled syringes reduces the risk of contamination and simplifies the surgical procedure.

Alternatively, a vial and syringe can be used. In this case, the rubber stopper of the vial should be moistened externally with an alcohol-based skin antiseptic without the addition of a residual-acting antiseptic (exposure time 1 min). The micron filter needle included in the outer carton is attached to the sterile 1-ml syringe equipped with a Luer-Lock adapter. Only after the skin antiseptic has completely dried should the needle be inserted centrally until the needle is fully inserted into the vial and the tip touches the bottom or lower edge of the vial. Under aseptic conditions, the entire contents of the vial are drawn up by holding the vial upright in a slightly tilted position. To prevent drawing in air, ensure that the beveled edge of the filter needle is immersed in the solution. Since only 50 μl are to be administered, the excess amount should be discarded before injection. After disposing of the filter needle, the injection needle is firmly screwed onto the Luer-Lock tip of the syringe (check for bubbles as above). The vial is also intended for single use only.

▶ A general postoperative antibiotic therapy is no longer recommended after an intravitreal injection (statement of the German Ophthalmological Society, the Retinological Society, and the Professional Association of Ophthalmologists Germany as of 09/2012).

3.5 Responsibility and Quality Management (QM)

▶ The practice owner is responsible for ensuring and maintaining hygienic standards.

The German Infection Protection Act [53] stipulates that the heads of facilities for outpatient surgery and medical practices must ensure that the measures required according to the state of medical science are taken to prevent nosocomial infections and to avoid the further spread of pathogens, especially those with resistance to antibiotics. The practice operator is obliged to comply with the laws and regulations for the protection of patients and employees. This also applies if he or she delegates corresponding activities, e.g., the reprocessing of medical devices, to knowledgeable personnel.

▶ In facilities for outpatient surgery, a medical staff member must have acquired the 40-hour training to become an infection prevention link physician based on the curriculum of the German Society for Hospital Hygiene [54].

The content and scope of the course must be recognized by a state medical association [55]. These courses are also offered as an electronic curriculum with only two days of face-to-face instruction.

▶ The heads of facilities for outpatient surgery must ensure that the occurrence of pathogens with specific antibiotic resistances and multiresistances, as determined by the Robert Koch Institute (RKI), is continuously recorded and evaluated as part of a Surveillance [56].

Based on this, conclusions regarding necessary preventive measures must be drawn and implemented together with the staff.

▶ In facilities for outpatient surgery, the establishment of antibiotic stewardship is required [53].

This includes qualified advice on clinical-microbiological and clinical-pharmacological issues based on a facility-specific antibiotic guideline and the at least annual recording and evaluation of antibiotic consumption and resistance situation, taking into account regional resistance data.

▶ The internal procedures for infection control of patients and staff must be defined in hygiene plans. Standard operating procedures (SOPs) are helpful for the implementation of specific measures.

The hygiene plan must regulate the following concerns in particular: hand hygiene, personal hygiene and personnel protection, hygiene measures in diagnostics and therapy, reprocessing of medical devices, use of disinfectants and environmental hygiene, hygiene in supply and disposal, reporting obligations according to IfSG, indications for microbiological diagnostics, collection and dispatch of examination material and training intervals.

The hygiene plan must be made known and explained to employees upon hiring. In the event of changes in the area of responsibility and the introduction of new work equipment or procedures, the hygiene plan must be adjusted. Training on the hygiene plan must be repeated and documented at least annually. External advice from hygiene specialists or the local health department is helpful in establishing hygiene management.

Monitoring compliance with the measures specified in the hygiene regulations includes, for example, operating procedure analyses and analyses of environmental and reprocessing safety. A checklist can support self-monitoring of the quality of reprocessing.

▶ Upon discharge of the patient, if measures are required to prevent transmissible pathogens, these must be communicated to persons involved in follow-up care, e.g., general practitioners, outpatient nursing services, and, if necessary, relatives involved in further care, based on the medical risk assessment in the transfer form.

Patients must be informed in advance about the transfer of information.

Literature and Further Reading

1. KRINKO (2018) Prävention postoperativer Wundinfektionen. Empfehlung der Kommission für Krankenhaushygiene und Infektionsprävention (KRINKO) beim Robert Koch-Institut. Bgbl 61:448–473
2. Kramer A, Wendt M, Assadian O, Zacharowski K, Bulitta C, Vakil R, Lippert H (2022) Klinische und ambulante Operationszentren, Herzkatheterlabor und Hybrid-Operationseinheit. In: Kramer A, Assadian O, Exner M, Hübner NO, Scheithauer S, Simon A (Hrsg) Krankenhaus- und Praxishygiene, 4th edn. Elsevier, München, pp 668–681
3. Kramer A (2020) Requirements for hygienically safe, environmentally friendly dispensers for hand disinfectants and hand washing preparations. GMS Hyg. Infect Control 15:Doc02. https://doi.org/10.3205/dgkh000337
4. Suchomel M, Leslie RA, Parker AE, Macinga DR (2018) How long is enough? Identification of product dry-time as a primary driver of alcohol-based hand rub efficacy. Antimicrob Resist Infect Control 7:65
5. Kramer A, Pittet D, Klasinc R, Krebs S, Koburger T, Fusch C, Assadian O (2017) Shortening the application time of alcohol-based hand rubs to 15 s may improve frequency of hand antisepsis. Inf Contr Hosp Epidemiol 30:1–5
6. Harnoss JC, Dancer SJ, Kaden CF, Baguhl R, Kohlmann T, Papke R, Zygmunt M, Assadian O, Suchomel M, Pittet D, Kramer A (2020) Hand antisepsis without decreasing efficacy by shortening the rub-in time of alcohol-based handrubs to 15 seconds. J Hosp Inf 104(4):P419–P424
7. Paula H, Krebs U, Becker R, Assadian O, Heidecke CD, Kramer A (2018) Wettability of hands during 15s and 30s contact intervals: a prospective, randomized cross-over study. Infect Control Hosp Epidemiol 46(9):1032–1035
8. Pires D, Soule H, Bellissimo-Rodrigues F, Gayet-Ageron A, Pittet D (2017) Hand hygiene with alcohol-based hand rub: how long is long enough? Infect Control Hosp Epidemiol 38(5):547–552
9. KRINKO (2016) Händehygiene in Einrichtungen des Gesundheitswesens. Empfehlung der Kommission für Krankenhaushygiene und Infektionsprävention (KRINKO) beim Robert Koch-Institut (RKI). Bgbl 59:1189–1220
10. Hübner NO, Kellner NB, Partecke LI, Koburger T, Heidecke CD, Kohlmann T, Kramer A (2011) Determination of antiseptic efficacy of rubs on the forearm and consequences for surgical hand disinfection. J Hosp Infect 78(1):11–15
11. TRBA 250. Biologische Arbeitsstoffe im Gesundheitswesen und in der Wohlfahrtspflege. 4. GMBl 2014, Nr. 10/11 vom 27.03.2014, letzte Änderung vom 2.5.2018, GMBl Nr. 15
12. TRGS 401. Gefährdung durch Hautkontakt Ermittlung – Beurteilung – Maßnahmen. GMBl 2011, S 175 [Nr. 9]
13. Harnoß JC, Brune L, Ansorg J, Heidecke CD, Assadian O, Kramer A (2014) Practice of skin protection and skin care among German surgeons and influence on the efficacy of surgical hand disinfection and surgical glove perforation. BMC Infect Dis 10(14):315
14. Kramer A, Assadian O (2016) Indications and the requirements for single-use medical gloves. GMS Hyg Infect Control 11:Doc01. https://doi.org/10.3205/dgkh000261
15. Assadian O, Leaper DJ, Kramer A, Ousey KJ (2016) Can the design of glove dispensing boxes influence glove contamination? J Hosp Infect 94(3):259–262. https://doi.org/10.1016/j.jhin.2016.09.005
16. Diedrich S, Scholz S, Below H, Baguhl R, Heidecke CD, Papke R, Seifert U, Kramer A (2020) Influence of Bio-sorb® cream on sweat production and efficacy of surgical hand antisepsis under surgical gloves. Surg Infect 21(3):293–298
17. KRINKO/BfArM (2012) Anforderungen an die Hygiene bei der Aufbereitung von Medizinprodukten. Empfehlung der Kommission für Krankenhaushygiene und Infektionsprävention (KRINKO) beim Robert Koch-Institut (RKI) und des Bundesinstitutes für Arzneimittel und Medizinprodukte (BfArM). Bgbl Gesundheitsforsch Gesundheitsschutz 55:1244–1310
18. Guerra RL, Freitas Bde P, Parcero CM et al (2012) An outbreak of forty five cases of pseudomonas aeruginosa acute endophthalmitis after phacoemulsification. Arq Bras Oftalmol 75(5):344–347
19. Hoffmann KK, Weber DJ, Gergen MF et al (2002) *Pseudomonas aeruginosa*-related postoperative endophthalmitis linked to a contaminated phacoemulsifier. Arch Ophthalmol 120(1):90–93
20. Pathengay A, Flynn HW, Isom RF et al (2012) Endophthalmitis outbreaks following cataract surgery: causative organisms, etiologies, and visual acuity outcomes. J Cataract Refract Surg 38(7):1278–1282
21. Chang DF, Mamalis N (2018) Guidelines for the cleaning and sterilization of intraocular surgical instruments. J Cataract Refract Surg 44(6):765–773
22. Mamalis N, Edelhauser HF, Dawson DG et al (2006) Toxic anterior segment syndrome. J Cataract Refract Surg 32(2):324–333. https://doi.org/10.1016/j.jcrs.2006.01.065
23. Verma L, Chakravarti A (2017) Prevention and management of postoperative endophthalmitis: a case-based approach. Indian J Ophthalmol 65(12):1396–1402

24. Roth K, Heeg P (2001) Überprüfung der Sterilität von wiederaufbereitbaren Schlauchsystemen für die Augenchirurgie. SMP GmbH, Tübingen
25. Lakkis C, Lian KY, Napper G, Kiely PM (2007) Infection control guidelines for optometrists 2007. Clin Exp Optom 90(6):434–444. https://doi.org/10.1111/j.1444-0938.2007.00192.x
26. Hong Y, Teska PJ, Oliver HF (2017) Effects of contact time and concentration on bactericidal efficacy of 3 disinfectants on hard nonporous surfaces. Am J Infect Control 45(11):1284–1285. https://doi.org/10.1016/j.ajic.2017.04.015
27. Omidbakhsh N (2008) Disinfectants and label claims. Realistically can contact times be met to achieve antimicrobial efficacy? Can J Infect Cont 23(1):49
28. RKI (2020) Aufbereitung von Medizinprodukten: Häufig gestellte Fragen und Antworten, Zur Frage der Validierbarkeit der abschließenden Desinfektion von semikritischen Medizinprodukten mittels Wischtüchern. Stand: 20.11.2020. Aus: http://www.rki.de/DE/Content/Infekt/Krankenhaushygiene/Aufb_MedProd/Aufb_MedProd_node.html. Zugegriffen am 11.03.2021
29. Eggers M (2016) Viruzide Desinfektion von Tonometer-Messkörpern sowie Laser- und Diagnostikgläsern mit einem apparativen Verfahren. In: Kramer A, Assadian O, Exner M, Hübner NO, Simon A (Hrsg) Krankenhaus- und Prxishygiene, 3. Aufl. Elsevier, München, 427–428
30. Rutala WA, Weber DJ, Healthcare Infection Control Practices Advisory Committee (HICPAC) (2008) Guideline for disinfection and sterilization in healthcare facilities, 2008. Centers for Disease Control and Prevention, Atlanta. https://www.cdc.gov/infectioncontrol/guidelines/disinfection/
31. Hawksworth N (2016) Ophthalmic instrument decontamination. Royal College of Ophthalmologists, London
32. Rehork B, Rüden H (1991) Untersuchungen zur chirurgischen Händedesinfektion. In: Häring R (Hrsg) Infektionsverhütung in der Chirurgie. Blackwell, Berlin, pp 65–74
33. Rändler C, Matthes R, McBain AJ, Giese B, Fraunholz M, Sietmann R, Kohlmann T, Hübner NO, Kramer A (2010) A three-phase in-vitro system for studying *Pseudomonas aeruginosa* adhesion and biofilm formation upon hydrogel contact lenses. BMC Microbiol 10:282. https://doi.org/10.1186/1471-2180-10-282
34. Kitazawa K, Sotozono C, Sakamoto M, Sasaki M, Hieda O, Yamasaki T, Kinoshita S (2016) Nasal and conjunctival screening prior to refractive surgery: an observational and cross-sectional study. BMJ Open 6(5):e010733. https://doi.org/10.1136/bmjopen-2015-010733
35. Kumar CM, Seet E, Eke T, Dhatariya K, Joshi GP (2016) Glycaemic control during cataract surgery under loco-regional anaesthesia: a growing problem and we are none the wiser. Br J Anaesth 117(6):687–691. https://doi.org/10.1093/bja/aew305
36. Grzybowski A, Kanclerz P, Huerva V, Ascaso FJ, Tuuminen R (2019) Diabetes and phacoemulsification cataract surgery: difficulties, risks and potential complications. J Clin Med 8(5):716. https://doi.org/10.3390/jcm8050716
37. Benton AH, Fulton LK, Marquart ME (2017) Exogenous *Streptococcus pneumoniae* endophthalmitis in diabetic rabbits. Sci Rep 7:46196. https://doi.org/10.1038/srep46196
38. Behrens-Baumann W, Augustin AJ, Dick B, Fabrian E, Huber-Spitzy V, Klauß V, Kramer A, Pitten FA, Pleyer U, Zeitz J (2003) Leitlinie zur Prophylaxe und Therapie von Endophthalmitiden. Leitlinie der Deutschen Gesellschaft für Krankenhaushygiene. Hyg Med 28(11):447–460
39. Behrens-Baumann W, Kramer A (2002) Prophylactic indications for eye antiseptics. In: Antiseptic prophylaxis and therapy in ocular infections. Development in ophthalmology, vol 33. Karger, Basel, S 212–222
40. Pervanidi A, Sonntag HG (1981) Infektionsgefährdung und Hygienemaßnahmen in der Augenheilkunde. Hyg Med 7:539–543
41. Amon M, Hirschl AM, Freyler H (1991) Unterschiede im Keimspektrum des Konjunktivalsackes vor und nach Tränenwegsspülung. Klin Monatsbl Augenheilkd 199:330–332
42. Behrens-Baumann W, Kramer A, Pleyer U (2022) Ophthalmologie. In: Kramer A, Assadian O, Exner M, Hübner NO, Scheithauer S, Simon A (Hrsg) Krankenhaus- und Praxishygiene, 4th eedn. Elsevier, München, pp 477–488
43. Speaker MG, Menikoff JA (1991) Prophylaxis of endophthalmitis with topical povidone-iodine. Ophthalmoly 98:1769–1775
44. Maeck CR, Eckardt C, Höller C (1991) Bakterizide Wirkung von präoperativ angewendetem Gentamicin im Vergleich mit PVP-Jodlösung. Fortschr Ophthalmol 88:848–851
45. Kramer A, Behrens-Baumann W (1997) Prophylactic use of topical antiinfectives in ophthalmology. Ophthalmology 197:68–76
46. Hansmann F, Kramer A, Ohgke H (2005) Lavasept as an alternative to PVP-iodine as a preoperative antiseptic in ophthalmic surgery. Randomized, controlled, prospective double-blind trial. Ophthalmology 102(11):1043–1046, 1048–1050
47. Hansmann F, Kramer A, Ohgke H, Strobel H, Müller M, Geerling G (2004) Polyhexamethylbiguanid (PHMB) as preoperative antiseptic for cataract surgery. Ophthalmology 101:377–383
48. Behrens-Baumann W, Frank U, Neß T (2010) Rationale Antibiotikatherapie in der Augenheilkunde. Ophthalmologe 107:323–327
49. Banker TP, McClellan AJ, Wilson BD, Juan FM, Kuriyan AE, Relhan N, Chen FV, Weichel ED, Albini TA, Berrocal AM, Sridhar J, Gregori NZ, Townsend JH, Flynn HW Jr (2017) Culture-positive

endophthamitis after open globe injuries with and without retained intraocular foreign bodies. Ophthalmic Surg Lasers Imaging Retina 48:632–637
50. Narang S, Gupta V, Gupta A, Dogra MR, Pandav SS, Das S (2003) Role of prophylactic intravitreal antibiotics in open globe injuries. Indian J Ophthalmol 51:39–44
51. NICE (2016) Hypothermia: prevention and management in adults having surgery. https://www.nice.org.uk/guidance/CG65
52. Hansmann F, Below H, Kramer A, Kramer A, Müller G, Geerling G (2007) Prospective study to determine the penetration of iodide into the anterior chamber following preoperative application of topical 1.25% povidone-iodine. Graefes Arch Clin Exp Ophthalmol 245(6):789–793
53. Gesetz zur Änderung des Infektionsschutzgesetzes und weiterer Gesetze (IfSGuaÄndG) (2011) BgBl 2011, Teil I, Nr. 41: 1622
54. Deutsche Gesellschaft für Krankenhaushygiene (2007) Definition des Arbeitsfeldes Hygienebeauftragter Ärztinnen und Ärzte sowie ihrer Aus- und Fortbildung. http://www.dgkh.de/informationen/informationsarchiv/144. Letzter Zugriff 3.4.2023
55. KRINKO (2009) Personelle und organisatorische Voraussetzungen zur Prävention nosokomialer Infektionen. Empfehlung der Kommission für Krankenhaushygiene und Infektionsprävention. Bgbl 52:951–962
56. KRINKO (2020) Surveillance von nosokomialen Infektionen. Empfehlung der Kommission für Krankenhaushygiene und Infektionsprävention (KRINKO) beim Robert Koch-Institut. Bgbl 63:228–241
57. Bundesvereinigung Deutscher Apothekerverbände (2021) Neues Rezeptur-Formularium. Govi, Eschborn
58. Kramer A, Behrens-Baumann W (2002) Antiseptic prophylaxis and therapy in ocular infections. Karger, Basel, S 223–232
59. Medizinproduktegesetz in der Fassung der Bekanntmachung vom 7. August 2002 (BGBl. I S. 3146), zuletzt durch Artikel 223 der Verordnung vom 19. Juni 2020 (BGBl. I S. 1328) geändert.
60. Boppre D, Exner M, Krüger CM, Schuler H, Wendt M, Harnoss JC, et al. Achieving room air quality of room class Ib in the aseptic area using a mobile sterile ventilation unit in a room class II surgical unit. GMS Hyg Infect Control. 2024;19:Doc66. https://doi.org/10.3205/dgkh000521
61. Kramer A, Seifert J, Abele-Horn M, Arvand M, Biever P, Blacky A, Buerke M, et al. (2024) S2k-Guideline hand antisepsis and hand hygiene. GMS Hyg Infect Control. 19:Doc42. https://doi.org/10.3205/dgkh000497.
62. Zwicker P, Opitz N, Harris J, Stahl A, Kellner U, Koelb-Keerl R, Muether PS, Hunold A, Kramer A. In vitro efficacy of aqueous PVP-iodine solution below 5% as alternative to preoperative antisepsis in ophthalmology as the basis for an in vivo studyJ Ophthalmic Inflamm Infect. 2025 Apr 2;15(1):35.

Equipment Knowledge "What Does a Surgeon Need to Know?"

4

Thomas Hammer, Erik Chankiewitz, Frank Wilhelm, Wolfgang Schrader, Arne Viestenz and Martin Miertsch

Contents

T. Hammer
Klinik und Poliklinik für Augenheilkunde, Universitätsklinikum Halle/Saale, Martin-Luther-Universität Halle-Wittenberg, Halle/Saale, Germany
e-mail: thomas.hammer@uk-halle.de

Augenarztpraxis, Augenzentrum "Frohe Zukunft", Halle/Saale, Germany

E. Chankiewitz
Augenklinik, Städtisches Klinikum Braunschweig gGmbH, Braunschweig, Germany
e-mail: erik@chankiewitz.de

F. Wilhelm (✉)
Universitätsklinikum Halle Saale, Greifswald, Germany

W. Schrader
Augenzentrum Würzburg, Würzburg, Germany
e-mail: mail@profschrader.de

A. Viestenz
Klinik und Poliklinik für Augenheilkunde, Universitätsklinikum Halle/Saale, Halle/Saale, Germany

M. Miertsch
Greifswald, Germany

Before the first work on the patient in the operating room, it is absolutely necessary for the surgeon to familiarize himself with the devices he will use during a procedure. At least, an introduction by other surgeons or experienced OR staff should take place during the first operation. Although not required in all facilities, it is a good option to be instructed by a service technician or representative of the manufacturing company. One should assume, when making personal contacts (considering the rules of advantage), that the employees of the manufacturers are interested in the proper use of their products and want to convey as much as possible during these introductory training sessions!

It is important in any case that a "to-do" list is provided on how to proceed in case of emergencies and that a failure management system exists.

F. Wilhelm (ed.), *Ophthalmic Surgery for Beginners*, https://doi.org/10.1007/978-3-662-70287-1_4

▶ Given the variety of medical-technical developments from different companies, only selected examples will be presented in the following chapters, with which the respective authors work. Since the functions of devices from other manufacturers are comparable, this does not constitute a rating!

After the initial instruction into the function of the devices, it is recommended for beginners to practice outside of the OR operation, i.e., under non-sterile conditions, to become familiar with the function in the OR situation.

4.1 Operating Microscope

Thomas Hammer, Erik Chankiewitz and Frank Wilhelm

Ophthalmic surgeries are now routinely performed using an operating microscope. The first devices were already used in 1921 by Carl-Olof Siggesson Nylèn for procedures in otology [1]. In ophthalmology, the establishment for routine use began in the 1950s when the company Zeiss introduced the first operating microscopes suitable for ophthalmic surgery. Later, other manufacturers followed (e.g., Leica, Möller-Wedel).

The development began with the use of a modified slit lamp [2] and continued, for example, with the establishment of the double microscope (usable simultaneously by the surgeon and assistant) [3]. The introduction of a stereo beam splitter was an important step, as it allowed the assistant to see a three-dimensional image.

Even though the essential components such as eyepiece, tube, magnification changer, and objective (Fig. 4.1) are still retained today, extensive innovations have been introduced in recent decades to meet the growing demands of ophthalmic surgery. With the integration of the OCT, for example, the finest membranous structures can be displayed intraoperatively both in the anterior and posterior segments of the eye (Fig. 4.2). Through the camera, it is also possible to connect multiple monitors, allowing everyone involved in the procedure to follow the progress directly.

The operating microscope is one of the essential tools for the ophthalmic surgeon to successfully perform a procedure on the eyeball. In the field of microsurgical specialties, very different microscopes have been developed in recent decades, individualized for the respective specialty. For the magnification of ocular structures that are smaller than the resolving power of the human eye allows, this is indispensable! Microscopes in the ophthalmic field are not high-performance microscopes in terms of their magnification but fulfill special demands on light control. Today's operating microscopes offer a 6- to 40-fold magnification and provide an upright and three-dimensional image. The ophthalmic operating microscope is a classic light microscope, which, similar to a camera, consists of a collection of lenses. With the operating microscope, it is essential that the resulting image is upright and not reversed. Since the highest possible resolution of a classic light microscope is 0.2 μm, which also depends on the wavelength of the light used, this is completely sufficient to achieve the necessary intraoperative magnifications.

The surgical microscope is referred to as a compound microscope (Fig. 4.1) because it consists of an objective lens (facing the surgical area) and an eyepiece (facing the surgeon). Stereomicroscopes with two eyepieces are used,

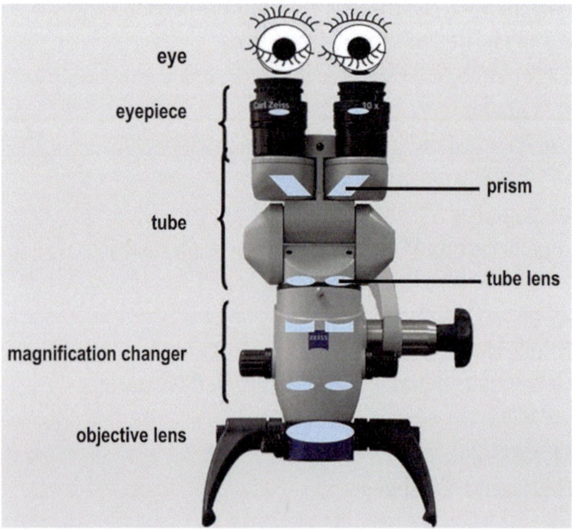

Fig. 4.1 Principle structure of the optical system of an operating microscope

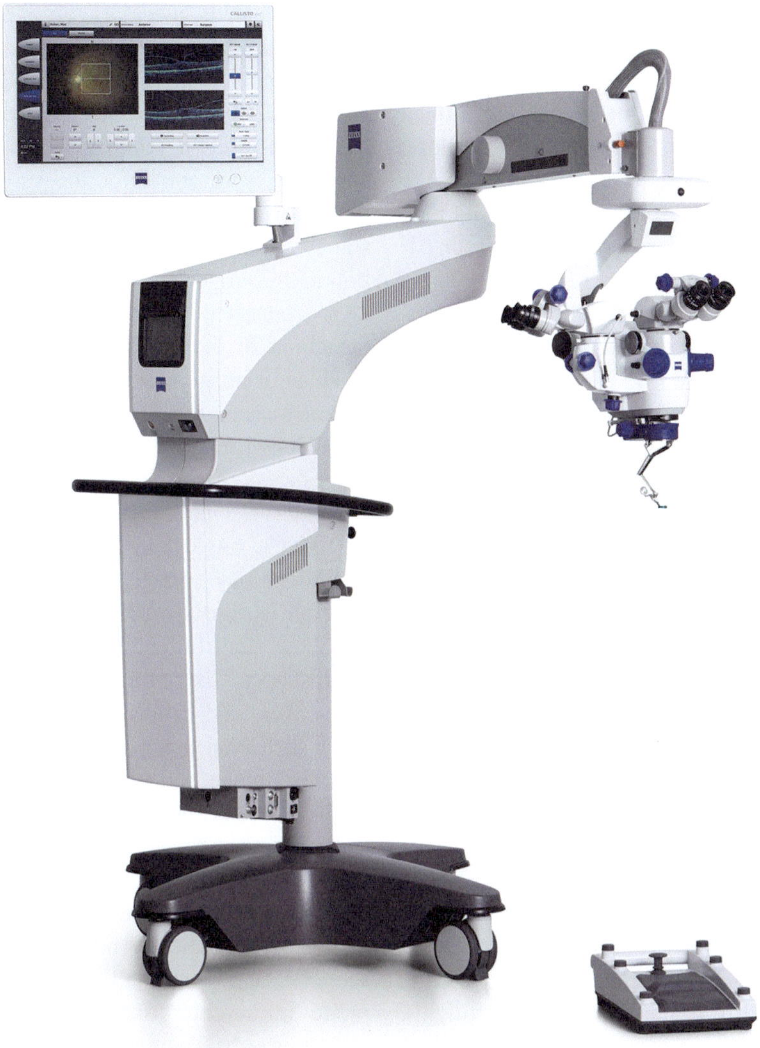

Fig. 4.2 Example of a modern operating microscope LUMERA700 with integrated OCT. (© Carl Zeiss Meditec AG)

allowing for three-dimensional capture and examination of ocular structures. We refer to this type of **reflected light microscopes** because the light falls on the object at a variable angle and not through the object as in transmitted light microscopy. Especially in cataract surgery, however, retroillumination is important for performing the operation, as it allows a good assessment of the lens opacity and a safe creation of the capsulorhexis. In retroluminescence, light shines parallel to the surgeon's line of sight into the eye and is reflected on the retina. Thus, the retina serves as an indirect light source. Since it is "indispensable today that a surgical microscope for ophthalmology has both lighting options" [4], microscopes used in the surgical field for cataract operations are combined with a coaxial illumination path in addition to lateral oblique illumination. Depending on the manufacturer, there is the possibility to add a coaxial light source in addition to two reflected light sources. In other models, both light sources illuminating the object include a coaxial component. Since the surgeon cannot change the objective lens intraoperatively, it is necessary to use a zoom control for magnification. Additionally, fine adjustment of the microscope position by hand is difficult intraoperatively. Therefore, control is now performed via a wired or wireless footswitch, which allows movement of both the x-y and z-axes of the microscope. This ensures precise positioning even intraoperatively. “Experience shows that if the unit is centered at the start of the operation, a possible deflection of 60-70 mm in all directions is sufficient” [5]. The magnification is also continuously motor-controlled.

The footswitches also integrate functions for light control. In devices from Zeiss, this can be switched via the footswitch so that the anterior segment illumination does not outshine the red reflex, making the rhexis more visible. This is also evident by the appearance of only two light source reflections (instead of three). This setting has proven particularly useful for performing capsulorhexis on eyes with brunescence lens nuclei.

Both halogen lamps and LED lights are used as light sources for the microscope. Modern microscopes are rather equipped with LED lights than with halogen lights, because LED last for about 25.000 hrs as compared to 800–2000 hrs (halogen lights). Another advantage is that modern LED light sources allow adjustment for color temperature (a lower temperature, e.g. 2700 K gives a warmer light, a higher color temperature, e.g. 4000–5000 K a cooler, more blueish light). In addition various color filters can be used to optimize the contrast of vessels and membranes to avoid the use of dyes. Surgeons who started operating with halogen lamps require a new learning phase. Various manufacturers also offer the option to produce the preferred light color by changing the appropriate color filters.

Surgical microscopes can be equipped with either a floor stand or a ceiling mount. The decision is usually based on cost and structural conditions, with additional selection criteria such as the elimination of extra cables on the floor with a ceiling mount versus the easier replacement of a floor stand device in case of emergency.

Most ophthalmic surgical microscopes today are configured with a beam splitter so that both a camera and an additional optic can be connected. This additional optic serves both the assistant and, if necessary, an experienced surgeon as a “teaching optic”. Depending on the microscope’s equipment, this additional optic can be designed as a stereo optic with two eyepieces or as a monocular system. The stereo optic is essential for the surgeon, and the degree of incoming light from the reflected light sources determines the quality of spatial orientation in the surgical situation.

A connected camera system enables documentation of the surgical situation. The control of video or image recordings is often realized via the microscope footswitch. In recent years, OCT technology has also been incorporated into microscopes (Sect. 21.2). The control of this additional imaging is also performed via the footswitch.

Today’s surgical microscopes typically offer magnifications between 6x and 40x and provide an upright and three-dimensional image. To allow easy intraoperative movement of the microscopes, they are equipped with sterilizable covers and handles. In some models, locking is achieved using a magnetic brake. These so-called brake balance systems allow for easy position changes without much effort and ensure a stable image for the surgeon. Surgical microscopes are now offered by Carl Zeiss Meditec, Leica Microsystems, Möller-Wedel, and other manufacturers. There is no right or wrong microscope; each surgeon will need to find the appropriate microscope for their surgical situation and approach. Therefore, it is strongly recommended that every beginning surgeon should test as many different models as possible to form his own opinion. This should be part of the training!

▶ The beginning surgeons should definitely know the model they are being trained on and practice handling it in advance—outside of the operating room!

Just as a pilot checks certain things on the aircraft before takeoff (“pre-flight check”), every surgeon should check the settings and functions of their microscope before each start. If sterile covers are on the handles and wheels, an adjustment can be made in the washed state; otherwise, settings and function changes are not completely sterile (see checklist).

Every ophthalmologist knows his individual interpupillary distance (PD) and adjusts it laterally on the eyepieces so that a comfortable, edge-free, and double-image-free view is possible in the surgical image. Usually, the adjustment range is between 55 and 85 mm. Additionally, both eyepieces can be adjusted separately with a fine scale in the plus and minus range. If there is "instrument myopia," the surgeon will notice that the image on the monitor is not always sharp when focused by the surgeon in the operating area. In this case, it is necessary to gradually turn the eyepieces towards the minus direction and refocus until a sharp image is achieved for both the surgeon and on the monitor. It is also important to know from which optical path (right or left) the camera derives the image. If surgery is to be performed without glasses, the corresponding refraction must be taken into account. The adjustment range is usually between −5 and +8 diopters. Some microscopes are also equipped with variable eyecups made of rubber or hard plastic, ensuring an optimal distance from the eye or glasses while limiting the amount of light entering from the side. In principle, one should be familiar with the working distance of the microscope, which is between 175 and 200 mm.

- The following aspects should be clarified by the surgeon before each procedure during the setup:

- What is my PD ("pupil distance") and where is it set? Usually, an eyepiece distance of 55 mm to 85 mm can be adjusted, resulting in an image for both eyes.

- What diopter setting (instrument myopia) do I have on the eyepieces and where is it set? Do not confuse this with the glasses prescription! The diopter number is set directly on the eyepieces (usually −5 to +8 dpt).

- Am I wearing glasses during the surgery? The eyecups must be folded in or out to have the optimal distance to the eyepieces.

- Are all adjustment wheels/buttons covered with sterile caps?

- Will I be working exclusively in the anterior or also in the posterior segment of the eye? If this is the case, appropriate technical requirements, including an inverter, are necessary.

- Which working distance will I be using (175 mm or 200 mm)?

- For cataract surgery, a red reflex is needed. Where is this set? (In some microscopes, it is set by default, in others, this setting must be selected separately).

- Is the XYZ setting in the zero position? It should be part of every procedure to trigger the residual function at the end!

To operate on the posterior segment of the eye, an additional optical system is necessary. Since no physical contact with the corneal surface results from its use and no assistance is needed for the permanent centering of the optics, the BIOM (and in recent years also EIBOS, RESIGHT, and others) has proven itself [6]. These are supplementary lens systems that cause an inverted image. Therefore, an inverter is additionally required to produce an upright image. If necessary, intraoperative switching between the anterior and posterior segments of the eye can be done.

While the positioning of the operating table must be adjusted with microscopes with ceiling stands, a stand microscope is more flexible. The two arms of the stand should be perpendicular to each other to retain as many degrees of freedom as possible. In most cases, the stand also carries the light source. On some models, the light sources can be easily swapped or defective bulbs replaced via a slide on the back.

When using a wireless footswitch, always ensure that charged batteries or the emergency connection cable are available. It is essential to know where the battery compartment or cable connections are located.

Many modern surgical microscopes can be individually configured and programmed. If the surgeon's name is stored, the saved presets can be easily retrieved repeatedly. It may seem cumbersome at first to find these settings, for example, to assign microscope handgrips and footswitches accordingly, but it will prove beneficial in the long run. For beginners, the easiest approach is to copy the settings of the instructor and later customize them.

4.2 Phacoemulsification Device

Wolfgang Schrader, Frank Wilhelm and Arne Viestenz

The **phacoemulsification** of the lens using ultrasound has been the gold standard in cataract surgery for over 30 years (Chap. 20). Precisely because it is the most frequently performed surgical procedure in medicine, every surgeon should know the device and its functionality. Given the multitude of available devices from various manufacturers, it is not possible to go into all the details here, especially since there are constant new developments, which is why the focus of this chapter is on the basic principles. Each phacoemulsification unit essentially consists of three components: the base unit, which contains the pump(s) and the control unit, the foot switch, and the phaco handpiece.

4.2.1 Base Unit

The base unit includes both the control and operating unit as well as the software, electronics, and the **fluidic circuit** with drives, pumps, and valves. It represents the central unit where the various functions for phacoemulsification are coordinated and, depending on the device configuration, additional options such as vitrectomy, endoillumination, and more (Chap. 19), are available.

It is responsible for coordinating the three actions that occur simultaneously during the phacoemulsification of the nucleus:

1. Fluid inflow (infusion or irrigation),
2. Aspiration, and
3. Application of ultrasound energy for nucleus fragmentation.

Depending on the device and settings, the fluid flow can be regulated intraocularly. Traditionally (historically), this was done passively: the height of the fluid level in the infusion bottle above the eye determines the infusion pressure (where 1 cm of water column corresponds to 1 mBar or 0.7356 mmHg), and the cross-section of the supply tubing and the phaco tip determines the flow rate. The **flow rate**, i.e., the volume of fluid that flows through the phaco tip per unit of time, can also be limited on the device, thereby determining the infusion-side flow rate.

▶ Before starting the operation, it must be checked whether there is enough fluid in the infusion bottle and (when using glass bottles) whether the air supply through the filter is ensured!

To minimize fluctuations in the anterior chamber depth, the use of active pressure infusions, which ensure a more stable anterior chamber, has recently become increasingly popular. Systematic monitoring of the vacuum can adjust the fluid inflow. Fluctuations in the anterior chamber depth are compensated. This is particularly significant when the suction abruptly increases after the end of an **occlusion** of the phaco tip opening!

The suction for intraocular aspiration of lens fragments is generated by the pump(s) integrated into the base unit. Their performance is defined by two parameters: the vacuum and the flow rate. The vacuum refers to the negative pressure or suction force exerted on the fluid in the suction line and in the eye. The smaller the suction opening, the higher the vacuum at a constant flow rate! Both criteria determine the suction performance of the pump and thus the amount of fluid exchanged during a procedure.

Both peristaltic pumps and venturi pumps have proven effective for use in phacoemulsification devices.

In a **peristaltic pump** (Fig. 4.3), a tube is compressed by massaging movements of small rotating rollers arranged around a disc. This rotating compression generates a flow and results in a vacuum. The rotation of the rollers moves the fluid in the direction in which the rollers turn. In phaco machines with such **roller pumps**, the rollers rotate in the direction in which the fluid is sucked away from the eye. Both the flow (usually

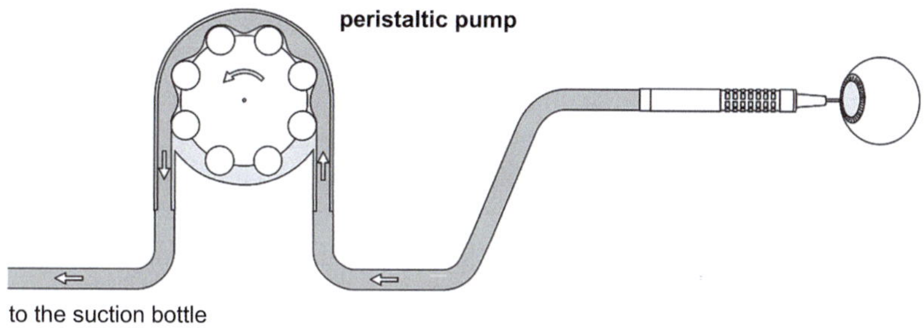

Fig. 4.3 Schematic representation of the functioning of a peristaltic pump. (Courtesy of Geuder Company)

up to 60 ml/min) and the vacuum (up to 650 mmHg) can be precisely dosed.

By reversing the rotation of the rollers, the flow direction can be changed, allowing for a reflux.

The operation of the Venturi pump is based on a completely different principle. The pneumatic Venturi system (Fig. 4.4) generates the vacuum through an air stream (usually compressed air) that is passed by a one-way valve. This creates a negative pressure at the one-way valve. The result is a suction that causes the liquid to be aspirated into an additional chamber (cassette).

In Table 4.1, the two pumps, as they have been used in intraocular surgery for almost 50 years, are compared in principle. While the pneumatic Venturi pump allows the rapid creation of a vacuum through the use of an additional chamber with compressed air, the electronically controlled peristaltic pump ensures a constant suction performance even when the vacuum increases. In a classic pneumatic Venturi pump, the vacuum was modulable and built up quickly, but the flow was not directly controllable. Although it allowed for quick operation, it was not finely modulable. This disadvantage of the Venturi pumps could be compensated by a system with small chambers and electronically controlled valves, so that the modified pump systems can build up a vacuum from 0 to 650 mmHg in 0.3 seconds and still ensure control of the flow with a precision of 0.1 ml. With this technology, the advantages of both pump systems are combined in modern control devices and their disadvantages are eliminated.

Especially for beginners and in time-consuming cataract surgery in complicated initial situations such as zonular weakness, phacoemulsification can be performed safely and without complications thanks to controlled irrigation and aspiration.

When the device is used for vitrectomy, the vitreous body can be removed particularly

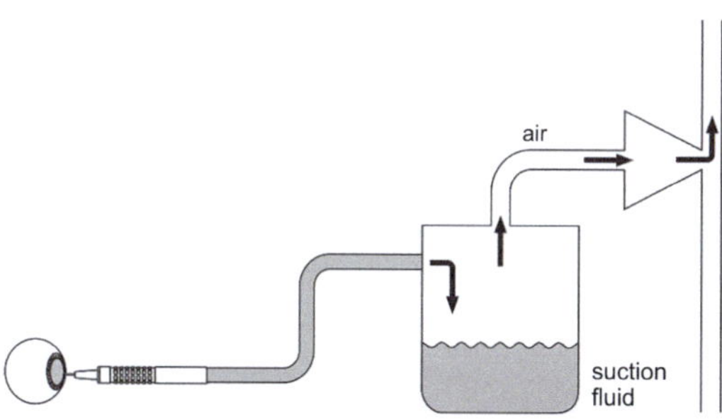

Fig. 4.4 Schematic representation of the operation of a Venturi pump with the use of an additional chamber. (Courtesy of Geuder Company)

Table 4.1 Comparison of peristaltic and Venturi pumps

Comparison Criteria	Peristaltic Pump	Venturi Pump
Vacuum Build-up	Gradual	Rapid
Suction Performance	Constant	Dependent on Vacuum
Compressed Air Connection Required	No	Yes
Additional Cassette Required	No	Yes
Reflux Function Possible	Yes	No

carefully and atraumatically in the retinal periphery with a function adapted to the classic roller pump. The vacuum level can be limited on the device by specifying a maximum value. The vacuum can then be varied linearly within the specified vacuum range using the footswitch. It is important to activate the linear function for the vacuum on the base unit! It can be said that the vacuum level represents the force with which the material to be aspirated is sucked into and transported away by the phaco tip. Linearly controlled vacuum is preferable to non-linear control (either 0 or maximum value).

▶ An individual instruction in the handling of the device by a technician from the manufacturer is just as essential as "dry runs" for operating the base unit, footswitch, and phaco handpiece (Chap. 1) before the first procedure. It has proven useful to have the individual parameters programmed on the device in a factory setting suitable for beginners and to coordinate these with the training colleague.

4.2.2 Foot Switch

In addition to the functions for performing phacoemulsification, this can include additional options for operation such as vitrectomy, endoilluminations, diathermy, and more. Here too, the assignment on the pedal should be coordinated with the other operators of the facility and should be as uniform as possible. To perform the phacoemulsification of the nucleus, three functions must be triggered via the foot switch: irrigation, aspiration, and ultrasound. Traditionally, these individual functions are triggered in three stages (linear axial). In recent years, the linear-dual operation, adopted from retinal-vitreous surgery, has increasingly gained acceptance. Today, most devices have the option to trigger the various functions either sequentially (linear axial) or in parallel (linear dual) depending on the setting (Fig. 4.5, phaco mode).

▶ In principle, irrigation is initially triggered. The phaco tip should always be introduced into the anterior chamber while dripping. This automatically checks this function! The introduction of disturbing air bubbles is thus prevented.

In the linear-axial mode, the functions are triggered sequentially in three stages by pressing down the pedal. This means that when the irrigation (stage 1) is activated, the foot switch is pressed down until the aspiration (stage 2) occurs. By further pressing down the footplate, the phacoemulsification (stage 3) is added (Fig. 4.5b).

In the linear-dual mode, irrigation (stage 1) is also started by pressing the pedal down, and in the same movement, the aspiration is triggered in the second stage through an extended pedal path. The phacoemulsification is added by a lateral deflection of the footplate (Fig. 4.5c). In this mode, aspiration and ultrasound effect can then be increased separately (i.e., independently of

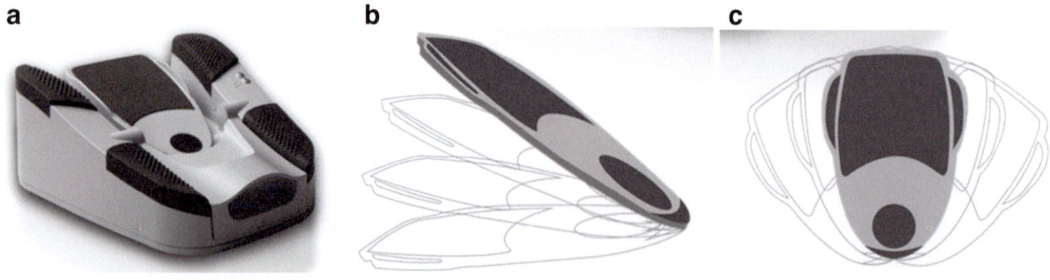

Fig. 4.5 (**a–c**) (**a**) Foot switch. (**b**) Linear-axial mode. (**c**) Linear-dual mode. (Courtesy of Bausch and Lomb)

each other) but simultaneously by extending the movement downwards or to the side.

4.2.3 Phaco Handpiece

The phaco handpiece is the component that transfers the various functions (irrigation, aspiration, emulsification) to the eye. These handpieces have become smaller and lighter over time. They have been ergonomically shaped so that they are almost as easy to handle as a fountain pen. Some operators prefer heavier handpieces that transmit less hand tremor to the eye. The phaco needle applies the ultrasound energy to the lens nucleus, and the fragmented lens parts are aspirated through its lumen. The phaco needle is beveled to be able to dig into the lens nucleus with the protruding part. It is surrounded by a silicone sleeve through which irrigation occurs (Fig. 4.6). The irrigation openings should be lateral so that the irrigation stream does not damage the corneal endothelium (Fig. 4.7). The moving phaco needle generates heat, which is dissipated by the surrounding infusion. A bare phaco needle can cause burns to the eye tissue!

▶ Before first entering the anterior chamber with the phaco tip, the correct positioning of the sleeve must be checked!

It is important to ensure that, on the one hand, the phaco tip is sufficiently free to create a groove in the nucleus, and on the other hand, the sleeve is pushed far enough onto the tip so that the fluid adequately covers and cools the needle during the ultrasound application to prevent damage to the surrounding area ("corneal burn"). To avoid direct fluid flow onto the endothelium, the irrigation ports must be correctly positioned laterally. If the silicone sleeve is too loose and shifts on the needle during intraocular manipulation, it must be replaced (Fig. 4.7)!

To understand the process of lens liquefaction and to assess the energy usage, every user should be aware in advance of what happens during phacoemulsification.

The phaco handpiece is connected to the base unit via three connections: the two tubes for irrigation (usually marked blue) and aspiration (usually marked red) and the electrical cable for controlling the piezoelectric crystal in the handpiece. The crystal sets the phaco needle

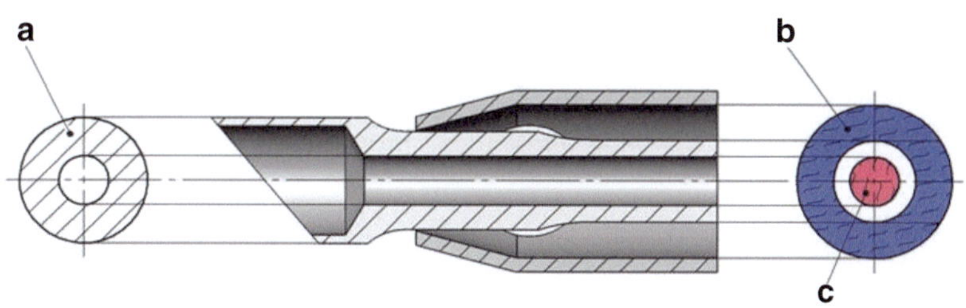

Fig. 4.6 (**a–c**) Section through a phaco tip (Oertli): (**a**) Phaco needle. (**b**) Lumen between phaco needle and sleeve for irrigation. (**c**) Lumen for aspiration

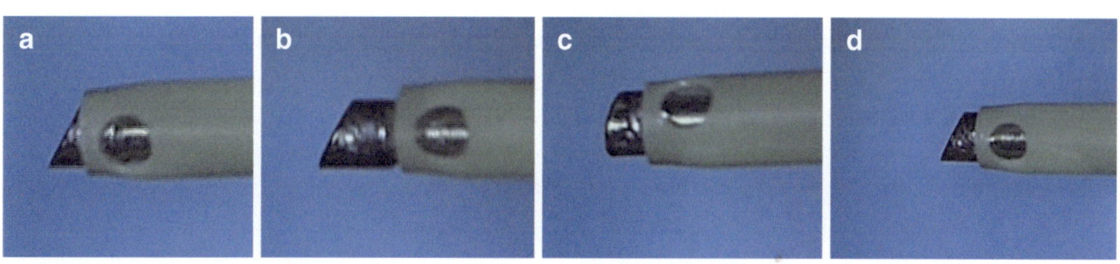

Fig. 4.7 (**a–d**) Phaco tip with sleeve. (**a**) Positioned too far forward. (**b**) Not pushed sufficiently over the phaco tip. (**c**) Without correct lateral positioning of the irrigation openings. (**d**) With optimally placed sleeve

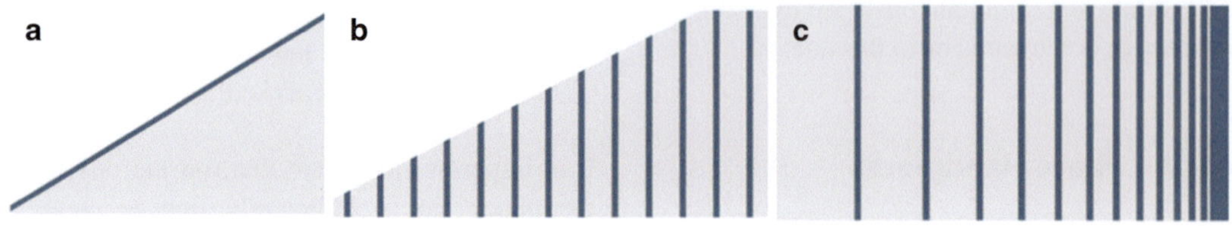

Fig. 4.8 (**a–c**) Types of ultrasound energy delivery. (**a**) Continuous. (**b**) Pulse modulation. (**c**) Burst modulation

into oscillations with frequencies between 20 kHz and 60 kHz (ultrasound oscillations). These vibrations are transmitted to the lens nucleus, causing it to be fractionated (or "emulsified") due to cavitations and mechanical disruptions, allowing the individual pieces to be aspirated. The oscillation of the phaco needle in the mentioned frequency range means friction and thus a risk of burns in the incision area. This highlights the particular importance of the cooling function and the stability of the anterior chamber of the eye with an intact sleeve.

When the technique was introduced, the ultrasound energy was initially supplied continuously, with the surgeon increasing the energy supply by pressing the foot pedal in position 3 (Fig. 4.8a). When using the pulsed mode, the phaco energy is delivered in pulse waves, thereby reducing the risk of thermal damage to the eye (Fig. 4.8b). By increasing the pressure on the foot pedal, the **pulse rate** can be increased. The wave-like energy supply at a constant frequency (28.5 kHz) further reduces the risk of coagulations in the tunnel area (Fig. 4.8b). Alternatively, the distance of the **phaco bursts** can also be varied (Fig. 4.8c).

▶ It is to be expected that additional torsional and longitudinal movements of the phaco needle will make nucleus fragmentation even more efficient. The use of lighter materials (titanium) allows for even more delicate intraocular manipulation with the phaco handpiece, and the technical parameters of the machines are further optimized. However, the key to the success of the operation is the surgeon's safe control of the phacoemulsification device!

4.3 Operating Chair and Surgeon's Seat

Martin Miertsch and Frank Wilhelm

The operating chair and the surgeon's seat serve to securely position the patient and the surgeon during the procedure. In addition to using the Operating Chair efficiently, surgeons should also practice physical exercise to make the back strong to avoid spine problems in future.

▶ It is absolutely necessary that every surgeon familiarizes themselves with all the functions of the devices through "non-sterile" practice BEFORE the first procedure [7, 8].

Operation is performed under sterile conditions, usually without visual contact with the control elements. This means that changes to the settings must be done "as ifasleep." Before the start of the first procedure in the OR program, the surgeon's seat is positioned so that the surgeon can work in a relaxed posture even during longer operations.

▶ The operating table is then adapted in the OR to the settings of the surgeon's seat and not vice versa!

In recent years, these requirements have been met by the development of functional and easy-to-use devices. The basics of the function will be explained here using the example of the company UFSK-International OSYS GmbH Heidelberg, representing products from various manufacturers.

The operating table should not only provide a comfortable position for the patient but also enable a smooth transition between the rapidly successive procedures [9]. It is adapted to the requirements of positioning and ergonomic and comfortable treatment of the patient. It features diverse setting options of the head, back, seat, and leg sections, as well as the overall chair height for treatment and surgery, including shock and flat positioning. A key requirement is the accessibility of the surgical field for the surgeon, taking into account that, for example, he must be able to position his knees under the headrest in such a way that he has enough space to operate the foot controls of the various devices.

All positions can be conveniently adjusted via a hand control (Fig. 4.9). Alternatively, the head and height adjustments can also be operated via a foot control. Thus, a surgeon can comfortably readjust a position even after surgical hand disinfection without having to disinfect again.

The adjustment functions are triggered by a light, central press of the buttons with the tip of the foot.

The head section (Fig. 4.10) is three-dimensionally adjustable and can be set for precise head positioning of the patient, which is especially important when used in eye surgery to align the head exactly horizontally. This prevents the accumulation of rinsing fluid in the inner corner of the eyelid.

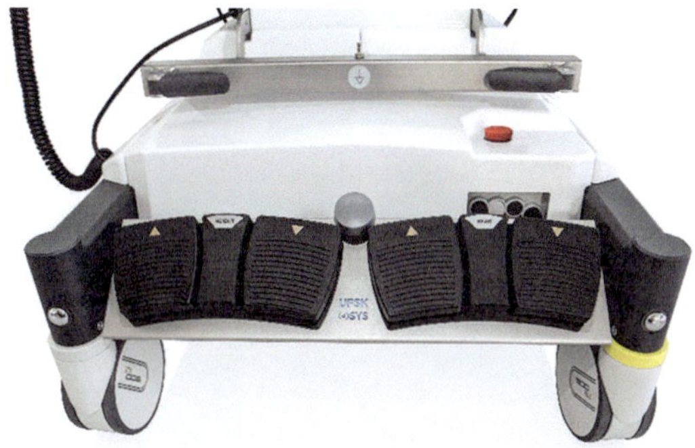

Fig. 4.9 Foot pedals for adjusting the height of the operating table and head section

The treatment chair is equipped with a mechanically operated brake on both sides and features directional wheel functions that facilitate controlled maneuvering of the chair by one person and ensure secure fixation in the operating room during the procedure.

The treatment chair is equipped with an emergency stop switch (Fig. 4.11). This is located on the top of the battery box at the back of the chair and is recognizable by its red signal color.

Activating the emergency stop switch immediately and directly cuts off all power supply to the device and instantly puts the chair in a safe state. This function is needed in daily practice, for example:

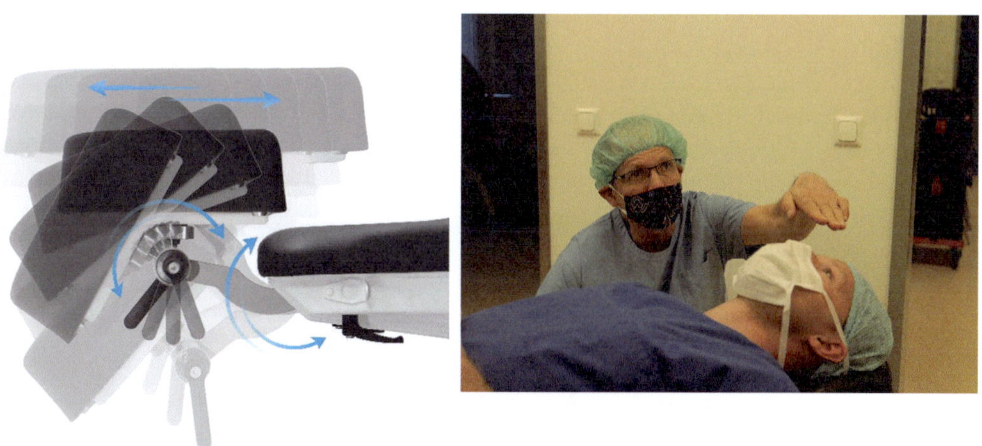

Fig. 4.10 The variable adjustment of the headrest allows for horizontal positioning of the eye surface

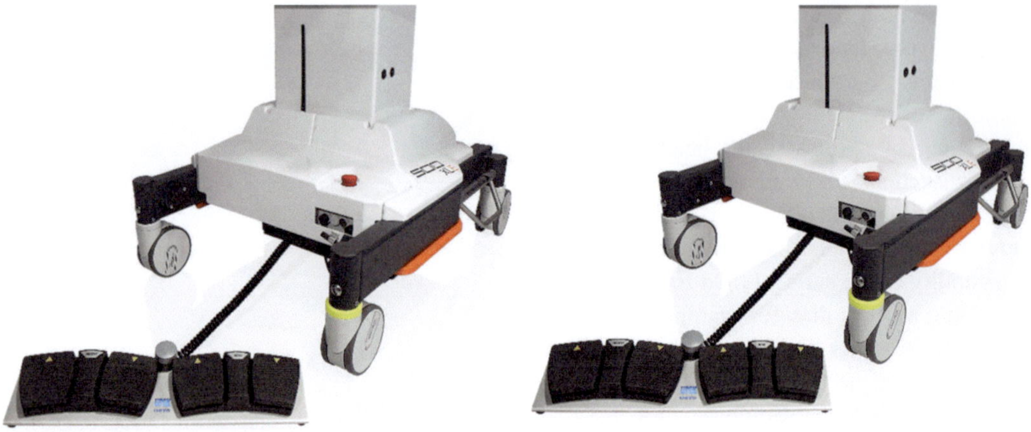

Fig. 4.11 Everyone working in the operating room must know the function of the red button as an emergency stop switch! On the left hand side, the button is not pressed, while on the right hand side the button is pressed.

- during the performance of a treatment or medical procedure to prevent any unwanted activation of adjustment functions or movements of the chair,
- in case of danger or to avert a hazard,
- during unsupervised rest periods of the patient to prevent unauthorized, self-initiated activation of adjustment functions or movements of the chair by the patient,
- for proper shutdown at the end of the workday.

The **surgeon's chair** is adapted to the requirements of relaxed and ergonomic sitting and features versatile adjustment functions for seat height, seat posture/backrest, and armrests (Fig. 4.12). Ideally, the chair should be easy to roll! Equipped with a mechanically operated brake on both sides, it features directional wheel functions that facilitate controlled maneuvering of the chair by one person [6].

The electric, stepless height adjustment can be effortlessly operated via the foot pedal (Fig. 4.13). The desired seat height can be adjusted within the range of 535 to 735 mm.

- Left foot (from the operator's perspective), press: The chair moves downwards.
- Right foot (from the operator's perspective), press: The chair moves upwards.

The ergonomically designed seating system of the operator's chair (Fig. 4.14) supports active, healthy sitting. The tiltable seat and the height-adjustable backrest allow individual adjustment to the surgeon's weight and size. The variable

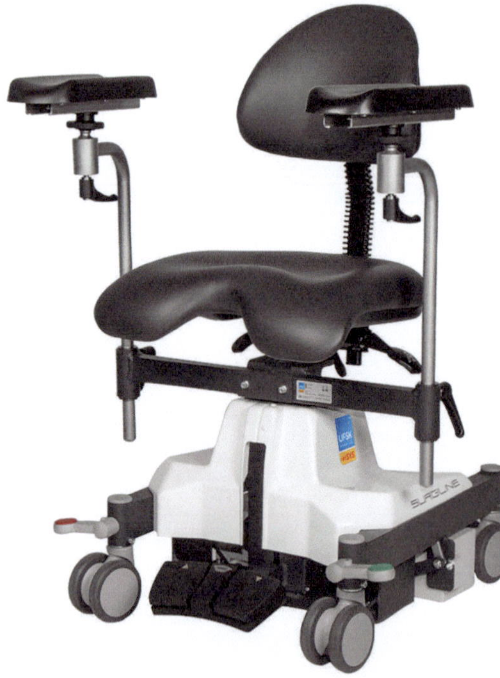

Fig. 4.12 The surgiLine surgeon's chair from UFSK-International OSYS GmbH exemplifies the diverse functions and adjustment options of a surgeon's seat

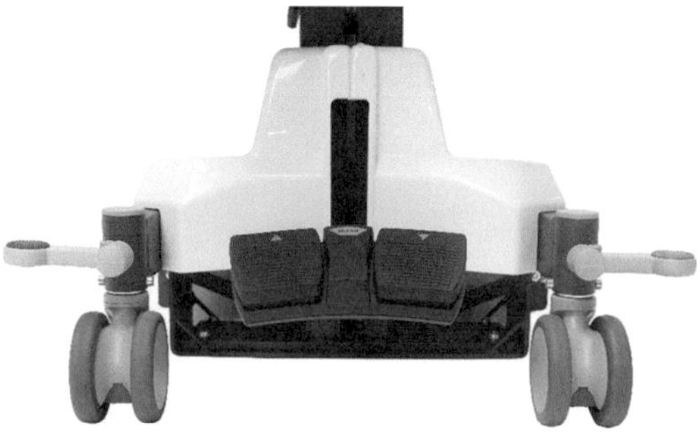

Fig. 4.13 Foot pedals for adjusting the seat height of the operator: 1 = upwards, 2 = downwards

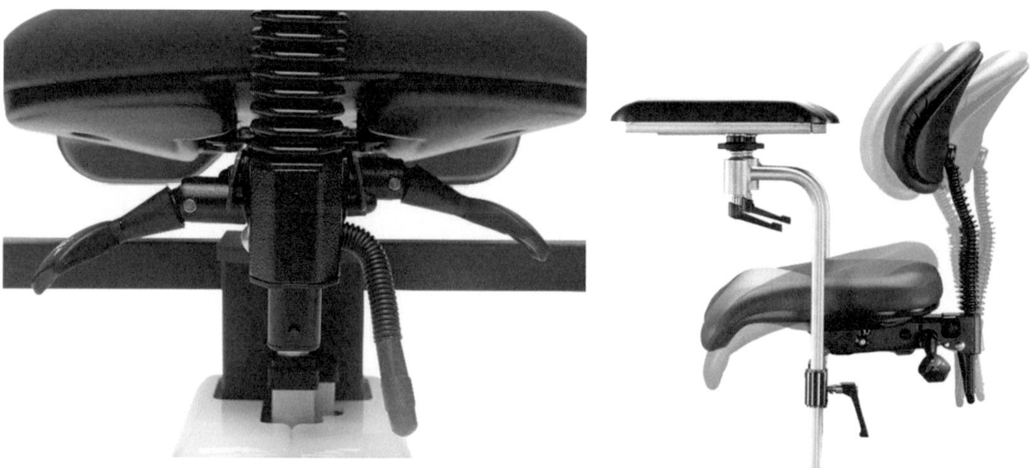

Fig. 4.14 The adjustments of the tilt of the seat and backrest as well as the height of the backrest can each be made separately

tilt of the chair's back axis optimizes the individual "sitting angle" and, in conjunction with the freely movable, body-pressure-responsive back cushion, prevents a posture that could be harmful to health in the long run.

The adjustment for the tilt angle of the backrest is made by operating the handle lever (1) on the right side of the chair. By pulling the handle towards the body, the backrest is released. The backrest is then brought to the desired position by simply leaning forward or backward with the back and fixed in this position by releasing the handle (1).

The same procedure is followed when adjusting the tilt of the seat. The handle lever (2) is loosened, the optimal seating position is found by shifting weight (forward or backward), and fixed by releasing the handle lever (2).

The overall height of the backrest is adjusted via the clamping lever (3). By slightly turning the lever, the backrest is loosened or fixed again by turning the lever in the opposite direction. It is important to ensure that the freely movable, body-pressure-responsive back cushion is positioned in an optimally adjusted position to the back, thus supporting the lumbar region in a back-friendly manner.

It is also important to ensure that the backrest is adjusted so that it just touches the operator's back. He should not lean against it! The seat height should be chosen so that, depending on the leg length under the operating table, he can still operate the foot switches of the microscope, phaco machine, operating table, and other devices without any impairments.

The desired height and swivel range of the armrests can be brought into the desired position via the joint arms (1). To do this, the corresponding clamping levers on the joint arm are loosened, and the arm is moved or rotated into the desired ergonomic position. Once the preferred setting is found, it is fixed by locking the clamping lever (Fig. 4.15).

▶ The secure fixation of the armrests in the desired position should be checked by the operator before the start of the operation day!

▶ For the novice operator, the armrests are generally helpful, but they gradually lose their importance with increasing experience.

The operator's chair also has an easy-to-use central brake that acts on all four wheels (Fig. 4.16).

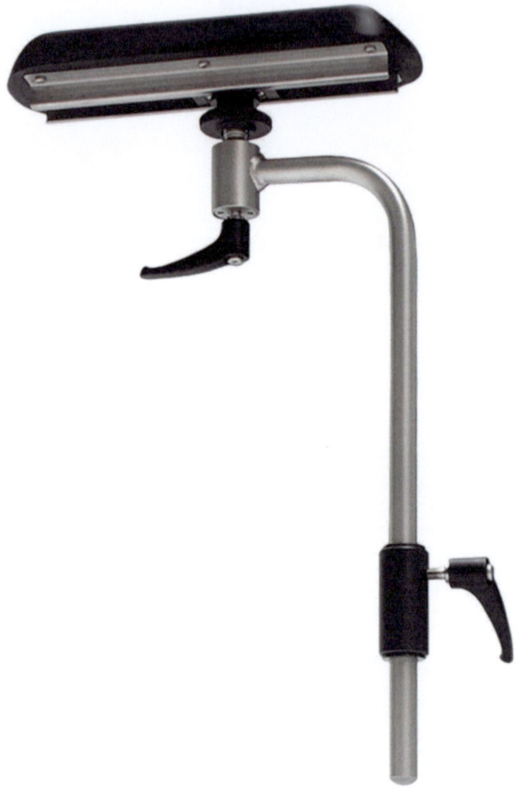

Fig. 4.15 The various joints and locks on the armrests allow optimal adjustment for each operator

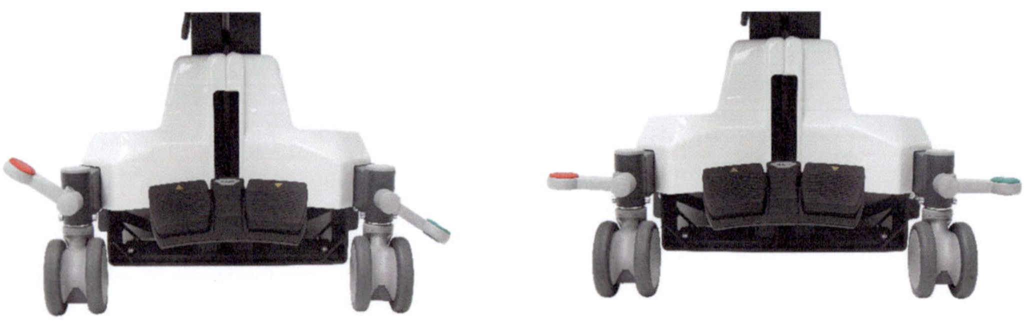

Brake released

braked

Fig. 4.16 To fix the operating seat with the brake, the red lever must be operated, and to release the brake, the green lever must be operated

References and Further Reading

1. Nylen CO (1954) The microscope in aural surgery, its first use and later development. Acta Otolaryngol Suppl 116:226–240
2. Littmann H (1963) Ein neues Operationsmikroskop. Klin Mbl Augenheilk 142:50–671
3. Harms H, Mackensen G (1989) Augenoperationen unter dem Mikroskop. Georg Thieme, Stuttgart, 291 S
4. Draeger J, Kirchner M (1988) Technische Ausstattung und Organisation einer ophthalmologischen Operationseinheit. In: Mackensen G, Neubauer H (Hrsg) Augenärztliche Operationen, Teil 1. Springer, Berlin, S 1–41
5. Draeger J, Garweg J (1990) Funktionelle Gesichtspunkte bei der Verwendung von Operationsmikroskopen. Ophthalmochirurgie 2:189–197
6. Kuhn F (2016) Vitreoretinal surgery: strategies and tactics. Springer, Berlin
7. Gebrauchs- und Serviceanleitung Version 11/2015 SN 352-1999. Operateurstuhl surgiLine. UFSK-International OSYS GmbH
8. Velhagen K (1964) Propädeutische augenärztliche Operationslehre. VEB Georg Thieme, Leipzig
9. Mackensen G, Neubauer H (1988) Augenärztliche Operationen, Teil 1, 3. Aufl. Springer, Berlin. ISBN 3-540-18267-5

5 Instrument Knowledge

Alexander Petzold and Frank Wilhelm

Contents

5.1 Introduction

An important prerequisite for working in the operating room is the knowledge of the instruments—the tools of every surgeon! The development of surgical instruments has been rapid in recent decades, as a look back in history shows (Fig. 5.1)

For modern surgical procedures, these are manufactured in microsurgical dimensions and must meet the highest standards.

Today, ophthalmic surgeons have a variety of different instruments at their disposal, which differ more or less in shape and material use [1]. High-quality instruments used in the medical field differ significantly from those produced in mass production. Tweezers or scissors are not just tweezers or scissors! The requirements for medical devices are generally very high, especially when used in ophthalmology.

▶ The specific functional characteristics of each surgical instrument and their specific application are prerequisites for the smooth running of an operation, and every aspiring ophthalmic surgeon must know and master "their" working material.

5.1.1 Quality Pays Off

The longevity of sensitive instruments is significantly influenced by external factors. A particular strain is posed by the high temperatures during the sterilization process of up to 134°C, contamination with blood and protein residues, as well as other chemicals, and the risk of corrosion due to constant moisture. Mechanical damages, which can be minimized by proper fixing

A. Petzold (✉)
Augenzentrum am Johannisplatz, Leipzig, Germany
e-mail: a-p@posteo.de

F. Wilhelm
Universitätsklinikum Halle Saale, Greifswald, Germany

F. Wilhelm (ed.), *Ophthalmic Surgery for Beginners*, https://doi.org/10.1007/978-3-662-70287-1_5

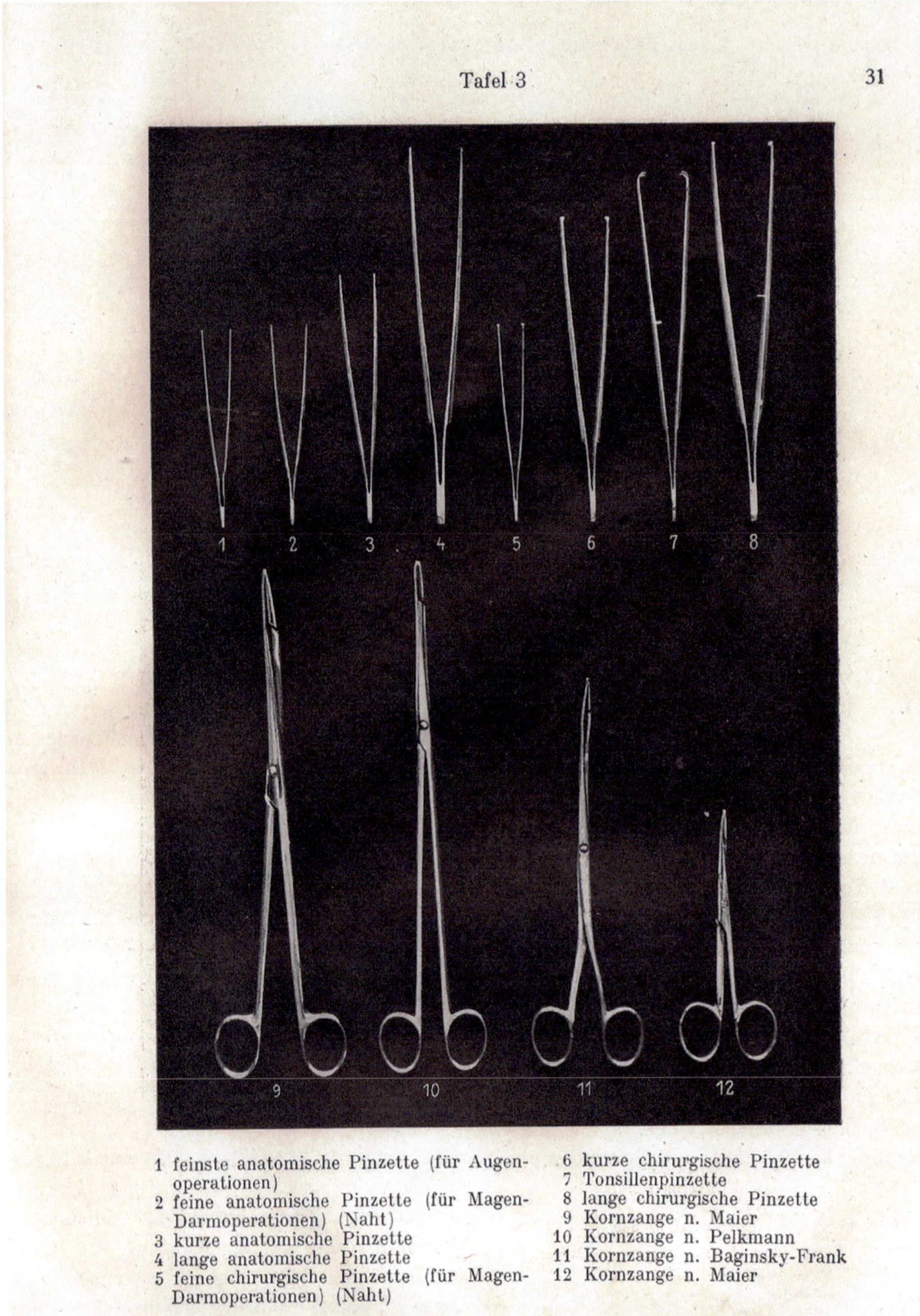

Fig. 5.1 Overview of available surgical grasping instruments—including eye forceps—in the operating room from the year 1943. ([3])

on the instrument tray and transport safeguards (to avoid damage to the surface protection layer of the instruments—also called the passive layer), should also not be neglected.

This results in high demands on the manufacturer regarding the correct selection and composition of materials. The material properties are significantly determined by the proportions of chromium and carbon.

The high prices compared to those from mass production can be explained by the high manual manufacturing effort under the microscope in the production of specific shapes.

▶ Before making a purchase decision, one should contact medical product advisors from well-known manufacturers and have the corresponding instruments demonstrated. Often, companies also offer the service of temporary practical testing.

5.2 European Medical Device Regulation (MDR)

The manufacturer is responsible for the medical use and the "placing on the market" of medical devices. Since May 25, 2017, the European Medical Device Regulation (MDR) has been in force together with the In-vitro Diagnostic Regulation (IVDR) [5]. The MDR must be applied mandatorily after a four-year transition period from May 26, 2021. It is expected that there will be delays in certification according to MDR for numerous medical devices used in eye surgery, which will lead to future supply shortages [8]. Therefore, every surgeon is required to prepare for this situation in the interest of their patients and to consider this in the planning of their surgical activities.

In principle, the MDR regulates the manufacture and placing on the market of medical devices for the entire EU, without the need for national legislation (as previously the Medical Devices Act—MPG).

What you should know about the new EU Medical Device Regulation:

- The EU Medical Device Regulation primarily provides for increased requirements for the placing on the market and monitoring of medical devices in the European Union.
- The definitions in the field of medical devices and active implantable medical devices have been significantly expanded and now also include products without a medical purpose, such as colored contact lenses, as well as implants and substances for aesthetic purposes.
- The introduction of a unique device identification (UDI) is intended to simplify the traceability of certain items within the supply chain for manufacturers and authorities, thus enabling the quick and efficient recall of medical devices that pose a safety risk.
- To comply with the new classification rules, manufacturers must examine their products according to risk, contact duration, and invasiveness and update their technical documentation accordingly.
- Stricter clinical requirements apply to Class III medical devices and implantable products.
- Country-specific regulations are to be governed by the German Medical Device Adaptation Act-EU (MPAnpG-EU) or the Medical Device Law Implementation Act (MPDG) [5].

▶ The European Medical Device Regulation (MDR) regulates the manufacture and placing on the market of medical devices and thus also for surgical instruments throughout the EU.

5.3 Medical Devices

Medical devices are all products with a medical purpose that are placed on the market by the manufacturer for use on humans. In contrast to pharmaceuticals, which act pharmacologically, immunologically, or metabolically, the primary intended effect of their use is achieved primarily through physical means. Medical devices also include products that contain a substance or preparations of substances or are coated with such, which, when used separately, are considered pharmaceuticals or components of a pharmaceutical (including plasma derivatives) and can exert an effect on the human body in addition to the functions of the product.

5.3.1 Active and Non-Active Medical Devices

A distinction is made between active medical devices, whose operation depends on a power source or another energy source, and non-active medical devices, which are not powered. The legislator imposes increased requirements on active medical devices to ensure that a high degree of protection is always guaranteed for patients, users, and third parties, and that the properties specified by the manufacturer are met at all times [6].

5.3.2 Medical Device Classification

The classification of medical devices is based on a risk-based system, which is oriented towards the "vulnerability of the human body" and the risk potential of the product, with the duration and location of the application of the respective medical device being decisive [10]. The longer the product is used or the deeper the product is brought into the body, the higher the classification and thus the risk. This risk increases stepwise from Class I to Class III. Class I products pose no or very low risk, while Class III products pose a very high risk to patients.

The classification of medical devices into one of the risk classes depends, among other things, on the duration of use (up to 60 minutes, up to 30 days, longer than 30 days), the degree of invasiveness (invasive, surgically invasive, implantable), and the application to the central circulatory system or the central nervous system.

▶ In the European Union, medical devices are divided into four main classes, which carry varying levels of risk potential (Table 5.1).

Table 5.1 Classification of Medical Devices

Class	Classification/Risk Potential	Examples
I	Low risk potential low degree of invasiveness temporary use (< 60 min)	Glasses, tongue depressors, urine bottles, neck braces, wheelchairs, walking aids, support stockings, bandages, mouth-nose protection
Is (sterile)	Products marketed in a sterile state	Protective equipment
Im (measure)	Devices with measuring function	Stethoscopes, thermometers
Ir (reusable)	Products that are reprocessed or reused	Reusable surgical instruments, endoscopes
IIa	Medium risk potential moderate degree of invasiveness short-term use (<30 days) in the body continuous/repeated use of the same product	Disinfectants (for instruments and devices), disposable syringes, hearing aids, contact lenses, bladder catheters, cannulas, surgical gloves, diagnostic ultrasound, MRI
IIb	Increased risk potential systemic effect non-invasive contraception long-term use (> 30 days)	Ventilators, defibrillators, peripheral vascular prostheses or stents, dialyzers, surgical lasers, nails and plates, external pacemakers, X-ray machines, condoms
III	High risk potential immediate application to the heart, central circulatory or nervous system implantable and/or highly invasive invasive contraception	Heart catheters, stents, artificial joints, pacemakers, heart valves, breast implants

Medical devices of class I are mostly non-invasive products that pose very low risk and have no impact on the human body. Class I products can be certified by the company itself. Class I contains three subclasses. Medical devices marketed in a sterile state are categorized as class Is (s = "sterile"). Products with a measuring function are designated as class Im (m = "measure") and products that can be reused or reprocessed are assigned to class Ir (r = "reusable").

The next risk class consists of class II products, with the two subclasses IIa (medium risk) and IIb (medium to high risk). Class IIa products are generally invasive (limited to natural body openings) and are often operated with the help of an external energy source or used for the diagnosis and monitoring of diseases. If these products are in any way potentially dangerous to a patient, they are automatically assigned to class IIb. Class IIb includes most surgically invasive or active products that are partially or fully implanted in the body.

The products with the highest risk for patients are classified as class III. These products either have life-sustaining functions and are therefore of significant importance to human health or pose a particularly high methodological risk of disease or injury.

5.3.3 CE Marking

The CE marking indicates the conformity of a product with the product safety regulations applicable in the Union. The abbreviation "CE" today means "Conformité Européenne," the French term for "European Conformity." The CE marking stands for EU-wide harmonized regulations that are intended to simplify European trade and serves as an "EU passport" for a product.

▶ The aim of the CE marking is to document the fulfillment of the essential safety requirements of the applicable EU regulations (e.g., for machinery or medical devices).

A product may only be placed on the market and put into operation if it complies with the provisions of all applicable Union regulations and if a corresponding conformity assessment procedure has been carried out. By affixing the CE marking, the manufacturer or its authorized representative established in the EU (for manufacturers outside the EU) confirms the conformity of the product with the applicable European regulations and the fulfillment of the essential requirements. Products with CE marking may be placed on the market in any member state within the EU (Fig. 5.2).

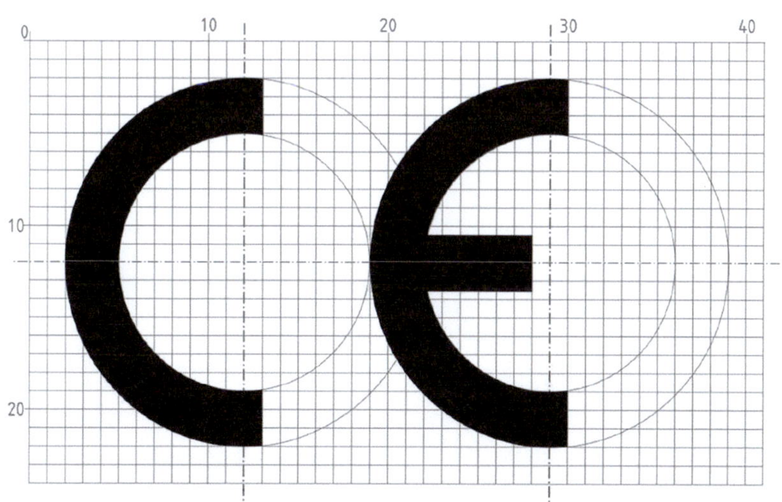

Fig. 5.2 Standard representation of the CE marking [9]

5.3.4 Ophthalmic Surgical Instruments

The anatomy of the eye places special demands on ophthalmic surgical instruments in terms of size, shape, and material selection. For example, instruments for the posterior segment of the eye are longer and tube-guided, in contrast to the instruments typically used in anterior segment surgery.

Thanks to rapid developments in materials science, instruments with new materials and refined surfaces are now used to improve corrosion resistance. Instruments made of titanium alloy are lightweight and resistant to corrosion, but more difficult to process and therefore more expensive. Other common materials include various types of steel and their alloys, natural and synthetic diamonds, ceramics, (temperature-resistant) plastics, silicone, rubber, glass, textiles, and nylon.

5.3.5 Disposable Instruments

Disposable instruments are being used more and more frequently. These are mass-produced plastic products that are usually manufactured by injection molding, with the functionally relevant parts made of high-quality materials (Chap. 14). Advantages of these single-use products include lower production costs with comparable quality and functionality. For many narrow-lumen instruments used in ophthalmic surgery, there are no validated reprocessing procedures classified as safe, so the use of disposable instruments can ensure the best possible infection prophylaxis. The labor-intensive reprocessing steps of reusable instruments, along with the associated costs, are also significantly reduced. Corrosion issues are practically irrelevant.

▶ The use of disposable instruments has proven effective. In the future, an increased environmental burden from disposable instruments and their packaging materials is to be expected.

5.4 Structure of an Instrument

Some of the most commonly used instruments, and of particular importance to the ophthalmic surgeon, are micro-surgical forceps. Using a pair of forceps (Fig. 5.3) as an example, the structure and terminology of an instrument will be explained [2]. There are often many variants of each instrument, with only slightly modified details, often named after their developer.

▶ Only the most commonly used instruments can be presented in this chapter. The surgeon can obtain information about the various individual designs from the manufacturers if needed.

5.4.1 Anatomical and Surgical Forceps

The legs of a pair of forceps are formed by the connecting plate, the spring, the mirror, as well as the grip and jaw surfaces. They can be straight, curved, angled, or crossed. The instrument is grasped and operated at the grip surfaces, which can be either smooth or transversely or longitudinally grooved. The jaw surface is part of the working end, which is used directly to grasp, hold, and cut tissue, organs, and medical aids. The dentition determines the profile of the different jaw types. A distinction is made between anatomical (Fig. 5.4) and surgical jaw types,

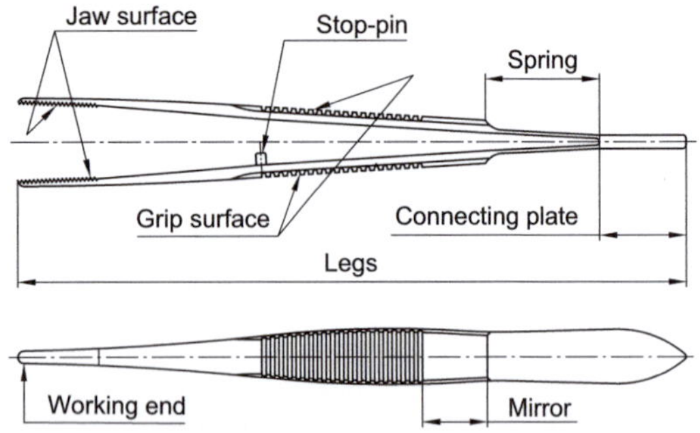

Fig. 5.3 Technical drawing (schematic) of an anatomical forceps (image courtesy of Geuder AG)

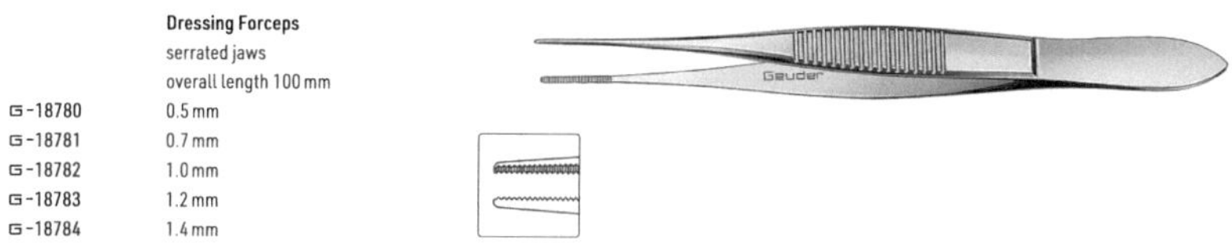

Fig. 5.4 Anatomical eye forceps with grooved branches (image courtesy of Geuder AG)

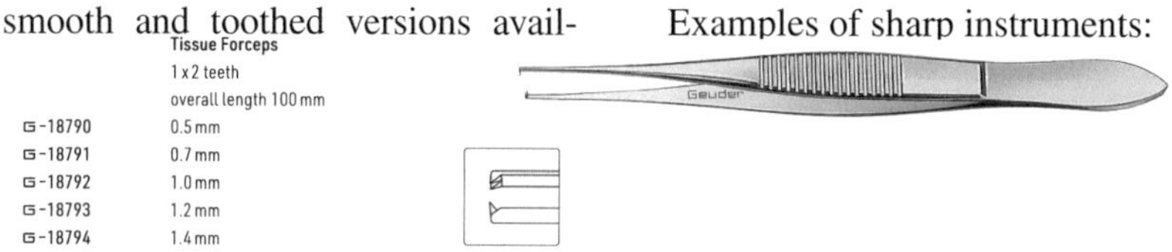

Fig. 5.5 Surgical eye forceps (image courtesy of Geuder AG)

with both smooth and toothed versions available. The interlocking, sharp teeth of surgical forceps (Fig. 5.5) allow for good fixation of the grasped tissue parts and enable stronger traction if needed. However, structures such as blood vessels are more easily injured. For this purpose, the more tissue-friendly anatomical forceps are more suitable, although they do not allow for stronger traction. Forceps are also available with a pin, a component that prevents the working end from deviating from a predetermined position, or with a lock to secure the instrument in a defined position. The version with an adjusting screw allows for variable fixation of the working end. Each instrument is available in almost any configuration of the individual components in terms of size, width, shape, and surface texture.

5.4.2 Classification

With regard to their function, surgical instruments can be classified as follows (Table 5.2 with examples of ophthalmic surgical instruments).

Sharp Instruments

This group includes instruments that have a cutting edge and can therefore be used to cut through tissue.

Examples of sharp instruments:

- Lances
- Knives of all kinds (diamond, disposable knives)
- Scrapers and spoon instruments
- Foreign body instruments
- Punches and chisels
- Circular knives
- Trephines

Scalpels are often used as disposable knives in ophthalmology. The blades of paracentesis knives are triangular and available in 15-degree or 30-degree variants (Fig. 5.6). Phaco lances and clear cornea knives are usually angled and available in various blade widths for different incision widths (Fig. 5.7). The beveling of the facets varies. For the preparation of a scleral-corneal tunnel, there are tunnel knives with different rounded blade shapes (Sect. 21.1).

Diamond knives (here the designation includes the material of the blade) are sharp with a correspondingly high risk of injury. The knives are very delicate and any unnecessary contact should be avoided, which is why transport in suitable boxes with blade protection has proven effective (Fig. 5.8). The acquisition and repair costs are very high. The companies' instructions

Table 5.2 Classification of surgical instruments based on their function

Function
Sharp (Knives, Threphines, Diamond knives)
Blunt (Spatulas, Hooks)
Cutting (Scissors, Vitrectome)
Grasping (Forceps)
Holding (Fixation instruments, Needle holders)
Spreading (Eye specula, Clamps)
Irrigation / Aspiration (Cannulas, I/A instruments)
Measuring and Marking (Calipers, Markers)

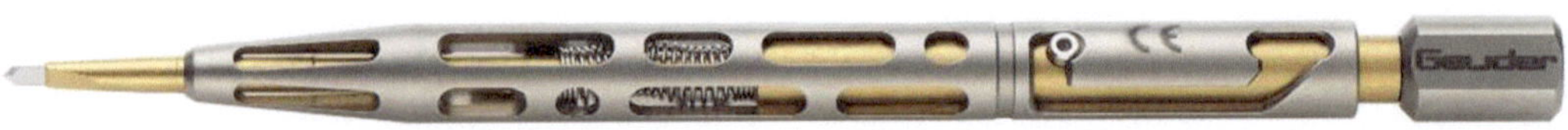

Fig. 5.6 Diamond paracentesis knife 1 mm

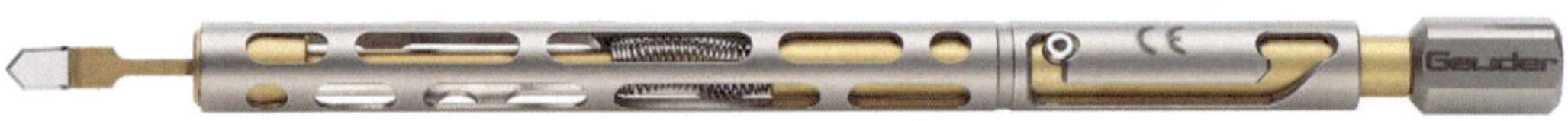

Fig. 5.7 Diamond phaco lance 2.4 mm

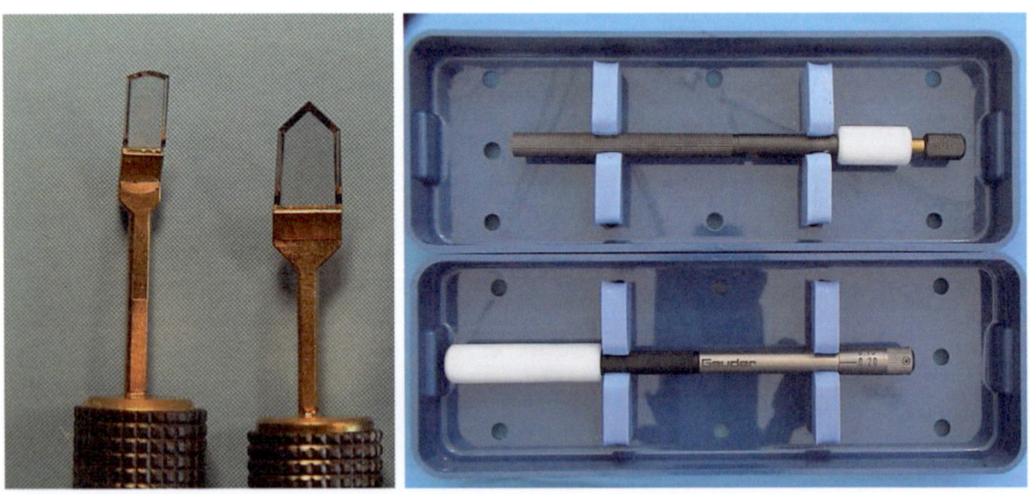

Fig. 5.8 Diamond knife in transport box and blade protection

regarding care and sterilization must be followed. These should only be carried out by appropriately trained personnel (Fig. 5.9 and 5.10).

5.4.3 Blunt Instruments

Blunt instruments are used for gentle manipulation of tissue and implants.

Examples of blunt instruments:

- Lens nucleus rotator
- Position hooks
- Iris hooks/retractors
- Spatulas (microsurgical)
- Loop instruments
- Strabismus hooks
- Probes
- Orbital spatulas
- Localizers

Lens nucleus rotators and nucleus splitters (Fig. 5.11) are found on every cataract tray. These instruments come in many variants, as single or double instruments. The iris hook according to Dardenne has a push-pull tip, while the

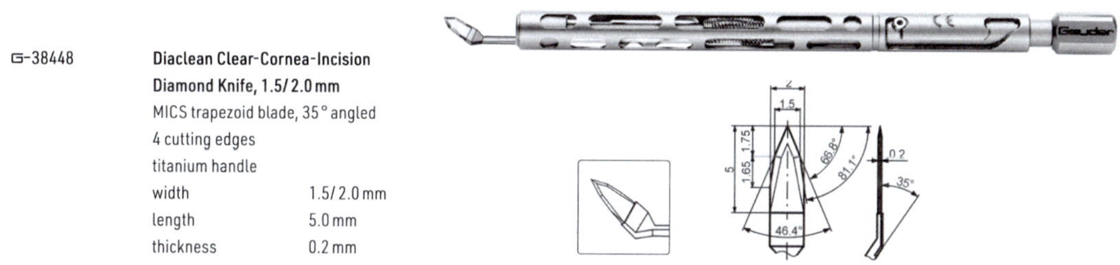
G-38448
Diaclean Clear-Cornea-Incision
Diamond Knife, 1.5/2.0 mm
MICS trapezoid blade, 35° angled
4 cutting edges
titanium handle
width 1.5/2.0 mm
length 5.0 mm
thickness 0.2 mm
1.5
5
1.65
1.75
66.8°
81.1°
46.4°
0.2
35°

Fig. 5.9 Diamond phaco lance with four cutting surfaces, angled at 35°, widths between 1.5 mm to 2.00 mm, but it can enlarge the incision to 2.2 mm or above when needed (image courtesy of Geuder AG)

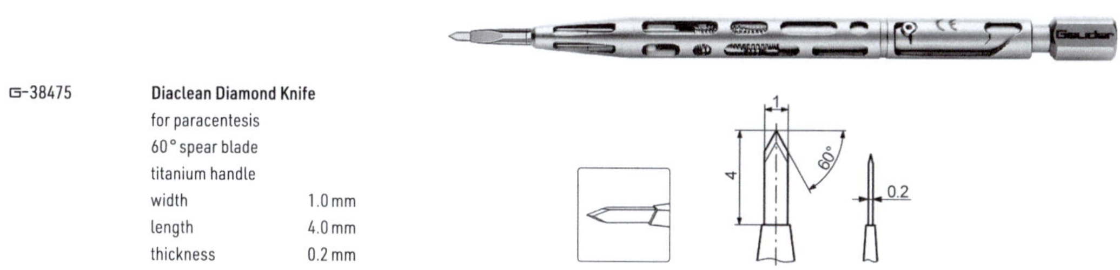

Fig. 5.10 Diamond knife for paracentesis, lance 1 mm (image courtesy of Geuder AG)

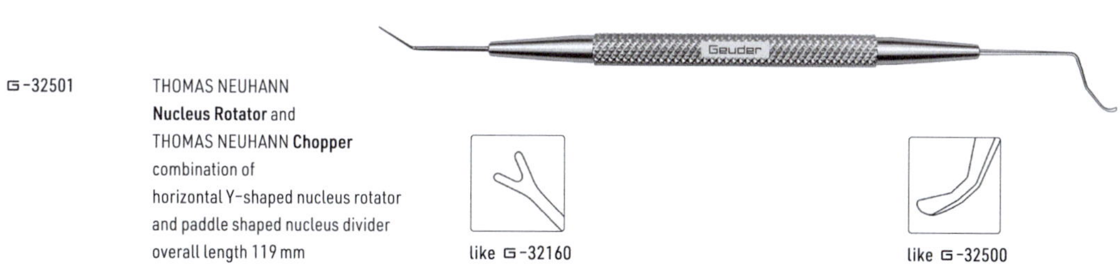

Fig. 5.11 Double instrument consisting of a horizontal Y-shaped lens nucleus rotator and a paddle-shaped nucleus splitter (image courtesy of Geuder AG)

version according to Lund has a button shape. The push-pull instrument (Fig. 5.12) can be used in many ways. Pulling, pushing, and also as a spatula when cracking the nucleus are possible uses of this instrument in cataract surgery (Fig. 5.13) (Chap. 18).

5.4.4 Cutting Instruments

This section summarizes instruments that usually have two blades.

Examples of cutting instruments:

- Eye scissors
- Spring scissors
- Corneal scissors
- Vitreous scissors

As a standard version, scissors with rings for opening and closing the blades are used. Examples of this version are the Stevens tendon scissors (Fig. 5.14), which can be used during an eyelid operation, or strabismus scissors. The enucleation

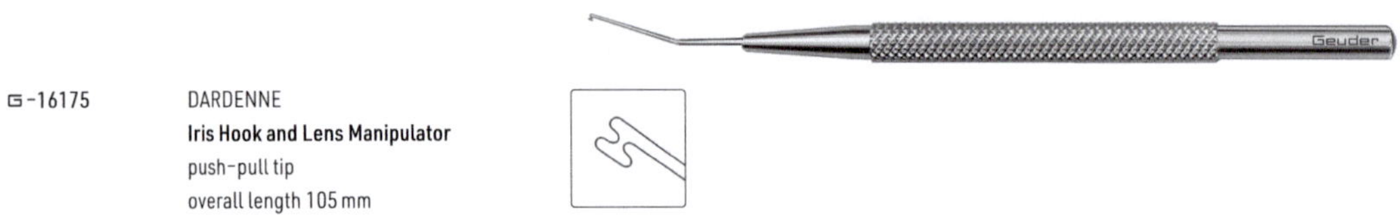

Fig. 5.12 Iris hook (push-pull instrument) according to Dardenne (image courtesy of Geuder AG)

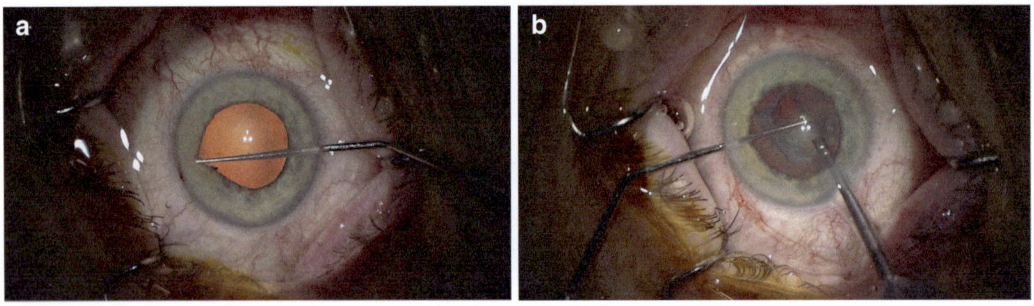

Fig. 5.13 **a**, **b** Examples of the use of an iris hook during cataract surgery. (**a**) Release of a posterior synechia. (**b**) Cracking a lens nucleus

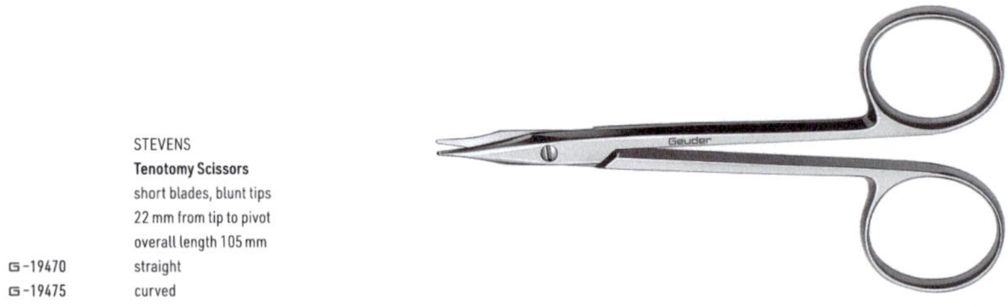
STEVENS
Tenotomy Scissors
short blades, blunt tips
22 mm from tip to pivot
overall length 105 mm
G-19470 straight
G-19475 curved
Geuder

Fig. 5.14 Stevens tendon scissors, short blade, blunt-blunt tip (image courtesy of Geuder AG)

scissors are used for cutting the optic nerve. Scissors whose blades are opened by spring force and closed by operating the handles are frequently used in eye surgery. The most well-known spring scissors include the Vannas capsulotomy scissors (Fig. 5.15), the Westcott spring scissors, and various iridectomy and corneal scissors, which are often used in anterior segment surgery.

The shape can be straight, angled, or curved (Fig. 5.16), while the blades can be pointed and blunt either alone or in various combinations. Instruments whose moving elements are "tube-guided" allow access through paracenteses in the anterior segment as well as through 20, 23, 25G, and even smaller incisions for procedures in the posterior eye segment.

5.4.5 Grasping/holding instruments

Examples of grasping and holding instruments:

- Corneal forceps
- Capsulorhexis forceps
- Cilia forceps
- Vitrectomy forceps

Since the colibri forceps (Fig. 5.17) are practically indispensable in microsurgery, this "multitalent" will be discussed in more detail here.

Due to the curved leg shape and the thereby ensured unobstructed view of the surgical field, it fulfills the function of fine surgical forceps when grasping with the tips, thus enabling secure tissue fixation. With the flat profile of the suture plate, the colibri forceps are also suitable as knot-tying forceps for grasping fine suture material, and in the closed state, they can be used as a fine spatula. A micro-colibri forceps can be easily felt at the recess in the grip area, even without having to take the eyes off the microscope. (Fig. 5.18 and 5.19)

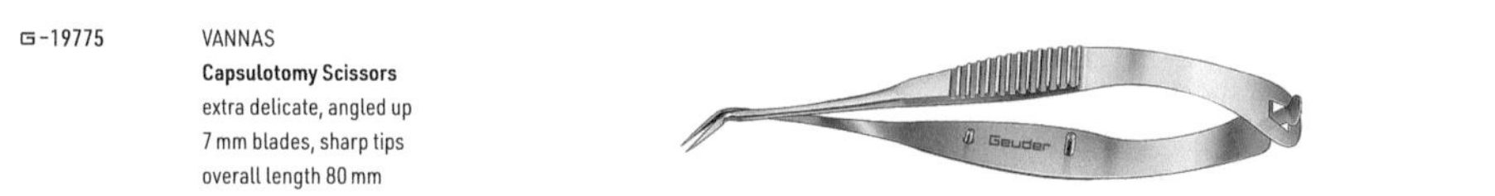
G-19775
VANNAS
Capsulotomy Scissors
extra delicate, angled up
7 mm blades, sharp tips
overall length 80 mm
Geuder

Fig. 5.15 Vannas capsulotomy scissors, extra fine, upward curved tip (image courtesy of Geuder AG)

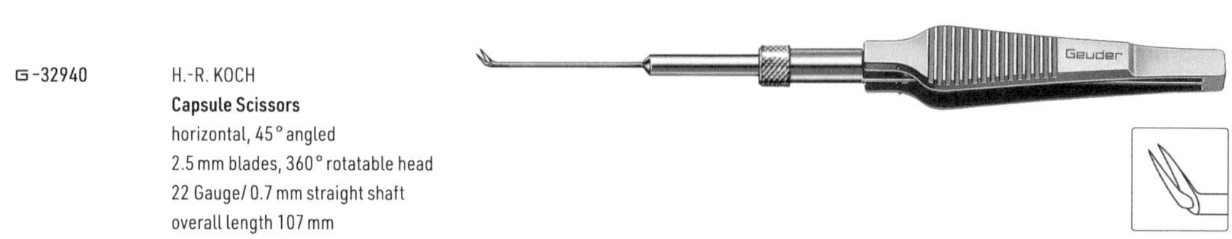

Fig. 5.16 Koch capsular scissors, horizontal, 45° angled, head 360° rotatable, 22 gauge (image courtesy of Geuder AG)

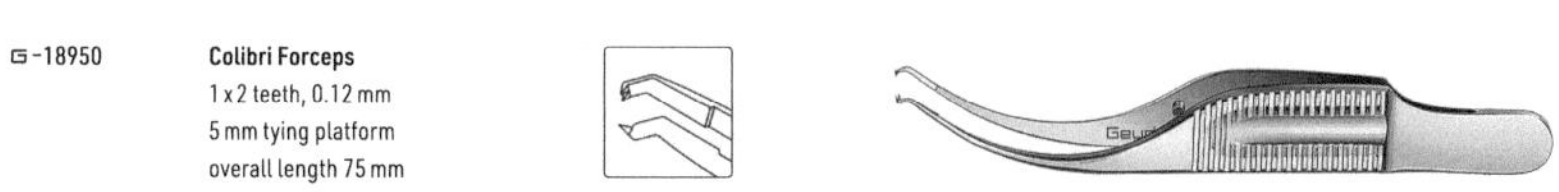

Fig. 5.17 Colibri forceps, surgical (image courtesy of Geuder AG)

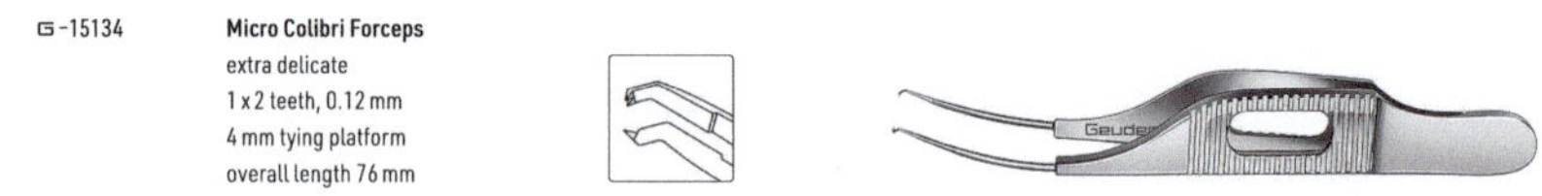

Fig. 5.18 Micro-colibri forceps, extra fine, surgical (image courtesy of Geuder AG)

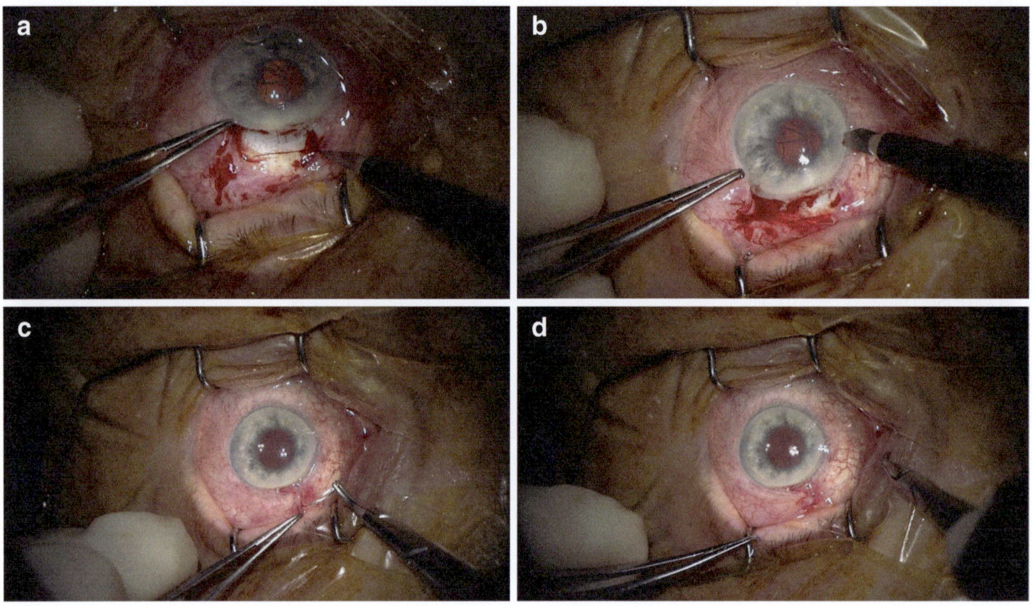

Fig. 5.19 Examples of the use of colibri forceps. (**a**) Fixation of the eyeball during the creation of a scleral-corneal tunnel. (**b**) Fixation of the eyeball with counterpressure during paracentesis. (**c**) Fixation and presentation of the conjunctiva. (**d**) Conjunctival suture

5.5 Instruments for pars plana vitrectomy

Special requirements must be met for instruments used in vitreous and retinal surgical procedures. They must be able to be introduced intraocularly through correspondingly small scleral openings and be longer than those used in the anterior segment to manipulate the posterior pole. Scissors and forceps for vitrectomy are therefore generally tube-guided (Fig. 5.20). Since a detailed treatment of these operations is not the concern of an introduction for beginners in ophthalmic surgery, reference is made here to the book "Vitreoretinal Surgery: Strategies and Tactics" by F. Kuhn.

5.5.1 Holding Instruments

Examples of blunt instruments:

- Needle holder
- Razor blade holder
- Artery clamps
- Towel clamps
- Dieffenbach clamps
- Position hooks
- Fixation rings

Needle holders (Figs. 5.21 and 5.22) are mainly used in eyelid and strabismus surgery. In addition to the various sizes, one can choose between straight and curved designs for the

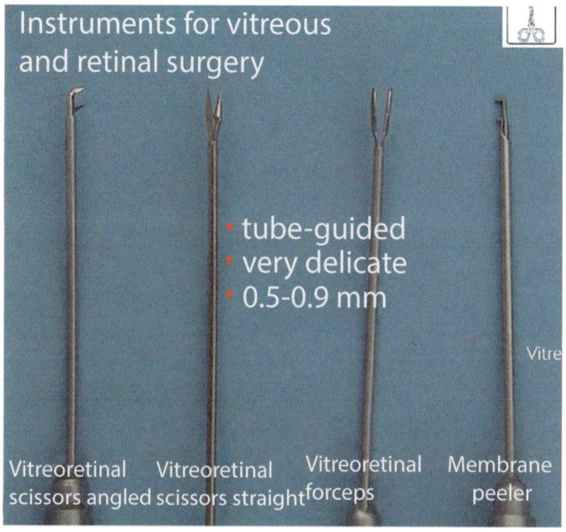

Fig. 5.20 Examples of instruments frequently used in vitreous/retinal surgery

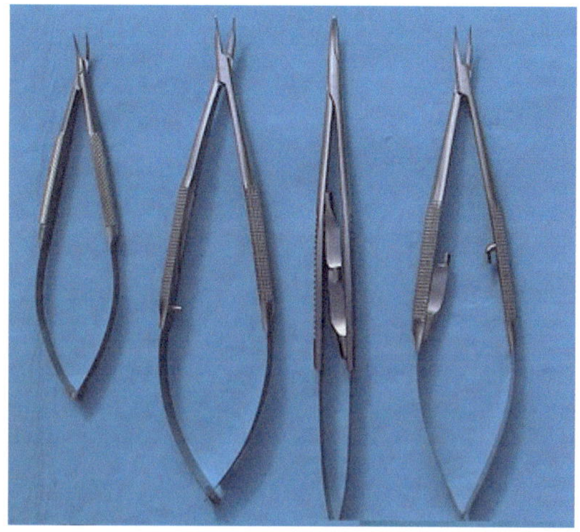

Fig. 5.21 Needle holders of various sizes, with and without lock

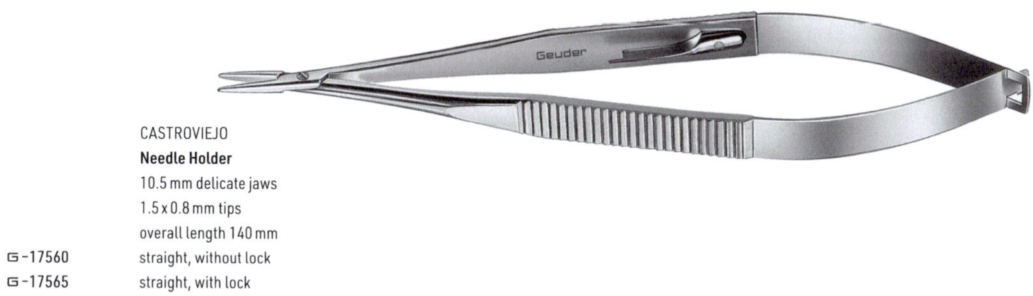

Fig. 5.22 Needle holder according to Castroviejo, fine jaw, with lock (image courtesy of Geuder AG)

jaw geometry. In ophthalmology, needle holders with a spring mechanism are generally used, optionally with or without a lock. When sewing with very fine threads, needle holders without a lock and with a curved tip have proven effective (Chap. 10).

5.5.2 Spreading Instruments

Examples of spreading instruments:

- Eyelid speculums
- Eyelid retractors
- Wound spreaders
- Wound hooks

Eyelid speculums (Figs. 5.23, 5.24, 5.25 and 5.26) are available in different sizes for use in infants, young children, and adults. The valves are fenestrated or closed and are manufactured in various shapes. In addition to the eyelid speculums with a simple spring mechanism, there are also adjustable ones that are either self-retaining or can be fixed with a locking screw. To remove excess fluid from the surgical area, eyelid specula with integrated suction can be used if necessary.

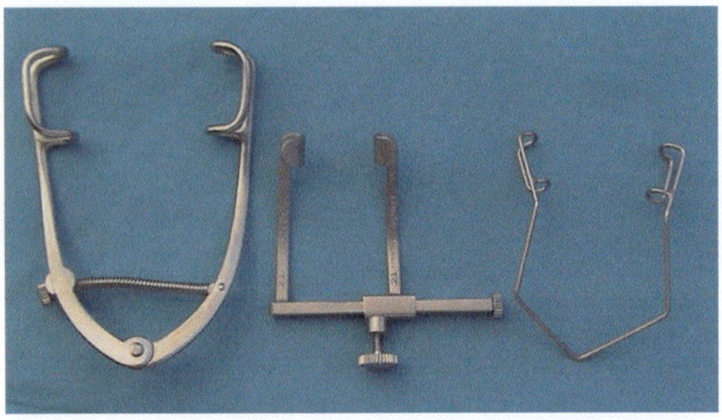

Fig. 5.23 Selection of commonly used models: Eyelid speculum according to Weiss (adjustable, with locking screw, open valves), Eyelid speculum according to Cook (adjustable, with locking screw, closed valves), Eyelid speculum according to Barraquer (fenestrated)

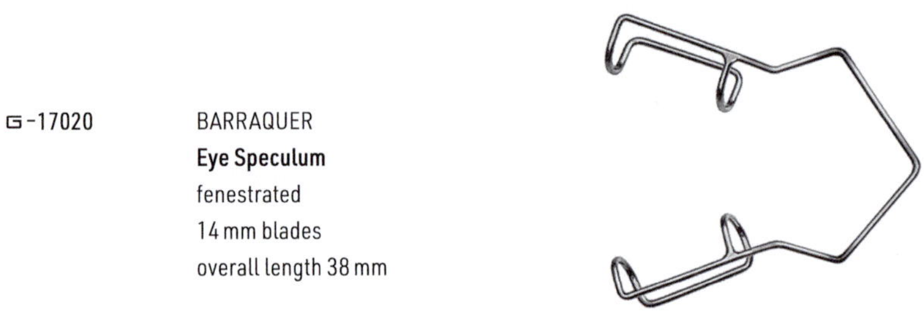
G-17020
BARRAQUER
Eye Speculum
fenestrated
14 mm blades
overall length 38 mm

Fig. 5.24 Eyelid speculum according to Barraquer (fenestrated) (image courtesy of Geuder AG)

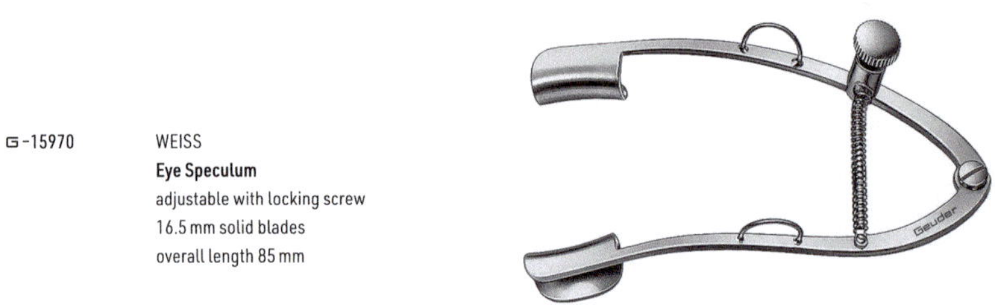

Fig. 5.25 Eyelid speculum according to Weiss (adjustable, with locking screw, closed valves) (image courtesy of Geuder AG)

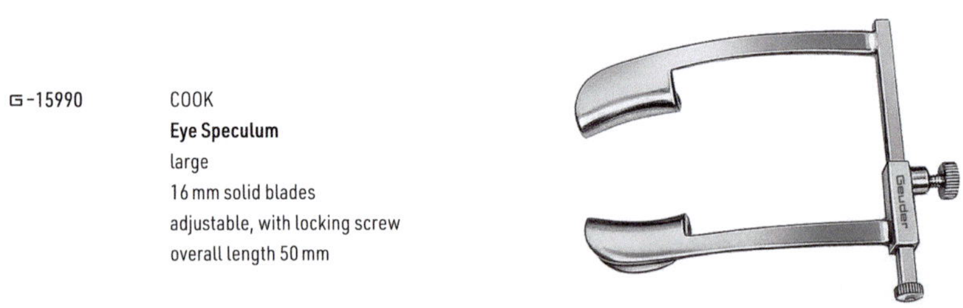

Fig. 5.26 Eyelid speculum according to Cook (adjustable, with locking screw, closed valves) (image courtesy of Geuder AG)

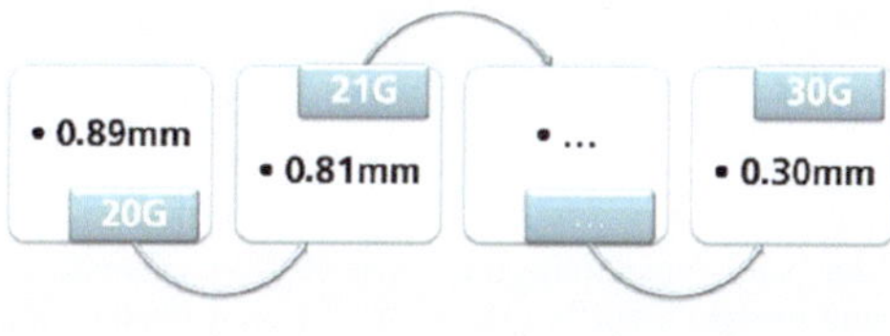

Fig. 5.27 The specification of the cannula tube's gauge is given in Gauge

5.5.3 Suction and Irrigation Instruments

Examples of suction and irrigation instruments:

- Irrigation cannulas for tear ducts
- Suction-irrigation handpieces

The specification of the cannula tube's gauge is given in "G" (Gauge). The higher the gauge value, the smaller the outer diameter of the cannula. The corresponding outer diameters of the cannulas in millimeters and the color coding are standardized in EN ISO 6009 and EN ISO 9626 (Fig. 5.27).

5.5.4 Measuring and Marking Instruments

Examples of instruments for measuring and marking:

- Compasses
- Measuring spatulas
- Rulers
- Measuring rings
- Depth gauges
- Keratometers
- Markers as positioning and suturing aids for the cornea

5.5.5 Sterilization Containers

The assembly of surgical instruments is done according to the individual preferences of the surgeon. If different procedures are performed, it is advisable to acquire various surgical trays (e.g., cataract tray, lid tray, glaucoma tray, etc.).

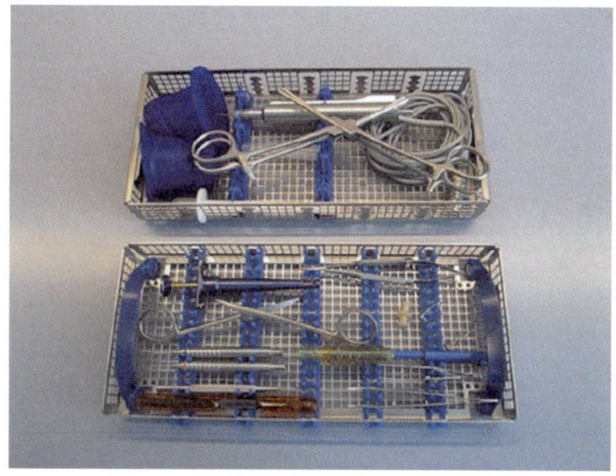

Fig. 5.28 Instruments on a surgical tray for cataract operations

The instruments are then stored in appropriately labeled, sterilizable containers, where they are fixed by silicone nubs, stored, and sterilized in one or more sieve trays (Chap. 1).

For a smooth and safe operation process, the instruments should always be stored on the trays in the same manner. Especially in larger surgical facilities, photographic documentation is useful as a guideline for uniform procedures and for training personnel (Fig. 5.28).

References and Further Reading

1. Blaskovics-Kettesy (1970) Eingriffe am Auge, Ferdinand. Enke, Stuttgart
2. DIN-Taschenbuch 100/1, Medizinische Instrumente 1, Grundnormen, Schneidende Intrumente, HNO-Instrumente und Wiederaufbereitung, 5th edn. Beuth
3. Kaboth B (1943) Lehrbuch der Instrumentenkunde für die Operationspraxis. Walter de DeGruyter &Co, Berlin
4. Kuhn F (2016) Vitreoretinal surgery: strategies and tactics. Springer, Berlin
5. Medizinprodukte-EU-Anpassungsgesetz – MPEUAnpG. https://www.bundesgesundheitsministerium.de/fileadmin/Dateien/3_Downloads/Gesetze_und_Verordnungen/GuV/M/Anpassung_des_Medizinprodukterechts.pdf
6. Neue EU-Verordnungen. https://www.bundesgesundheitsministerium.de/themen/gesundheitswesen/medizinprodukte/neue-eu-verordnungen.html

7. Normgerechte Darstellung der CE-Kennzeichnung. https://upload.wikimedia.org/wikipedia/commons/thumb/f/ff/CE_with_grid.svg/440px-CE_with_grid.svg.png
8. Osterloh F (2024) drohen Engpässe. Dtsch Ärztblatt 118(22):1094–1095, 4.Juni 2021
9. Verordnung (EU) 2020/561 des europäischen Parlaments und des Rates vom 23. April 2020 zur Änderung der Verordnung (EU) 2017/745 über Medizinprodukte hinsichtlich des Geltungsbeginns einiger ihrer Bestimmungen: https://eur-lex.europa.eu/legal-content/DE/TXT/PDF/?uri=CELEX:32020R0561&from=EN%20_blank. Zugriffsdatum Mai 2021
10. Was sind Medizinprodukte? https://www.bundesgesundheitsministerium.de/themen/gesundheitswesen/medizinprodukte/definition-und-wirtschaftliche-bedeutung.html

Suture Material

6

Erik Chankiewitz and Martin Knorrn

Contents

Healing requires contact! Traumatic or surgically created interfaces should come into contact with each other using suitable suture material, because only then will a "restitutio ad integrum" – a complete healingresult. The healing of wounds is a highly complex cascade in the interplay of cell biological mechanisms such as inflammatory reactions, debridement, cell migration, and fibroblast activity. A wound is considered healed when it withstands all natural mechanical stresses and no inflammation is present. In the eye, a satisfactory result is always associated with the physical-optical, mechanical, or biological function. For example, a single corneal suture can completely seal a corneal incision and bring about healing, but make vision imperfect due to suture-induced astigmatism. A poorly treated eyelid wound can lead to an ectropion and have serious effects on the corneal surface, up to blindness. The correct choice of suture material, as well as the proper handling of it, is particularly important for the treatment of wounds on the eye.

E. Chankiewitz (✉)
Augenklinik, Städtisches Klinikum Braunschweig gGmbH, Braunschweig, Germany
e-mail: erik@chankiewitz.de

M. Knorrn
Augenzentrum am Johannisplatz, Leipzig, Germany

6.1 Suture

The surgical suture material to be used must meet high-quality standards to ensure controlled healing. Nowadays, suture material is used exclusively as a strictly certified medical product.

Depending on the area of application and task, the suture material must temporarily or permanently take over the mechanical bridging function to replace the lost tissue integrity. This determines the choice of the right suture and requires knowledge of its physical and biological properties. Sutures made from organic materials have been largely replaced by synthetic ones.

In ophthalmic surgery, sutures made of polyglactin, polydioxanone, polypropylene, polyester, and polyamide are predominantly used. Silk, as a material of organic origin, is still used. Steel wire is mentioned here only for completeness and is no longer really used in the eye.

F. Wilhelm (ed.), *Ophthalmic Surgery for Beginners*, https://doi.org/10.1007/978-3-662-70287-1_6

Properties such as sterilizability, compatibility, high tensile strength, secure knot stability, good knot run, good tissue glide, and the smallest possible capillarity are prerequisites for use in surgery. Additionally, good visibility when handling under the microscope is a particular challenge in ophthalmology.

The properties of the suture can also be influenced by the type of processing. Thus, the suture structure can be fundamentally distinguished as monofilament and polyfilament.

A monofilament suture, consisting of only one filament, is characterized by a smooth surface with low capillarity, without a sawing effect, with good tissue passage, good knot glide properties, but poorer knotting ability and easier tissue passage (Fig. 6.1). A disadvantage is often the stiffness in handling and the poor knotting ability, which requires some practice and experience for secure knot placement. Examples of available and often used monofilament sutures are made from materials such as polyamide, polypropylene, and PVDF (polyvinylidene fluoride).

A polyfilament—or also referred to as "multifilament"—suture consists of a braided suture structure, similar to a rope (Fig. 6.2). The filaments are intertwined, twisted, or both. This results in very high tensile strength, optimal flexibility, and secure knot stability, while tissue passage is more traumatic due to the surface texture compared to the monofilament suture. Typical examples of polyfilament sutures are those made from silk and polyglycolic acid.

Another classification of suture material describes the absorption property. A fundamental distinction is made between absorbable and non-absorbable. A material is considered absorbable if it can be completely broken down. The absorbable thread gradually loses its tensile strength in the process. The **absorption time** is, by definition, the time in which the thread loses 50% of its knot tensile strength and should not be confused with complete material breakdown. The breakdown occurs enzymatically in animal materials into protein chains and amino acids or hydrolytically in synthetic materials into lactic acid (lactate), glycolic acid (glycolate), water, and carbon dioxide. Non-absorbable materials remain almost unchanged in the tissue. Depending on the material properties, they are incorporated into the scar tissue and remain or must be removed after sufficient wound adaptation. For example, suture removal in the eyelid area can occur after five to ten days. Even longer-lasting non-absorbable threads can undergo changes due to degradation by light and fluid, but complete breakdown does not occur.

A suture function exists only as long as the tensile strength is present. Therefore, "a loose thread is without function and should always be removed or replaced." In the same proportion as the tensile strength decreases, the strength of the wound should increase.

The **half-life** of an absorbable thread is understood to be the time in which the tensile strength has decreased to half of the original tensile strength.

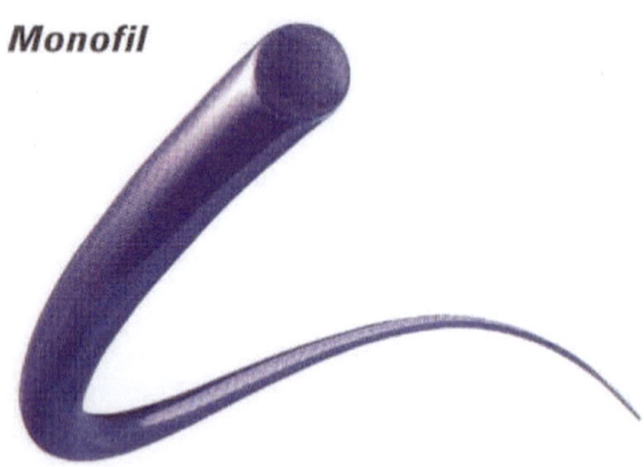

Fig. 6.1 Monofilament suture

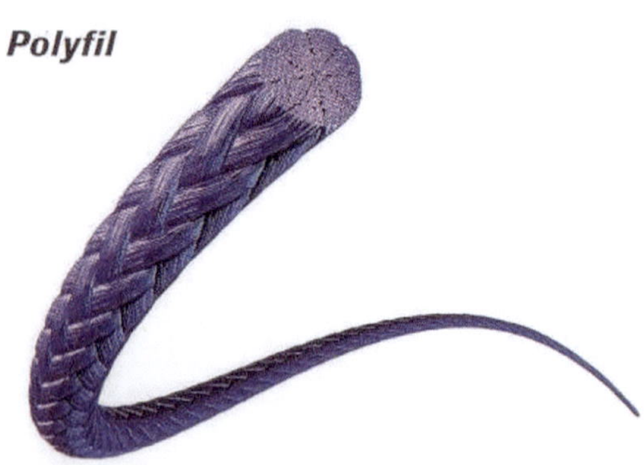

Fig. 6.2 Braided polyfilament suture

Table 6.1 Comparison of the different specifications for the thread thickness of the suture material

USP	PH.Eur. metric	mm range
11–0	0.1	0.010–0.019
10–0	0.2	0.020–0.029
9–0	0.3	0.030–0.039
8–0	0.4	0.040–0.049
7–0	0.5	0.050–0.059
6–0	0.7	0.070–0.079
5–0	1	0.100–0.149
4–0	1.5	0.150–0.199
3–0	2	0.200–0.249
2–0	2.5	0.250–0.299
1–0	3	0.300–0.349
0	3.5	0.350–0.399
1	4	0.400–0.499
2	5	0.500–0.599
3+4	6	0.600–0.699
5	7	0.700–0.799
6	8	0.800 0.899
7	9	0.900–0.999
8	10	1.000–1.099

The suture thickness (see Table 6.1) is defined by the American and European compendiums of standards for the quality of pharmaceuticals, medical devices, and individual medical products. While the American designation is largely used in everyday surgical practice (USP: United States Pharmacopeia), the underlying metric specification forms the basis of the European designation (Ph.Eur.: European Pharmacopeia). The following table lists the two designations for suture thickness with the corresponding millimeter specifications.

6.2 Needle

In modern ophthalmic surgery, only atraumatic needles, i.e., needles that are firmly connected to the thread at the end in a sleeve (thus armed), are used. There are threads with one needle (single-armed) or with two needles (double-armed).

The most important requirements for surgical needles are absolute rust resistance, high bending strength, high fracture strength, good piercing and cutting ability, optimal penetration, and secure fit in the needle holder.

In addition to the mentioned properties of the material, there are form-specific features for the needle cross-section, arc length, and needle curvature, as well as the needle tip, depending on the area of application.

Most commonly, needles are used in 5/8, 1/2, 3/8, and 1/4 circles (Fig. 6.3). The choice of length is determined by the spatial possibilities, the tissue load, and to some extent the preferences of the surgeon.

The following will discuss the more commonly used needles.

The **cutting needle** (Fig. 6.4a) has a distinctly sharp tip with long cutting edges that are perpendicular to the direction of insertion. After the long round body follows a secure shaft for holding the needle. Very firm tissue, such as the epidermis, can be sutured with minimal trauma.

The **cutting needle with micro tip** (Fig. 6.4b) has a shorter, sharp tip that is flat to the direction of insertion. Firm and loose tissue, such as eyelid skin or conjunctiva, can be sutured with maximum tissue preservation.

The pointed **round-bodied needle**(Fig. 6.4c) has a round tip and thus no cutting edge. The puncture is microscopically always a crater-like tear. It is suitable for loose tissue of all types.

The **spatula needle** (Fig. 6.4d) is a small needle and has a sharp tip with a long cutting edge. The puncture is atraumatic, i.e., without tearing the tissue, and allows for secure and precise guidance without high penetration pressure. It is suitable for firmer tissue in the eye, such as the cornea and sclera.

The **blunt round-bodied needle** (Fig. 6.4e) has no tip. A puncture is not possible (or very traumatic) and is only suitable for looping eye muscles or vascular ligatures, for example, in temporal artery biopsy.

The **straight needle** (Fig. 6.4f) is thin and without curvature. It has a slightly rounded tip. The puncture is traumatic. Its application in the eye involves guiding the long needle across the entire width of the anterior chamber to adapt iris tissue or to suture secondary intraocular lenses.

The so-called **skin needle** (Fig. 6.4g) is a long, thin needle with a slight bend at the end and a slightly rounded tip. The puncture is traumatic. Its application in the eye also involves

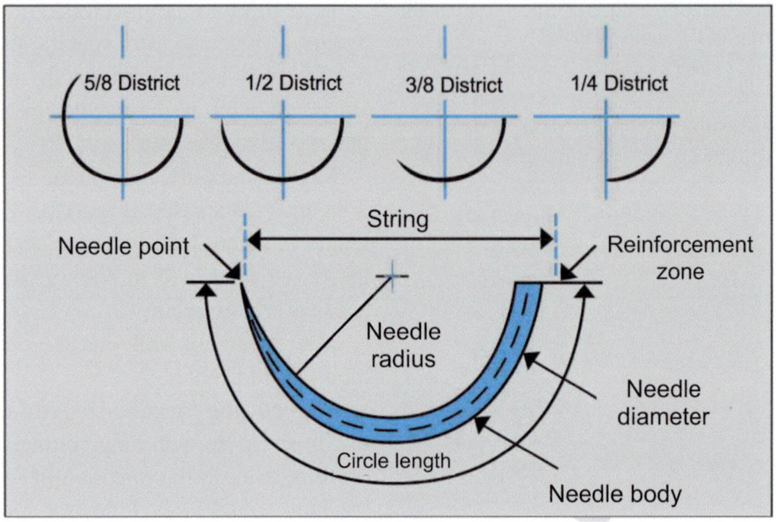

Fig. 6.3 Circle length and needle structure

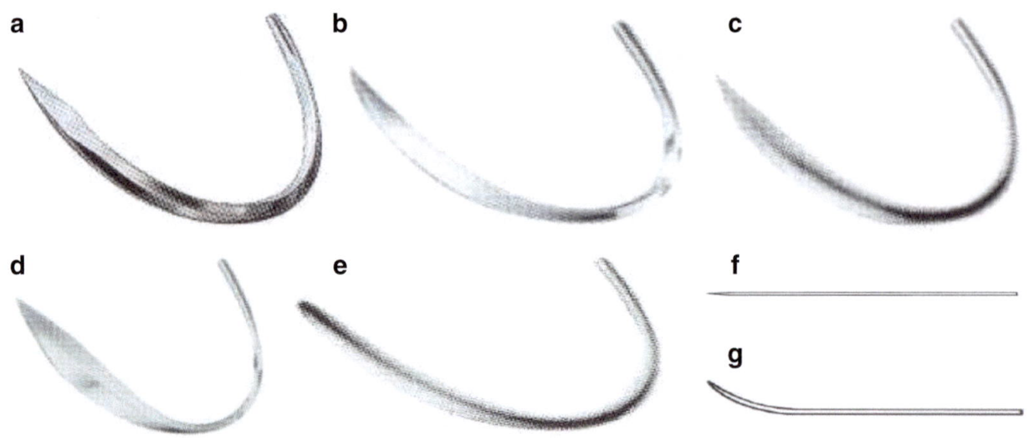

Fig. 6.4 (**a**–**g**) (**a**) Cutting needle. (**b**) Cutting needle with micro tip. (**c**) Round-bodied needle. (**d**) Spatula needle. (**e**) Blunt round-bodied needle. (**f**) Straight needle. (**g**) Skin needle

guiding the needle through the anterior chamber when suturing iris tissue or secondary lenses.

6.3 Packaging and Coding

Safe and quick handling in the operating room is an important prerequisite for a complication-free, successful procedure. Based on the color coding, the suture material can be immediately identified. The other properties mentioned above are clearly marked on the packaging (Fig. 6.5).

The following table (Table 6.2) is intended to provide a recommendation for selecting the appropriate suture material for each procedure.

▶ The given recommendations can only serve as a guideline for choosing the appropriate suture material. Ultimately, the decision is made based on the individual experiences of the surgeon and the specific conditions in the surgical area.

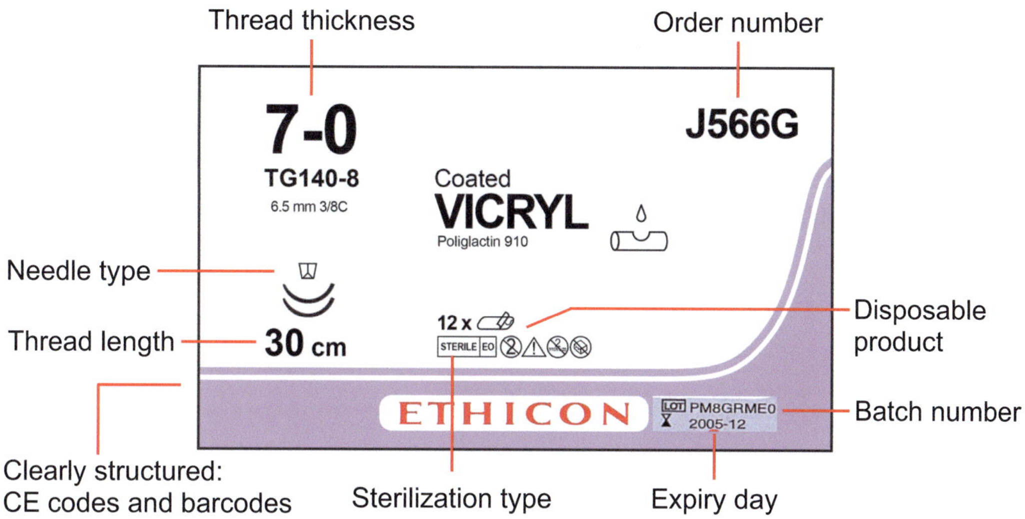

Fig. 6.5 Packaging labels using the example of an original package from the company Ethicon

Table 6.2 Recommendations for the selection of suture material

Anterior Segment	Indication	Material	Strength
	Conjunctiva	Polyglactin	7/0–8/0
	Glaucoma	Polyglactin	10/0
		Polyamide	10/0
	Cornea	Polyamide	10/0
	Iris Suture	Polypropylene	10/0
	IOL Lens Fixation	Polypropylene	10/0
Strabismus		Polyglactin	6/0
Eyelid and Plastic Surgery	Blepharoplasty	Polypropylene	7/0
		Polyglactin	6/0–7/0
	Chalazion	Polyglactin	6/0–7/0
	Levator Resection/ -Folding	Polypropylene	7/0
Retinal Detachment Surgery	Scleral Buckling and Cerclage Suturing	Suturamid	4/0

7 Preparations as a Surgeon

Frank Wilhelm, Karlheinz Hannig, Martin Knorrn, Gerd U. Auffarth and Hyeck-Soo Son

Contents

7.1 Introduction

The previous chapters served to summarize the basic knowledge for starting in eye surgery. In this chapter, possibilities will be presented on how the aspiring ophthalmic surgeon can prepare as practically as possible for the first procedure.

First and foremost, the study of specialized literature is required, for which the present book, with the literature references in the individual sections, provides additional hints. F. Kuhn recommends in his "To-Do" list for aspiring retinal-vitreous surgeons to read the most important books on this topic in preparation for surgical activity, with the mentor necessarily assisting in the selection.

Participation in surgical courses and conferences also offers the opportunity to obtain targeted information. In addition to discussing the specialist lectures with the speakers, direct collegial exchange can take place. It also makes sense for beginners to gather additional information about products used in surgery at the industry exhibition and to receive well-founded advice from the company representatives in personal conversations.

In recent years, video training has proven effective, enabling the novice in surgery to learn and analyze the course of a procedure in detail. This is possible on the occasion of corresponding events, but can also take place in a small group in the clinic or individually in the home office. In this context, surgical videos from one's own institution can be used, as well as those downloaded from relevant portals on the internet (Fig. 7.1).

F. Wilhelm (✉)
Universitätsklinikum Halle Saale, Greifswald, Germany

K. Hannig
MTS-the wetlab company GmbH, Mötz, Austria
e-mail: karlheinz@mts-wetlab.com

M. Knorrn
Augenzentrum am Johannisplatz, Leipzig, Germany

G. U. Auffarth · H.-S. Son
Augenklinik, Universitätsklinikum Heidelberg, Heidelberg, Germany
e-mail: gerd.auffarth@med.uni-heidelberg.de

F. Wilhelm (ed.), *Ophthalmic Surgery for Beginners*, https://doi.org/10.1007/978-3-662-70287-1_7

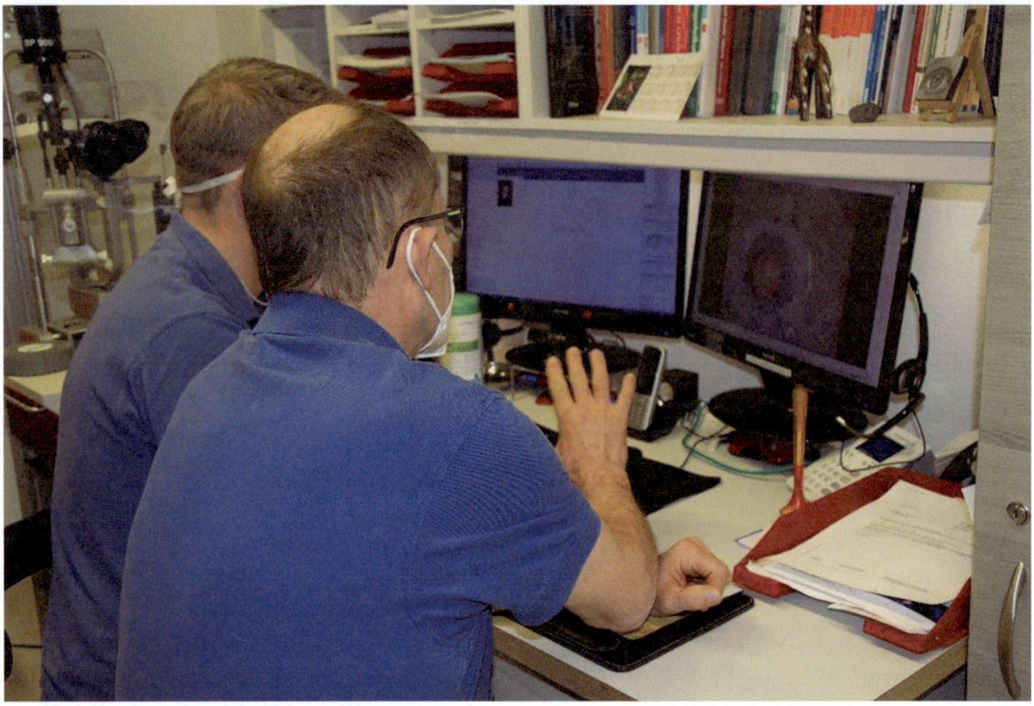

Fig. 7.1 Using video sequences from the operating room of the training institution, both the preparation for the planned procedure and the postoperative analysis can be carried out in great detail

The analysis of one's own surgical activity is particularly valuable. Every surgeon should take advantage of this opportunity to question and optimize their surgical approach. For beginners, it makes sense to discuss performed procedures subsequently in this way together with the mentor.

In 1970, D. Vörösmarthy wrote verbatim in the introduction to the fourth edition of Blascovics' surgical teaching:

> If a maneuver does not succeed immediately for the young colleague, he should practice it, for which operating on a cadaver offers the best conditions. [1]

Implementing this advice is impossible today, not least for ethical reasons—its validity, however, is not lost. Therefore, possible alternatives are presented in this chapter.

In practical work in the wet lab and on the surgical simulator, the surgical procedure itself can be practiced. This allows for gaining a feel for microsurgical work and orientation under the microscope.

7.2 Practice in the Wet Lab

Karlheinz Hannig, Frank Wilhelm and Martin Knorrn

The importance of training in a wet lab ("wet laboratory") in the training of ophthalmic surgeons has increased in recent years [2]. This is reflected in the structure of this book by placing it immediately before the start of surgical activity on patients.

Even surgically experienced course participants who want to further develop their surgical skills often repeatedly take advantage of this opportunity for "life-like surgery" practice. The focus in the wet lab is most often on learning and practicing cataract surgery. In addition to treating eye injuries, operations on the posterior segment of the eye [3] or new techniques of corneal transplantation and refractive surgery procedures are increasingly the subject of such courses. The modern wet lab also prepares for successful operations on the human eye, such as lens implantations and glaucoma implants, which come closest to the reality in the operating room. A special emphasis is placed on the undisturbed practice (Fig. 7.2) under the microscope, where the operator does not look directly at the surgical field, to train the hand eye ("oculodogital") coordination.

The need to train surgical techniques in a practical manner exists among ophthalmologists worldwide [4, 5] (Fig. 7.3). In clinics, outdated surgical microscopes, instruments, and phaco machines are provided to assistants for this purpose (Fig. 7.4). Then, attempts are made to improvise more or less successfully, which can be an option. However, often only compromise solutions result, which generally significantly limit the effect of practicing in the wet lab.

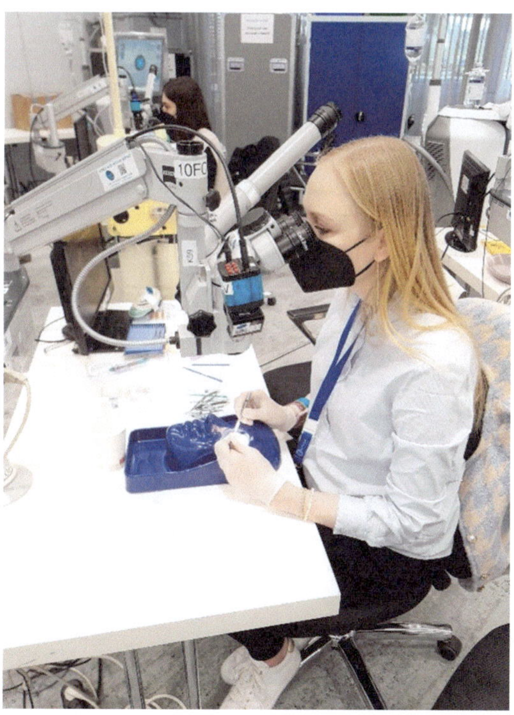

Fig. 7.2 Undisturbed practice

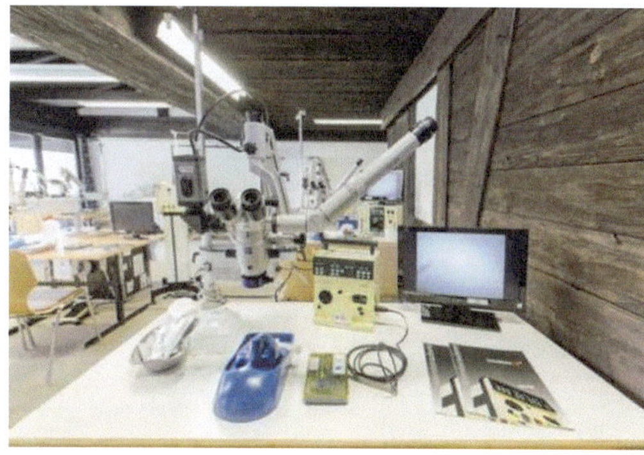

Fig. 7.3 Training surgical techniques in a practical manner

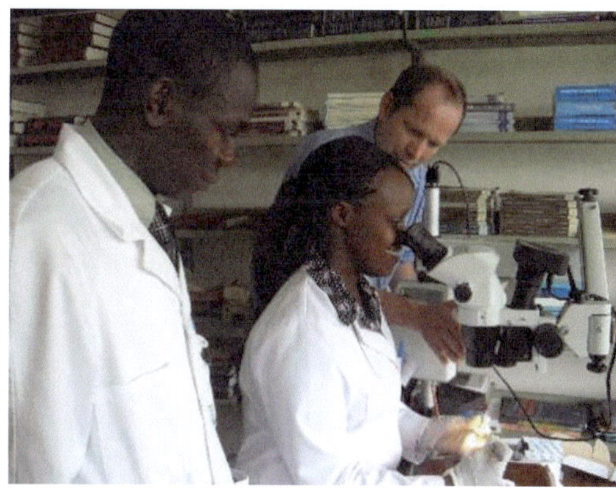

Fig. 7.4 Practical training

The purpose of wet labs is to learn, practice, and deepen individual surgical steps. In doing so, important skills for the safe execution of ophthalmic surgery should be developed and improved during training [6]. With professionally equipped wet labs, didactically experienced course instructors, and the right eye models, the craft of microsurgical operating can be automated to a certain extent, and learning curves can be drastically shortened (Figs. 7.5 and 7.6).

The psychological component during the first surgeries still represents a significant hurdle for beginners, the weight of which can be reduced through particularly realistic training in the wet lab.

Before registering to participate in an organized wet lab, it is highly recommended to familiarize oneself with the "basics."

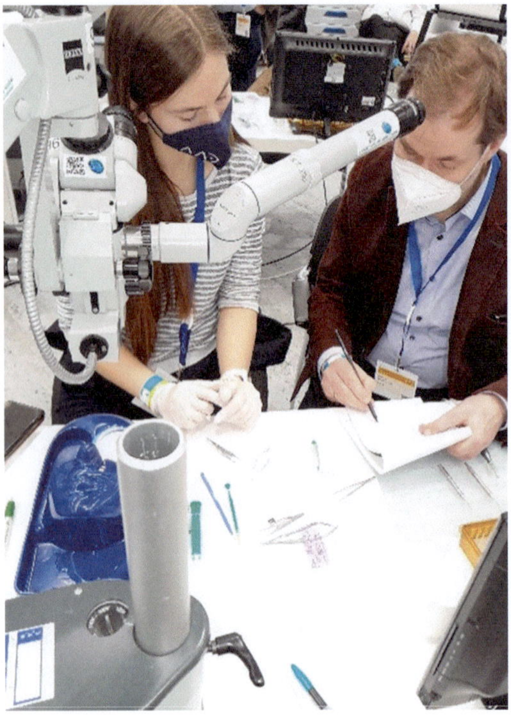

Fig. 7.5 Microsurgical operating

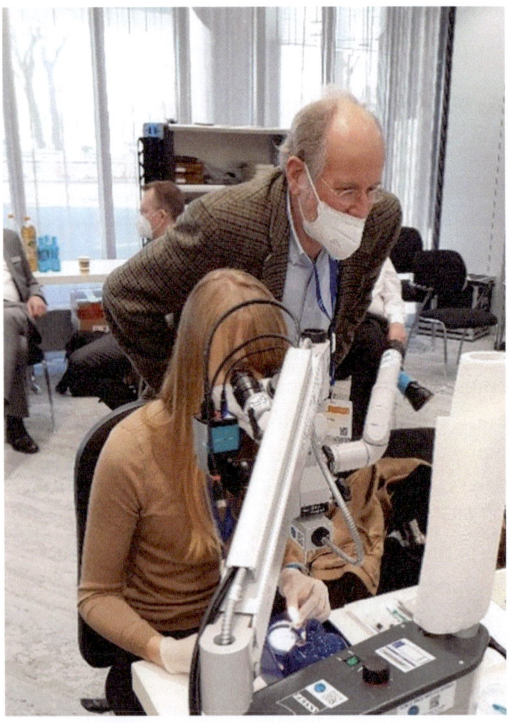

Fig. 7.6 Microsurgical operating

For preparation, Chaps. 1 to 5 as well as 11 and 12 of this book can be used. Since organizing these courses requires a lot of effort, it is frustrating for all involved when valuable practice time is wasted explaining, for example, the handling of suture material or discussing the names and use of individual instruments.

The prerequisites for the successful execution of wet lab training are summarized as follows:

Regarding the spatial conditions for training under surgical-like situations, it is important to ensure that there is sufficient space for each aspiring surgeon as well as for the extensive equipment, while also ensuring that communication with the tutor can be maintained over short distances (Fig. 7.7). Under extreme conditions (e.g., when distance rules must be observed during the coronavirus pandemic), this presents a particular challenge!

The devices used in the wet lab primarily include the **surgical microscope and the phaco/vitrectomy machine** (Fig. 7.8, Chap. 4). In this situation, competent supervision and instruction by trained personnel (from the organizer or present company representatives) are particularly important, so that the beginner can familiarize themselves with the given parameters and find their individual settings. To ensure uninterrupted practice, regular maintenance of this equipment is carried out for professional courses.

Especially for colleagues who want to practice various procedures for the first time, it is

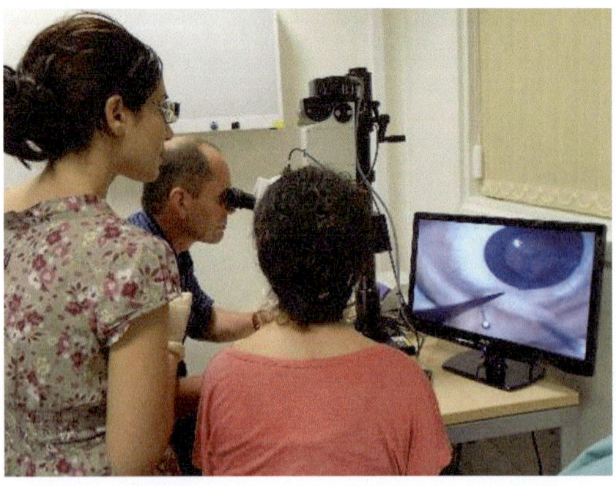

Fig. 7.7 Communication with the tutor

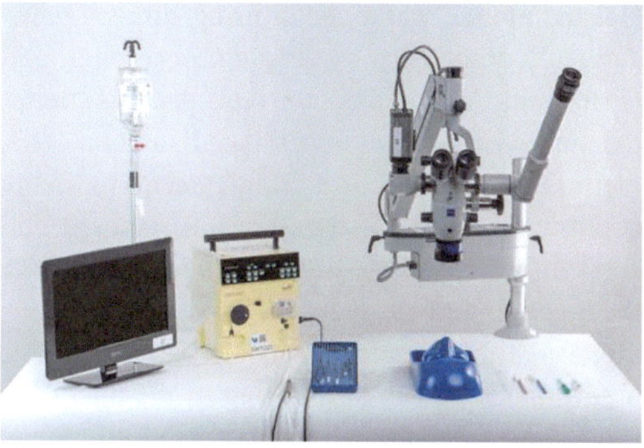

Fig. 7.8 Surgical microscope and the phaco/vitrectomy machine

important to work with suitable instruments that are of good quality (Fig. 7.9). Due to the high sensitivity of these costly **microinstruments**, this is often only possible to a limited extent in individually equipped wet labs.

- The use of various **consumables** is indispensable for practical training under laboratory conditions. For this purpose, for example, remnants of viscoelastics or already used disposable knives from the ongoing surgical program are used. For hygienic reasons and to have sufficient material available, unsterile samples from manufacturers are usually used in professionally organized courses.
- Since human donor eyes are not an option for wet labs for ethical reasons, the pig eye has proven itself as a **practice object** due to its similarity to the human eyeball and its good availability.

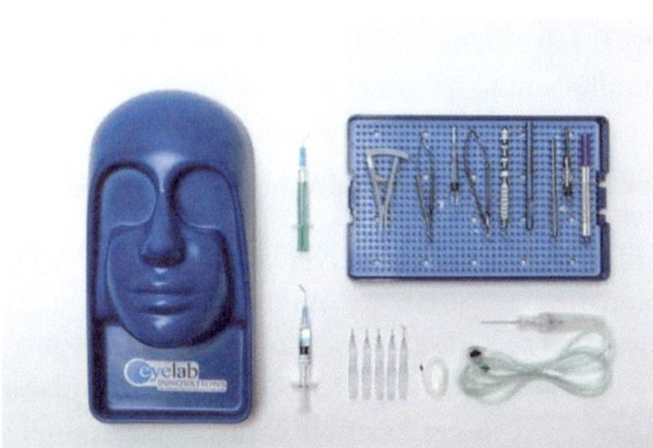

Fig. 7.9 Microinstruments

- The provision of well-preserved pig eyes with clear corneas for practice purposes is laborious, requiring experience and care. Freshly enucleated and, very importantly, not scalded! pig eyes are best suited.
- This also includes the fixation of the practice eyes with the appropriate equipment (Figs. 7.10 and 7.11).
- In various countries, it may be necessary (e.g., for religious reasons) to switch from the pig eye model to another species (sheep, goat, rabbit) [7, 8]. Despite the proven use of pig eyes, there are indeed limiting differences compared to the human eye. For example, the tissues of the eyeball wall are significantly tougher than in humans. The cornea of the pig not only has a much larger diameter, but it also lacks a Bowman's membrane [9, 10] and, like the sclera, is considerably thicker. A cataract, which would be desirable for practice purposes, is generally not found in the pig eye. This can be simulated by treating the eyes in a microwave. Increasingly, artificial eyes are being used in practice courses [11].
- Ensuring safety and hygiene is a fundamental requirement for a wet lab. To protect students and instructors as well as staff and representatives, sufficient surgical gloves, disinfectant

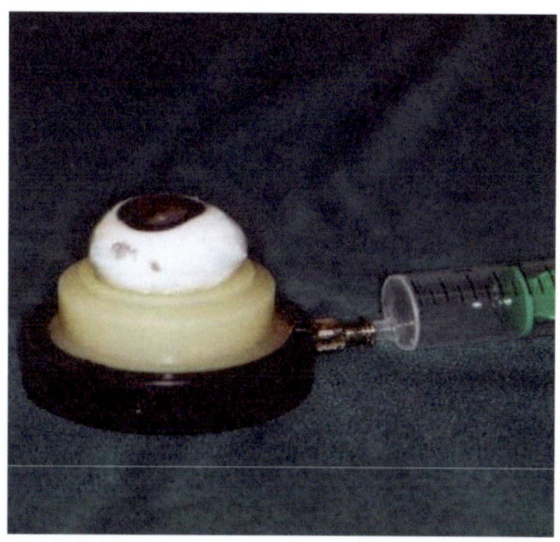

Fig. 7.10 Fixation

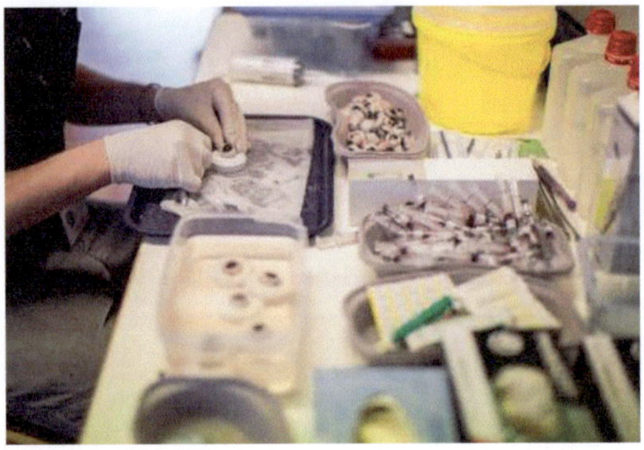

Fig. 7.11 Fixation of the practice eyes

solution, and protective gowns, if necessary, must be available.

- A prerequisite for imparting important knowledge to the aspiring ophthalmic surgeon is guidance by **tutors** during the course. Not every good surgeon is experienced in training in the wet lab and may also not be able to convey their clinical knowledge and skills to beginners. For this reason, it can be particularly useful for beginners to be guided through the first steps within the framework of a professionally organized course. Guidance by colleagues who have experience in wet lab training is usually particularly appreciated [4].

This list of mandatory prerequisites demonstrates the requirements placed on wet lab training, which can usually only be met with significant limitations in an individually designed lab.

At the end of an established course with a wet lab, participants particularly emphasize the value of exchanging ideas with colleagues at a comparable training level during the course.

7.3 Surgical Simulator

Gerd U. Auffarth and Hyeck-Soo Son

7.3.1 Introduction

Historically, surgical training in ophthalmology has been primarily based on the traditional Halsted model, where the aspiring surgeon gains surgical competence by reading, observing, and performing operations on real patients under the supervision of an experienced surgeon. This method of training is still prevalent in many countries; however, it is often unstructured and carries the risks of a high complication rate at the beginning of the learning curve for the aspiring surgeon. Concerns about patient safety, high financial costs of teaching in the operating room, and the demand for increased efficiency were the main factors driving the development of alternative training methods.

7.3.2 Virtual Simulation

Virtual reality can be broadly defined as the use of computer methods to immerse users in a multimedia environment that simulates reality. By combining human-computer interfaces, the user can immerse themselves in an artificial environment and interact with it.

The concept of virtual simulation was born in 1929 when Edward Link developed a mechanical flight simulator, known as the "Blue Box," to reduce the frequency of catastrophic flight accidents. Since then flight simulation has dramatically improved the quality of flight training and has become an indispensable part of pilot training.

In medicine, the first surgical simulator with a model for operations on the lower extremities was developed in 1990. Just three years later, the first simulator for eye surgery was introduced [12]. Today, almost all surgical specialties, including general surgery, neurosurgery, and ENT, have adopted virtual reality training as a supplement to the basic training curriculum.

A surgical simulator offers a controlled, reproducible environment for surgeons to practice in. It is available at any time, and the significant time and effort typically associated with preparing a wet lab are eliminated by the on/off switch. The virtual simulation of a surgical procedure is harmless to the patient and promises, when used in conjunction with current training methods, to reduce complication rates through an improved training experience.

7.3.3 EyeSi®-Surgical-Simulator

In ophthalmology, the EyeSi®-Surgical (VRmagic GmbH, Mannheim, Germany) is currently the most widely used simulator for surgical training, and numerous studies have already investigated and demonstrated its construct validity and effectiveness [13–18]. The simulator consists of a computer system that connects a model head with a virtual eye, two foot pedals (for controlling the microscope and phaco machine), and an operating microscope that provides a three-dimensional stereoscopic image (Fig. 7.12).

Through the simulator's microscope, trainees see the virtual surgical field in stereo and high resolution while operating with lifelike surgical instruments. The handheld probes, ranging from forceps, cystotome, scissors to the phaco handpiece, simulate virtual instruments when inserted into the virtual eye. An integrated sensor system is capable of providing quantitative and qualitative feedback on the position of the surgical instruments. The focus and zoom can be adjusted via the microscope's foot pedal. The highly realistic simulation of real-time tissue interaction enhances the trainees' surgical experience without any risk to patients.

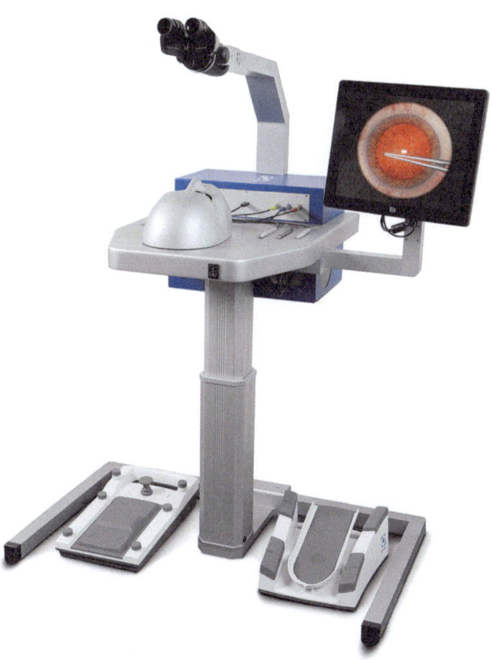

Fig. 7.12 The EyeSi®-Surgical simulator consists of a model head with a virtual eye, two foot pedals, and an operating microscope

The EyeSi Surgical features interfaces for cataract and vitreoretinal surgery as well as preinstalled course software. Starting with basic skills, the courses guide trainees step by step to mastering cataract and retinal surgery.

7.3.4 Cataract Surgery

Cataract surgery requires a good sense of stereopsis and spatial visualization, combined with excellent hand-eye coordination and the ability to use all four limbs simultaneously, as foot pedals are used to control the operating microscope or the ultrasound energy of the phaco handpiece.

The most common intraoperative complication of cataract surgery is posterior capsule rupture, which is widely regarded as a benchmark for assessing surgical quality. After a posterior capsule rupture, there is a significantly increased risk of retinal detachment and endophthalmitis, leading to vision loss. While certain ocular or systemic comorbidities may also be associated with an increased risk of capsule rupture, the surgeon's surgical skill and experience are among the most important risk factors for the occurrence of posterior capsule rupture.

The simulator's cataract course offers a variety of training modules to improve surgical skills and avoid such intraoperative complications. Initially, trainees must complete abstract simulation tasks such as anterior segment navigation, forceps, and anti-tremor training, which allow them to practice microsurgical motor skills, hand-eye coordination, and microscope handling, and help them understand the spatial boundaries within the anterior chamber (Fig. 7.13). After completing each training, the software provides a detailed performance summary that reflects the trainee's accuracy and efficiency. Various parameters related to instrument and microscope handling, surgical efficiency, and tissue treatment are recorded by the training system, allowing trainees to focus on their weaknesses and systematically improve their skills. Such standardized and objective skill assessment provides direct feedback to the trainee and helps them practice in a controlled and reproducible manner.

Since trainees must practice until they reach certain scores and only then are allowed to proceed to the next steps, the simulator also enables a uniform training experience.

The abstract modules are then followed by procedural training modules for cataract surgery, such as capsulorhexis, hydrodissection and hydrodelineation, phacoemulsification, irrigation/aspiration, and intraocular lens (IOL) insertion (Figs. 7.13 and 7.14). For advanced trainees, there is also the option to practice inserting a Malyugin ring or performing an anterior vitrectomy in simulated cases of a ruptured posterior capsule.

7.3.5 Capsulorhexis

In general, capsulorhexis is considered the most important step in cataract surgery. If an intact capsulorhexis is not achieved, the capsular bag is not only susceptible to tears during the operation, but there is also an increased risk of posterior capsule rupture and vitreous loss.

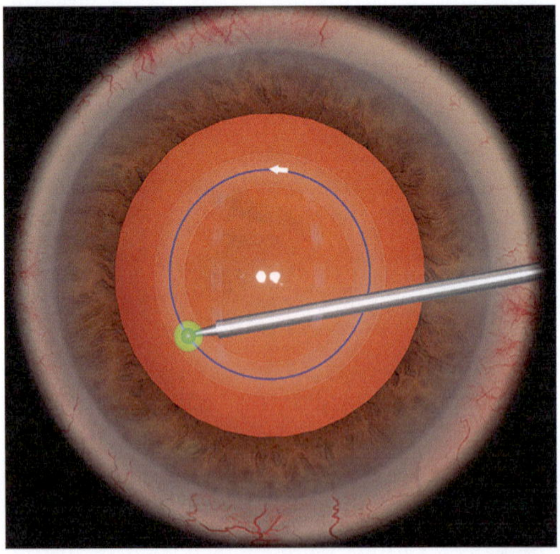

Fig. 7.13 The anti-tremor module allows one to practice microsurgical motor skills and hand-eye coordination

With the help of the simulator's capsulorhexis module, trainees can practice creating a round capsulorhexis (Fig. 7.14a). The trainee can choose whether to use a cystotome or forceps and adjust the setting so that, for example, a guiding circle with a diameter of 5 mm is displayed to visualize the optimal size.

The modules are presented with increasing complexity and difficulty: Once trainees have mastered the basic capsulorhexis modules, they are confronted with more challenging cases, such as eyes with highly tense capsules, capsule tears, anterior capsule plaques, or zonular dehiscence. The evaluation system for the capsulorhexis module is essentially based on the centering, roundness, and diameter of the rhexis, so that trainees can understand and learn what constitutes a good capsulorhexis.

McCannel and colleagues investigated the impact of intensive capsulorhexis training with the EyeSi® Surgical Simulator on the rates of faulty capsulorhexis in prospective residents and found that incorporating virtual reality simulation into surgical training led to a significant reduction in the rate of faulty capsulorhexis by 68% [19].

Similarly, Bisol and colleagues showed that training on the surgical simulator also effectively contributed to improving trainees' performance in creating capsulorhexis on high-tension capsules [20].

7.3.6 Phacoemulsification

The most demanding part of cataract surgery is the removal of the lens nucleus using phacoemulsification. Ultrasound energy must be used with caution: Although surgeons need it to emulsify and aspirate the lens nucleus, phaco energy can also damage delicate ocular structures such as the corneal endothelium. As ophthalmologists develop more advanced phaco skills, they must learn to minimize the amount of ultrasound energy introduced into the eye, as even small incorrect movements or the application of too much ultrasound energy or vacuum can lead to serious injuries.

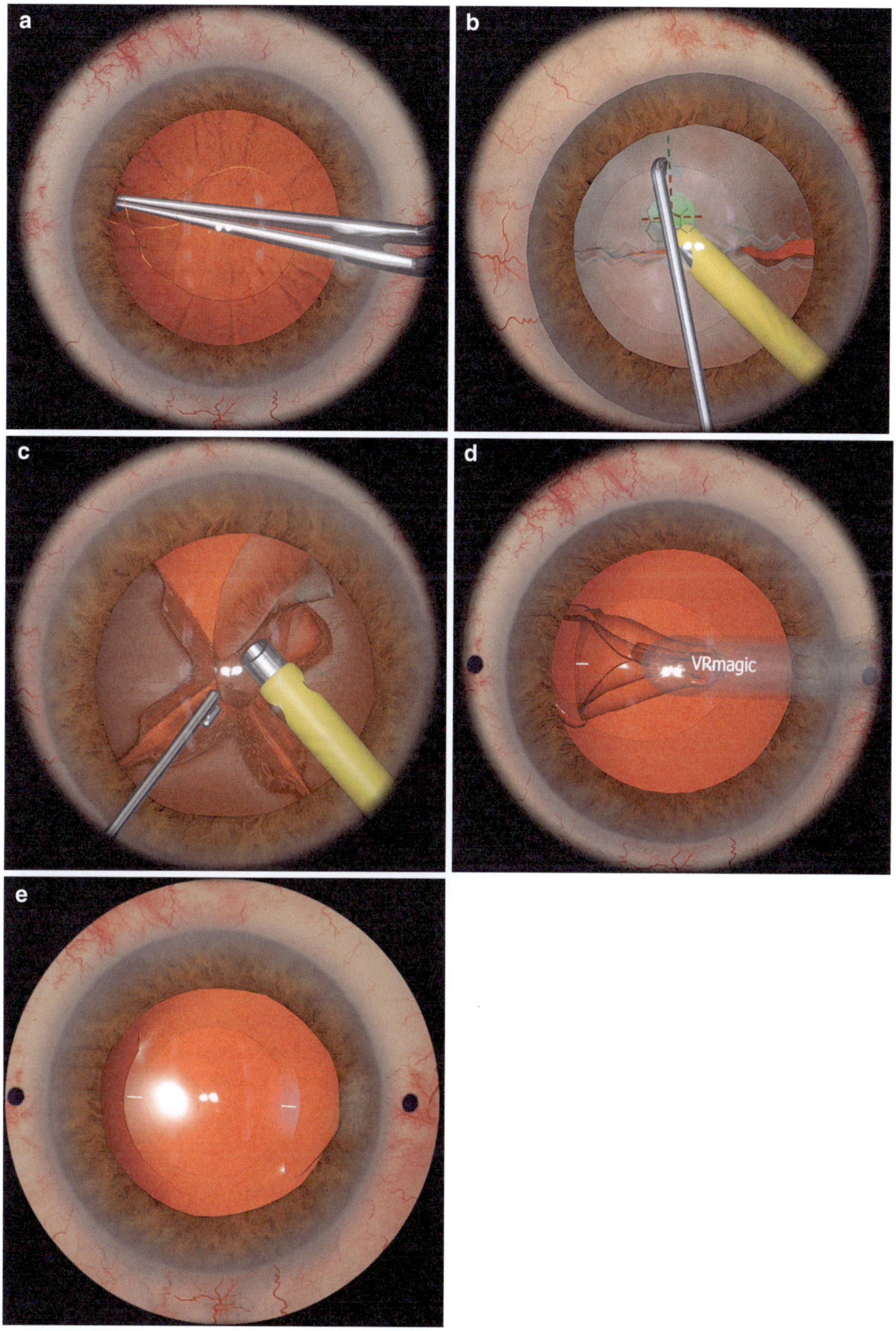

Fig. 7.14 (**a–e**) Training modules for cataract surgery: (**a**) Capsulorhexis. (**b**) Phaco-Chop. (**c**) Divide-and-Conquer. (**d**, **e**) Insertion of a toric intraocular lens (IOL)

With the integrated phaco machine and a biaxial phaco foot pedal, trainees can learn to control fluidics and select appropriate phaco parameters to safely and effectively disassemble and remove the lens nucleus (Fig. 7.14c). The simulator's cataract course consists of divide-and-conquer and chopping training exercises, emulsification of soft and hard nucleus, and cortex aspiration.

In a comparative case series, Belyea et al. reported that residents trained on the OR simulator performed phacoemulsification faster, used less power and had fewer intraoperative complications [21]. Pokroy also showed that training on the virtual simulator shortened the learning curve for the first 50 phacoemulsification cases and that less experienced residents seemed to benefit the most from virtual training [22].

7.3.7 Retinal Surgery

Vitreoretinal surgery is technically demanding and requires mastery of complex visuospatial techniques. Any mistake during the learning curve can lead to irreversible damage to the delicate structures of the retina.

The retina training module of the EyeSi® Surgical allows the development of essential vitreoretinal surgical skills and manual dexterity. Since the simulator is equipped with an instrument set for posterior segment surgery training and a vitreoretinal eye interface including a BIOM/SDI hardware mimic that functions like a real BIOM in the operating room, trainees can practice in a realistic environment.

For the purposes of this book, the current chapter focuses only on the simulation of cataract surgery and will not delve into the details of retinal surgery.

7.3.8 Limitations

Despite the proven effectiveness of the surgical simulator, it is important to acknowledge its limitations. For example, since the model eye already has puncture sites through which the trainee can insert the instruments, it is not possible to practice the paracentesis or the main incision. Additionally, despite the realistic simulations, there is no tactile feedback of "real tissue" as in the wet lab. The high cost of the simulator can also pose a financial burden for some training centers. However, Ferris and colleagues have argued that training trainees to cause fewer intraoperative complications, such as a posterior capsule rupture, through the investment in and use of the simulator can be more cost-effective in the long run than bearing the costs associated with additional surgical instruments and outpatient visits that may be necessary in cases of retinal detachment or endophthalmitis following a capsule rupture [13].

7.3.9 Conclusion

The training of an eye surgeon requires a comprehensive approach that should include knowledge of anatomy and surgical techniques, surgical judgment, and the development of manual skills. This last requirement can only be achieved by practicing movements and maneuvers, with better results when performed in a controlled environment, with evaluation and correction of errors between task repetitions.

Surgical simulators with virtual reality help bridge this gap in surgeon training by providing a reproducible scenario for safe, repeated practice, adding assessment feedback for performance correction, and offering the possibility to create a structured curriculum with exercises for standardized training.

As a computer-based simulator, it offers the possibility to develop various tasks for manual skills training and a curriculum of activities with an educational structure. The ability to perform surgical steps countless times without additional costs per attempt makes this a unique training opportunity. Although there is a high initial investment, there are no further costs (software updates are free), making this modality cost-effective in the long term.

When simulator training is implemented into a systematic training plan, it has the potential to improve both surgical and patient outcomes.

References and Further Reading

1. Blaskovics-Kettesy A (1970) Eingriffe am Auge. Enke, Stuttgart
2. Henderson BA, Grimes KJ, Fintelman RE, Oetting TA (2009) Stepwise approach to establishing an ophthalmology wet laboratory. J Cataract Refract Surg 35:1121–1128
3. Smolik I (2008) Im Wetlab netzhautchirurgische Fertigkeiten am Schweineauge trainieren. Spektrum Augenheilkd 22(3):195–197
4. Binder S (2007) Chirurgisches Training gestern und heute. Spektrum Augenheilkd 21(4):211
5. Inama H, Asif N, Sohail AA, Fatimia SH (2020) Wet labs: a useful tool in training surgical residents in a third world country. Ann Med Surg 57:137–139
6. Alwadani S (2018) Cataract surgery training using surgical simulators and wet-labs: course description and literature review. Saudi J Ophthalmol 32(4):324–329
7. Dada VK, Sindhu N (2000) Cataract in enucleated goat eyes: training model for phacoemulsification. J Cataract Refract Surg 26(8):1114–1116
8. Karadayi K, Gültekin Ç, Aytaç E (2018) Bimanual capsulorhexis using a new hand tool: an experimental study in sheep eye. Kafkas Univ Vet Fak Derg 24(5):769–774
9. Heydenreich A (1968) Mikroskopisch –histologische Untersuchungsmethoden unter besonderer Berücksichtigung des Sehorgans. Thieme, Leipzig, 419 S
10. Reme C, Müller FO, Bamasch P (1972) Der Einfluss von Konservierung durch Lufttrocknung auf die Feinstruktur von Schweinehornhautlamellen. Albrecht v Graefes Arch Clin Exp Ophthalmol 185:189–205
11. Observer (2017) Künstliche Augen für die Medizinerausbildung. Mediplast 13:2–4
12. Hunter IW, Doukoglou TD, Lafontaine SR et al (1993) A teleoperated microsurgical robot and associated virtual environment for eye surgery. Presence 2:265–280
13. Ferris JD, Donachie PH, Johnston RL et al (2020) Royal College of Ophthalmologists' National Ophthalmology Database study of cataract surgery: report 6. The impact of EyeSi virtual reality training on complications rates of cataract surgery performed by first and second year trainees. Br J Ophthalmol 104(3):324–329
14. Jacobsen MF, Konge L, Bach-Holm D et al (2019) Correlation of virtual reality performance with real-life cataract surgery performance. J Cataract Refract Surg 45(9):1246–1251
15. Staropoli PC, Gregori NZ, Junk AK et al (2018) Surgical simulation training reduces intraoperative cataract surgery complications among residents. Simul Healthc 13(1):11–15
16. Thomsen AS, Bach-Holm D, Kjærbo H et al (2017) Operating room performance improves after proficiency-based virtual reality cataract surgery training. Ophthalmology 124(4):524–531
17. Thomsen AS, Smith P, Subhi Y et al (2017) High correlation between performance on a virtual-reality simulator and real-life cataract surgery. Acta Ophthalmol 95(3):307–311
18. Privett B, Greenlee E, Rogers G et al (2010) Construct validity of a surgical simulator as a valid model for capsulorhexis training. J Cataract Refract Surg 36(11):1835–1838
19. McCannel CA, Reed DC, Goldman DR (2013) Ophthalmic surgery simulator training improves resident performance of capsulorhexis in the operating room. Ophthalmology 120(12):2456–2461
20. Bisol T, Bisol RAR, Rezende F (2016) Efficacy of Eyesi surgical simulator training in improving high-tension capsules capsulorhexis performance. Rev Bras Oftalmol 75(5):376–379
21. Belyea DA, Brown SE, Rajjoub LZ (2011) Influence of surgery simulator training on ophthalmology resident phacoemulsification performance. J Cataract Refract Surg 37(10):1756–1761
22. Pokroy R, Du E, Alzaga A et al (2013) Impact of simulator training on resident cataract surgery. Graefes Arch Clin Exp Ophthalmol 251(3):777–781
23. Kuhn F (2008) Ocular traumatology. Springer, Berlin
24. Velhagen K (1964) Propädeutische augenärztliche Operationslehre. VEB Georg Thieme, Leipzi

Preparation of the Patient in the Operating Department

8

Susan Schmitz-Gießler, Anke Habermann and Christiane Wiederhold

Contents

To ensure a smooth process in the operating room, it is important that all procedures are fundamentally adhered to and all preparatory measures are consistently carried out. All information on the surgery schedule must be checked! The surgeon must be able to fully concentrate on the procedure, especially if the surgeon is a beginner.

If important information is missing in the medical history and thus for the surgery schedule (for example, that it is a trauma or PEX eye), this can potentially lead to unexpected problems. Especially in such complicated cases, the surgeon must be able to adjust to the special initial situation (Sect. 21.1).

8.1 Documentation and Data Protection

Counceling usually takes place at least two weeks before (excluding emergencies and injuries) the operation in the practice. During the medical history, the patient is asked about eye diseases, general illnesses, surgeries, allergies, and medications, especially blood thinners and tamsulosin. After a thorough examination, the patient is explained the procedure of the operation and possible complications are discussed. Furthermore, they are informed about the possibility of implanting various intraocular lenses (monofocal lens, toric IOL, multifocal lens). If the patient cannot decide yet and wishes to have some time to think, they must contact the practice at least one week before the operation by

S. Schmitz-Gießler (✉)
Augenzentrum Leiterstraße, Magdeburg, Germany

A. Habermann
Augenzentrum “Frohe Zukunft”, Halle/Saale, Germany

C. Wiederhold
Augezentrum Sangerhausen, Augenärztliche Gemeinschaftspraxis, Sangerhausen, Germany
e-mail: wiederhold@augenarzt-sangerhausen.de

F. Wilhelm (ed.), *Ophthalmic Surgery for Beginners*, https://doi.org/10.1007/978-3-662-70287-1_8

phone or email so that the lens to be implanted can be ordered if it is not in stock.

> In case of language-related communication problems, the counceling must be conducted in the presence of a local language speaking family member or a certified interpreter. The patient is also informed that they must appear for the operation on an empty stomach, meaning the last food intake must be 6 hours prior. Clear fluids can be consumed up to 2 hours before the operation. The intake of regular medications is possible, but blood thinners (Chap. 9 and Table 8.1) and antidiabetics must be discontinued in consultation with the general practitioner.

The intake of oral antidiabetic drugs may also need to be paused temporarily (Chap. 9 and Table 8.2).

> Diabetics who are on insulin therapy must not administer it on the morning of the surgery day, as food intake is contraindicated, for example, due to the planned analgesia!

All important (and) discussed matters are documented on the surgery consent form. If there are no further questions, it is signed by the patient and the informing doctor. The file notes what should appear on the surgery schedule, such as the eye to be operated on, as well as special conditions like PEX syndrome, cornea guttata,

Table 8.1 Overview of blood thinners and anticoagulants to be considered

Drug group	Drug, trade name	Intake pause (whole days before surgery)	Active ingredient
Platelet aggregation inhibitors	ASS 100, Acesal, Godamed, Aggrenox, Axanum	4 days	Acetylsalicylic acid
	Iscover, Plavix, Clopigamma, Clopidolut, Clopidogrel	7 days	Clopidogrel
	DuoCover, DuoPlavin	Cannot be paused, always drip anesthesia	Clopidogrel + ASS
	Tiklyd	10 days	Ticlopidine
	Brilique	7 days	Ticagrelor
	Efient	7 days	Prasugrel
	Pletal	7 days	Cilostazol
Anticoagulants			
NOAC (new oral anticoagulants) **No** bridging with heparin	Pradaxa	2 days	Dabigatran
	Xarelto	2 days	Rivaroxaban
	Eliquis	2 days	Apixaban
	Lixiana	2 days	Edoxaban
Vitamin K antagonists Bridging with heparin	Falithrom, Phenpro	Quick > 50%, INR < 1.5	Phenprocoumon

Table 8.2 Overview of oral antidiabetic drugs to be recorded preoperatively are

Antidiabetics			
Metformin	Glucophage, Siofor, Metformin, Eucreas, Icandra, Janumet, Komboglyze, Velmetia, Competact, Diabesin, Espa-formin, Glucobon, Juformin	2 days	Metformin (pure or in combination)
All other antidiabetics ("sugar tablets")	Glimepiride, Acarbose, Glucobay, Galvus, Jalra, Januvia, Onglyza, Xelevia, Enyglid, NovoNorm, Starlix, Actos, Maninil, Diamicron	Do not take on the day of surgery	Others

narrow anterior chamber, post-trauma condition, oculus ultimus situation, the intake of blood thinners, diabetes medications, and medications that can cause floppy iris syndrome. The latter only needs to be known by the surgeon; a temporary discontinuation has no effect (Table 8.3).

The surgery schedule is created in advance. It must include, in addition to the patient's name, the planned surgery, the eye to be operated on, and, if applicable, the lens to be implanted, as well as any special features that are important for the surgeon (see Sect. 8.1), the chosen form of anesthesia, and the health insurance. The surgeon completes the surgery schedule, checks the side of the eye to be operated on, and the strength of the selected intraocular lens. If the patient desires a special lens, the calculation of the lens parameters and the order from the respective company are carried out in advance. In Table 8.4, an example of a surgery program is presented in anonymized form as follows:

Table 8.3 Medications that can lead to floppy iris syndrome [5]

Medication	Mechanism of action	Application	Medication	Mechanism of action	Application
Tamsulosin	Selective α1-receptor blocker	BPH	**Phentolamine**	Non-selective α-receptor blocker	Hypertension in pheochromocytoma Erectile dysfunction
Terazosin	Selective α1-receptor blocker	BPH	**Yohimbine**	α2-receptor blocker Affinities for serotonin receptors	Erectile dysfunction
Alfuzosin	Selective α1-receptor blocker	BPH	**Clomipramine**	α1-receptor blocker, serotonin and norepinephrine blocker	Depressions, anxiety disorders, obsessive-compulsive disorders
Silodosin	Selective α1-receptor blocker	BPH	**Duloxetine**	Affinity for α1-, α2-, dopamine, serotonin receptors	Depressions, anxiety disorders, polyneuropathy
Doxazosin	Selective α1-receptor blocker	BPH, hypertension	**Risperidone**	Dopamine and serotonin receptor antagonist,	Schizophrenia, schizoaffective disorders
Indoramin	Selective α1-receptor blocker	BPH, hypertension	**Quetiapine**	Histamine, dopamine, and serotonin receptor antagonist, NAT	Depressions, schizophrenia, obsessive-compulsive disorders,
Prazosin	Selective α1-receptor blocker	Hypertension	**Zuclopenthixol**	Dopamine and serotonin receptor antagonist	Psychoses
Urapidil	Selective α1-receptor blocker	Hypertension	**Imipramine**	α- and serotonin receptor antagonist	Depressions
Labetalol	α1-, β1- and β2-receptor blocker	Hypertension	**Mianserin**	α1-, α2- and serotonin receptor antagonist	Depressions
Carvedilol	α1-, β1- and β2-receptor blocker	Hypertension, angina pectoris	**Ergotamine**	Affinities for α1- and α2-, dopamine and serotonin receptors	Migraine
Phenoxybenzamine	α1- and α2-receptor blocker	Hypertension in pheochromocytoma	**Finasteride**	Selective 5α-reductase blocker	Androgenic hair loss, BPH

Table 8.4 Example of a surgery schedule (excerpt)

Surgery schedule for (date) Name of the surgeon									
Time	Last name, First name	Date of birth	Anesthesia	Surgery	Eye	Lens	Strength	Remarks	HI
07:00	Test, Otto	01.01.1930	Topical	Phaco+IOL	RA	EyeCeeOne	+24.0	po. Glaupax,	Technician KK
07:15	Sample, Hagen	02.02.1940	Topical	Phaco+IOL	RA	Panoptix	+21.5	Cave PEX	AOK Saxony-Anhalt
07:30	Hahn, Hildegard	03.03.1950	Topical	Phaco+IOL	RA	TIOL	+22.0 T3	C. guttata, HH protection!	Nuremberg BKK
07:45	Prof. Prima, Klaus	04.04.1960	Peribulbar	Phaco+IOL	RA	Polytech	+27.5	Very anxious, head tremor	**Self-payer**
08:00	Blume, Blumhild	05.05.1960	GA	ECCE	LA	Hoya	+25.0	Post-trauma, mature cataract	**Self-payer**
08:30	Klemm, Klemmhild	06.04.1970	Topical	Phaco+IOL	RA	SN60WF	+29.5	Target refraction—2.5 D Eliquis discontinued	AOK Halle

The schedule is to be placed everywhere in the OR department depending on the established procedures where it is needed—among other places at the OR counter, furthermore in the preparation room, at the anesthetist's workstation, in the OR at the microscope (clearly visible to the surgeon) as well as at the phaco machine (for the instrument nurse).

▶ It must be ensured in advance that all crucial data are correctly included (checked by the surgeon) and can be quickly and clearly captured by him during the OR program ("at a glance"). Only then can the surgeon fully concentrate on the procedure.

At the practice registration, the patient receives their surgery appointment, the duplicate of the consent form, a list of behavioral rules after the operation, the documents for the general practitioner, as well as an anesthesia consent form, which they bring filled out and signed to the operation. This form asks about previous surgeries and anesthetics and any possible complications (Chap. 8).

If the patient appears with all documents on the day of surgery at the practice, the patient is asked again at the surgery registration whether they are fasting and have discontinued the specified medications. Furthermore, they are asked for their health insurance card and the referral from the treating ophthalmologist, and the filled out and signed anesthesia form is collected. If the patient wishes for a special lens, it is checked whether a signed cost agreement is available.

If the patient has had breakfast or the general practitioner's findings are incomplete, consultation with the anesthetist and the surgeon is held to decide whether the type of anesthesia needs to be changed or the procedure postponed (Chap. 9).

8.2 Medication Pre-treatment

After the nurse at the surgery counter has ensured that the patient's name and the eye to be operated on are correct and no allergies to eye drops are known, mydriatics (Cyclopentolate®, Mydrum®, and Neosynephrine®) are instilled several times. Additionally, the eye to be operated on is superficially anesthetized with Novesine drops. The additional application of Xylo-Gel is also possible (Chap. 9).

▶ The eye that will be operated can be marked with a colored pencil or a cross of adhesive tape on the forehead to ensure the correct side for the operation. Regardless, the correct side of the surgery and the patient's identity must be checked multiple times.

8.3 Admittance to the Operating Room

The patient is provided with a head cap and shoe covers. Personal belongings are stored in a locker. This also definitely applies to the mobile phone! Jewelry should be removed for hygienic reasons. Then the patient is received by the anesthetist in the operating room admittance area and led into the operating room. Here, the patient is positioned and the anesthesia is prepared (Sect. 4.3 and Chap. 9). It is important to attune the patient to the procedures in the operating room and simultaneously convey a sense of security. Playing suitable music in both the preparation room and the operating room has proven effective. A randomized study with 330 patients in 2021 demonstrated the positive effect of music during the operation process. For this, systolic and diastolic blood pressure values were monitored [4].

8.4 Positioning

It is crucial that the patient lies comfortably [3]! They should not feel any pain in the back or neck, as this could make them restless during the operation. Pressing while breathing results in a "vis a tergo" (increased vitreous pressure), leading to a flattening of the anterior chamber. Additionally, all patients are positioned with a knee roll, which relieves the lumbar spine and is perceived as very comfortable. Neck discomfort can be alleviated with a small, rolled-up towel [2]. The head is loosely fixed by positioning it in a headrest (Sect. 4.3).

If the patient has a head tremor, the head can be fixed to the headrest of the operating table with tape after consultation. The upper body should be slightly elevated, but the head should be placed flat so that the cornea takes a horizontal position. This provides the surgeon with an optimal view during the procedure.

▶ The patient's head should be tilted so far temporally that the irrigation fluid can always drain well and does not accumulate in the nasal canthus!

8.5 Documentation after the Operation

In the surgery protocol (also surgery report), the patient's name, date of birth, surgery times, and any special features of the procedure are noted. After approval by the surgeon, the instrumenting and the non-sterile ("runner") assistant, the protocol can be inserted (scanned) into the patient's file. The batch stickers of the medical products used are utilized for documentation in the patient's file. For the implanted IOLs, these are collected on a form that is sent to the supplier at the end of the surgery day for replacement orders.

8.6 After the Procedure

During the postoperative observation in the recovery room (for approximately 10 minutes, Chap. 9), the operated patient is provided with a a beverage to drink.

In the case of performed cataract surgery, the patient is given their "lens passport" (with the names of the patient and surgeon, the surgery date, as well as the lens type, manufacturer, and strength of the implanted IOL) as well as a letter and a referral back to the continuing ophthalmologist. Additionally, they will receive the contact details of the practice with a phone number to reach the surgeon in case of complaints within the first 24 hours after the operation [1].

- If the patient feels subjectively well and free of complaints, they may leave the practice **only in accompaniment** .

References and Further Reading

1. Gerl G (1997) Ambulante Operationen in der Augenheilkunde. Hippokrates, Stuttgart
2. Kuhn F (2016) Vitreoretinal surgery: strategies and tactics. Springer, Berlin
3. Liehn M, Lengersdorf B, Steinmüller L, Döhler R (Hrsg) (2021) OP-Handbuch. Springer, Berlin/Heidelberg
4. Muddane SK et al (2021) Preoperative and perioperative music to reduce anxiety during first-time phacoemulsification cataract surgery in the high-volume setting: randomized controlled trial. J Cataract Refract Surg 47:471–475
5. Wilhelm U, Kohlhaas M, Weitschies W, Wölfelschneider P (2016) Welche Medikamente induzieren eine „Floppy Iris" bei der Kataraktoperation? Vortrag, gehalten 2016 in Dortmund, 30. Kongress der DGII

Anesthesia in Ophthalmology

9

Alexandra Stein, Frank Zimmermann and Frank Wilhelm

Contents

9.1 Which Anesthesia Methods are used for which procedures in ophthalmology?

In ophthalmic surgery, outpatient procedures have proven successful in recent years, also due to improved surgical techniques and consequently shorter procedure times. However, general anesthesia still has its place in the field of eye surgery. According to a representative survey, the current distribution of various anesthesia techniques in Germany is as follows: 43% topical methods, 46% retro- or peribulbar injections, 12% sedation or ITN anesthesia [1].

The ophthalmic surgeon is responsible for deciding which method is preferred in each individual situation [2].

A. Stein (✉)
Pampow, Germany

F. Zimmermann
Greifswald, Germany

F. Wilhelm
Universitätsklinikum Halle Saale, Greifswald, Germany

According to Velhagen:

> Everything the patient does wrong is primarily the doctor's fault and not the patient's, even if the patient appears foolish, such as suddenly standing up.

The demand for "a thorough general examination before an operation" [3], to "particularly consider the patient's general physical condition" [4], is important in close and collegial cooperation with the anesthetist and the patient's general practitioner.

The introduction of the electronic patient record may simplify the recording of patients' medical histories in the future. Important aspects of a comprehensive medical history can be found in Table 9.1.

The preoperative consultation with the patient should be used by the surgeon to assess the expected intraoperative compliance and to incorporate this into the decision when selecting the anesthesia method.

An example of a preoperative preparation form for the general practitioner is presented in the following overview:

F. Wilhelm (ed.), *Ophthalmic Surgery for Beginners*, https://doi.org/10.1007/978-3-662-70287-1_9

Table 9.1 Important Anamnestic Parameters

Medications	e.g., Tamsulosin, ASA, Xarelto, Falithrom, Metformin
Diseases	e.g., immune deficiencies, hepatitis C, HIV, diabetes, anxiety disorders, mental impairments
Special Treatments	e.g., chemotherapy
Allergies	e.g., antibiotics, local anesthetics
Laboratory	CBC, coagulation
ECG	

General practitioners report on surgical preparation of the patient

Dear colleagues,

In order to make the planned operation as safe as possible for our patient,

we would like to ask you for some additional information.

Underlying diseases:

Current medication:

Current relevant findings:

Yours sincerely

Gel anaesthesia with analgesia	Peribulbar anaesthesia with analgesia	General anaesthesia
Preparation according to EBM 31011-13	Preparation according to EBM 31011-13	Preparation according to EBM 31011-13
Leave anticoagulants	Change anticoagulant (rapid value 60%)	Change anticoagulant (rapid value 60%)

9.2 Local Anesthesia in Ophthalmic Procedures

The number of surgeries performed in ophthalmology has significantly increased due to improvements in diagnostic and therapeutic options, from the treatment of cataracts as one of the oldest procedures to vitrectomy and glaucoma surgeries, and the introduction of IVOM. Today, established forms of anesthesia methods in ophthalmology include general anesthesia, para- or peribulbar anesthesia, and surface anesthesia methods. Surface anesthesia is becoming increasingly important. Its application became standard with 28.1% in 2008 and 71.7% in 2017. This is due to the reduced operation time and the predominantly outpatient nature of the surgery in partially multimorbid patients.

9.2.1 Pain and Local Anesthetics

Pain is defined as an unpleasant sensory and emotional experience associated with actual or potential tissue damage or described in terms of such damage.

Local Anesthetics block pain perception at the neuronal level in a localized area. This means a primary specific blockade of fast voltage-gated sodium channels of the axon, preventing the formation of an action potential.

In clinical use, local anesthetics are mostly hydrochloride solutions with a pH value of 4–7. These are highly water-soluble and tissue-compatible. Since only the basic form can diffuse to the site of action, an extracellular bicarbonate buffer is necessary. Therefore, the effect of local anesthetics is significantly reduced or nullified in an acidic pH (e.g., inflammation).

9.2.2 Anesthesia Procedures in Cataract Surgery

The established local anesthesia procedures for the eye are defined by their anatomical application site. A distinction is made between injection and non-injection procedures.

Non-Injective Procedures

These include the various forms of surface anesthesia, where anesthesia of the eye surface is achieved by means of carrier media or the application of drops.

Surface Anesthesia

In topical anesthesia, analgesia of the cornea and conjunctiva is achieved with a reduction, but not elimination, of reflex movements (Fig. 9.1). It is established for smaller and short procedures where akinesia is not absolutely necessary, such as in contact lens examinations, tonometry, foreign body removals, IVOM, or in cataract surgery.

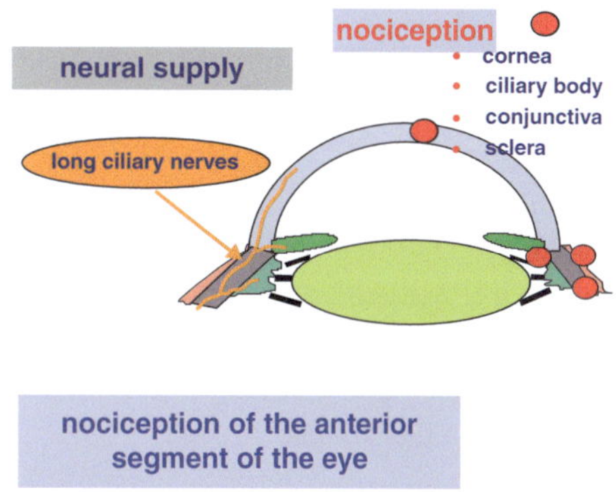

Fig. 9.1 Pain receptors in the anterior segment of the eye. (From [5])

The substances used require a short onset time of 30 to 60 seconds and have an effective duration of 10–20 minutes. By instilling surface-anesthetizing eye drops or applying a soaked carrier (e.g. swab), a uniform wetting of the cornea and conjunctiva is achieved (Fig. 9.2). The first application initially causes an unpleasant sensation (e.g. burning), after which the application is no longer perceived as such. The eyes must then be kept closed to prevent drying of the corneal epithelium and thus a reduced view into the eye during the procedure.

Medication Application Using the Example of Gel Anesthesia

- Start with the administration of eye drops to dilate and anesthetize the eye

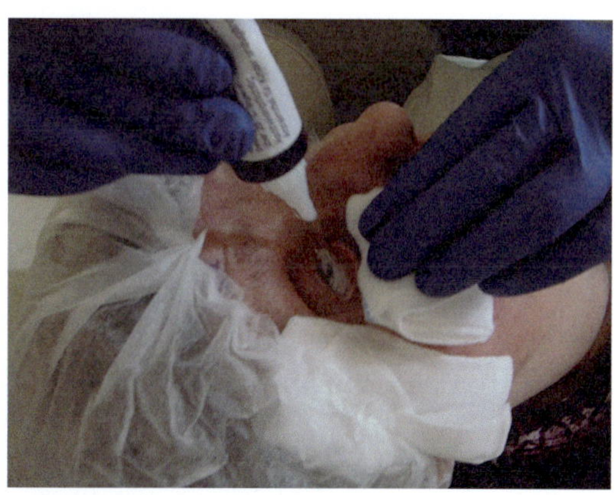

Fig. 9.2 Clinical image of the application of topical anesthesia by the preparation nurse

Drops are administered in three "rounds" at intervals of 10 minutes each, per round:

- 1 vial of Conjuncain
- 1–2 drops of Mydrum, Neosynephrine, and Cyclolat
- finally, the Xylocaine gel

The patient must be instructed to keep their eyes closed between the rounds.

Injective Procedures
In these forms of anesthesia, a local anesthetic is administered to interrupt impulse conduction in peripheral nerves in the sense of a conduction anesthesia. In ophthalmology, para- or peribulbar anesthesia and sub-Tenon anesthesia are mainly used as procedures. Retrobulbar anesthesia is losing significance due to higher complication rates.

Para- or Peribulbar Anesthesia
The para- or peribulbar anesthesia is essentially an orbital infiltration anesthesia, as it primarily results in a desired spread of the local anesthetic in a large area of the orbit. In the original technique by Davis and Mandel, two injections, one temporal lower and one nasal upper, were performed in the primary position either transcutaneously or transconjunctivally. The cannula is advanced parallel to the orbital floor. An intraconal administration is thus not possible. The rapid lowering of the upper eyelid is considered as direct success control. Today, usually only one injection is performed temporal lower (Fig. 9.3a, b). After that, an ocular pressor (40 mmHg for 15 min) may be placed to reduce vitreous pressure. The intraocular pressure rises, achieving a volume reduction in the ocular compartments. After removing the ocular pressor, the intraocular pressure drops, leading to a deepening of the anterior chamber. Additionally, this results in better tissue penetration of the local anesthetics.

▶ The opening of the cannula bevel should face the globe to minimize the risk of perforation. Additionally, fixing the cannula between two fingers while simultaneously applying pressure to the orbital tissue has proven to be very helpful.

Retrobulbar Anesthesia
This is the oldest regional anesthesia method. In the technique by Atkinson, the cannula is inserted transcutaneously through the temporal lower eyelid and advanced parallel to the orbital floor until it reaches behind the equator. Then, the direction is changed by slightly tilting towards the orbital apex. After overcoming slight resistance, the injection can be performed within the retrobulbar muscle cone. Subsequently, the procedure is the same as for para- or peribulbar anesthesia, and an ocular pressor is applied.

Sub-Tenon Anesthesia
In this procedure, the local anesthetic is to be introduced into the sub-Tenon space to block the nerve conduction at the eye as it passes through. Usually, the conjunctiva is opened temporally upper or nasally lower in the muscle-free area, and the local anesthetic is injected behind the equator with a curved blunt needle.

9.2.3 Possible Complications

Since important anatomical structures in the orbital area are closely situated, there is a risk of complications due to injury with the cannula tip, especially in injection procedures.

Retrobulbar Hematoma
With a probability of about 1%, it is the most common serious complication. This can lead to venous or arterial bleeding behind the eyeball. In this case, one can attempt to achieve hemostasis through pressure (oculopressor, finger). If this is not successful and a central retinal artery occlusion is present ophthalmoscopically, a decompression via a canthotomy must be performed, and the patient must be presented as quickly as possible to a department where further decompressive steps can be taken.

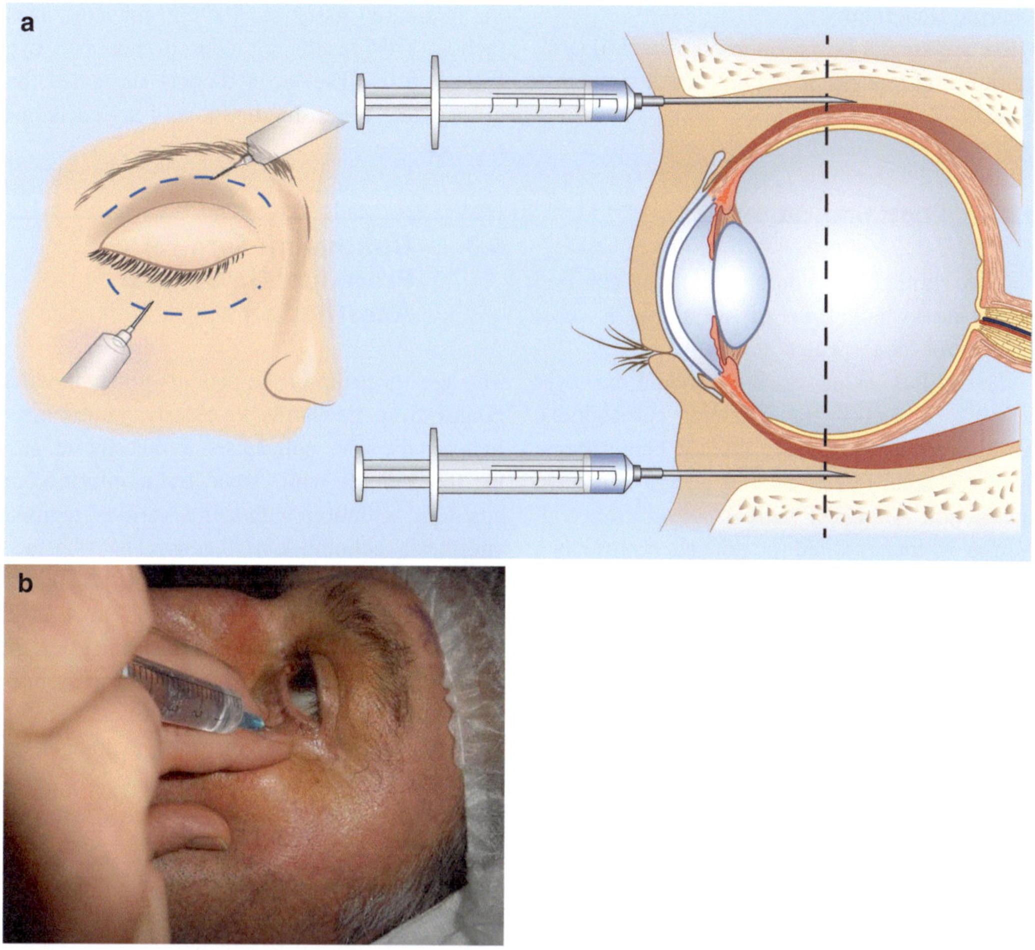

Fig. 9.3 (**a**, **b**) (**a**) Schematic representation of the parabulbar injection of anesthesia from "Practice of Anesthesiology" [6]. (**b**) Clinical image of a parabulbar injection: The index finger marks the injection site

Eyeball Perforation
The risk for this is about 0.075%. The patient usually reports pain, vision loss, or flashes as initial symptoms. The injection is difficult, and there is an increase in intraocular pressure, bleeding, or retinal detachment. Patients with a long eyeball, during follow-up injections, or after indentation procedures are more likely to experience perforation.

Muscle Paresis
These are caused by direct trauma with the cannula, hematomas, or toxicity of the local anesthetic. They can occur in up to 4% of cases after retrobulbar anesthesia.

Central Venous Reactions
These occur rarely in ophthalmology and usually only with intravascular injections or amounts >10 ml (i.e., retrobulbar anesthesia or follow-up injections). These include restlessness, vomiting, visual disturbances, numbness of, for example, the mouth and tongue, as well as seizures, respiratory arrest, and coma.

Allergic Reactions
These are known skin changes such as urticaria, pruritus and redness or swelling in the injection area.

9.2.4 Contraindications

For any surgical procedure, it must be clarified in advance which form of anesthesia is most suitable for the respective patient.

The Quick value or INR should be over 50–60% or <1.3 for injection procedures. Absolute contraindications include hemorrhagic diathesis, local infections and allergies to local anesthetics. A lack of patient cooperation with the risk of uncontrolled movements represents a relative contraindication. This includes psychiatric or neurological disorders as well as young patients. A previous indentation surgery with altered anatomy, a long eyeball due to high myopia, optic atrophy, oculus ultimus situation and recent intraocular surgeries or perforating injuries represent further relative contraindications.

9.2.5 Medications Used

Commonly used medications are listed below:

Local Anesthetics

- Ropivacaine: e.g., Naropin
- Oxybuprocaine Hydrochloride: e.g. Conjuncain EDO AT
- Lidocaine Hydrochloride: e.g. Xylocaine 2% Gel

Hyaluronidase
The enzyme hyaluronidase (e.g. Hylase Dessau) increases permeability by dissolving the interstitial tissue barrier, e.g. for local anesthetics. This results in more pronounced eyeball akinesia. The onset time is shortened, but at the same time, the duration of action is also reduced.

9.3 Ophthalmic Surgical Procedures in General Anesthesia

The age spectrum of the patients to be cared for ranges from newborns to elderly, multimorbid individuals. The colleagues in anesthesia care for the patients with "stand by/monitoring," in analgesic sedation with/using various regional anesthesia techniques up to general anesthesia.

In preparation for the operation, the patients present themselves to the general practitioner and are informed in a timely manner by the surgeon about the necessary surgical measures. Subsequently, the anesthetist provides information about the sedation treatment or general anesthesia.

During the procedure, the patients receive continuous monitoring with oxygen saturation control, electrocardiography, blood pressure measurement and an intravenous access.

ECG monitoring is indispensable for detecting a possible oculocardiac reflex.

General anesthesia is performed as balanced anesthesia or TIVA explain with airway management using a laryngeal mask or intubation, standard monitoring with continuous carbon dioxide measurement.

A special consideration for the anesthetist's work in the eye operating room is that there is no access to the patient's head during the surgical procedure, or it is severely restricted. Therefore, preoperative definitive and careful securing of the airway is all the more important.

Specialized Aspects of Anesthesia in Eye Surgery. (According to [7])

1. High proportion of pediatric and geriatric patients
2. Immobilization of the eye for microsurgical reasons
3. Interaction of positioning and anesthesia management with intraocular pressure and volume conditions
4. The oculocardiac reflex and its complications
5. Systemic effects of locally applied substances
6. Safety requirements due to special positioning and covering conditions
7. Special patient monitoring recommended

Causes of Triggering the Oculocardiac Reflex. (According to [7])

1. Traction on extraocular muscles
2. Globe pressure
3. Retrobulbar hematoma
4. Injuries to the eye and/or orbit
5. Retrobulbar injection
6. Iris manipulation in iris prolapse
7. Manipulations at the orbital apex during exenteration and enucleation

9.4 "What should be considered?"—Advantages and disadvantages of the procedures and complications

In principle, topical anesthesia is considered the most gentle and least stressful for the patient. It requires the least effort for the surgeon and carries the lowest risk of complications from the anesthesiological side. Additionally, after each procedure under local anesthesia, there is less tendency for nausea and vomiting, disturbances in endocrine regulations and electrolyte balance can be reduced, there is less tendency to bleed and with faster mobilization after the procedure, the care effort is lower and the outpatient performance of the procedure is safer [2].

- The surgeon must be aware that this procedure cannot be used for every surgical intervention and patient. Therefore, general anesthesia should definitely be preferred in the following situations:

- Surgeries on children, infants and mentally retarded patients, where appropriate behavior under local anesthesia cannot be reliably expected;

- Patients who fear (reject) a procedure under local anesthesia and therefore express a desire for general anesthesia—unless the general condition prohibits general anesthesia;

- Extensive surgeries such as tumor removals, procedures on the orbit, a treatment of bulbous trauma with lacerations, complicated retinal surgery, perforating keratoplasties, long-lasting procedures where infiltration of the surgical area is disruptive.

For globe-opening procedures, the decision for or against a peribulbar injection depends on the experience and requirements of the surgeon. A major advantage, besides the lower stress for the patient, is the avoidance of the risk of scleral perforations and bleeding that can be caused by the needle puncture. Furthermore, anticoagulant medications do not need to be discontinued. However, the ophthalmic surgeon must be aware that globe motility is preserved. In difficult situations, converting topical local anesthesia to peribulbar is not easily possible ([8])!

Tips and tricks for a smooth surgical procedure

1. Mark the surgical area preoperatively
2. Use checklists
3. The staff introduces themselves by name to the patient
4. Calm and openly communicating work atmosphere
5. Use of soothing music
6. Numerical surgical plans of the patients to be treated
7. Fixed surgical procedures and responsibilities
8. Postoperative discussion of the workday
9. Positive error culture

References and Further Reading

1. Wenzel M et al „Intraokulare Operationen: Ergebnisse der Jahresumfrage 2019/20" v. DGII, DOG
2. Mackensen G, Neubauer H (1988) Augenärztliche Operationen 1. Springer, Berlin, 660 S
3. Fasanella RM (1968) „Komplikationen in der Augenchirurgie und ihre Behandlung", Enke Stuttgart, 592 S
4. Barraquer J, Troutman RC, Rutllan J (1965) Die Chirurgie des vorderen Augenabschnittes. Enke Stuttart 515 S
5. Weindler J, Weindler M, Ruprecht KW (2004) Lokalanästhesie in der Ophthalmochirurgie. Ophthalmologe 847–865
6. Hemping-Bovenkerk A, Möllmann M (2017) Anästhesie in der Augenheilkunde. In: Wilhelm W (Hrsg) Praxis der Anästhesiologie. Springer, Berlin/Heidelberg. https://doi.org/10.1007/978-3-662-54568-3_59
7. Heuser D, Decker K. Anästhesie bei Eingriffen am Auge. Das Buch heißt: Anästhesie für Operationen im Kopfbereich, von E. Rügheimer, aus der Buchserie: Klinische Anästhesiologie und Intensivtherapie, Springer Verlag , Kapitel: Anästhesie bei Eingriffen am Auge, D. Häuser und K. Deckel, Seite 154–171
8. Kohnen S (2020) Umwandlung der Operation unter Tropfanästhesie und CCI ist schwierig. Ophthalmochirurgie 32:37–40
9. BVA und BDOC (2020) In: Pfeiffer N et al (Hrsg) 34. Kongress der DGII. TZ Verlag Print GmbH, Roßdorf, pp 55–58
10. van Aken, „Lokalanästhesie, Regionalanästhesie, Regionale Schmerztherapie" Thieme Verlag, 3. vollständig überarbeitete und erweiterte Auflage von 2010
11. H. Wulf, 3., vollst überarb u. erw. Aufl. „Lokalanästhesie, Regionalanästhesie, Regionale Schmerztherapie",Thieme Verlag, 3. vollständig überarbeitete und erweiterte Auflage von 2010
12. Naumann GOH, Lang GK (1988) Anästhesie in der Augenheilkunde. Pathophysiologische und operationstechnische Besonderheiten aus der Sicht des Ophthalmochirurgen. Springer, Berlin
13. Meyer-Bothling U, Jörgensen JS, Mann M (1998) Tropfanästhesie, Alternative zur Retro- oder Parabulbäranästhesie in der Kataraktchirurgie. Springer, Ophthalmo-Chirurgie, pp 204–208
14. Velhagen K (1964) Probedeutische Operationslehre. Springer, Thieme Leipzig, 257S
15. Lundström M et al (2021) Changing practice patterns in European cataract surgery as reflected in European Registry of Quality Outcomes for Cataract and Refractive Surgery 2008–2017. J Cataract Refract Surg 47:373–378

Intraocular Lenses—An Overview

10

Dirk Ehrich, Christine F. Kreiner and Frank Wilhelm

Contents

10.1 Introduction

A central element of any cataract surgery is the selection of a suitable intraocular lens. At the beginning of surgical training, the selection initially focuses on the correct lens strength according to the desired target refraction from an existing consignment stock. Depending on the training facility, only one or several lens types are likely available for selection. Their properties, especially their always present specific implantation peculiarities, may not necessarily be suitable for beginners, as the selection of the consignment stock is the responsibility of the management level, where often other premises exist.

- It makes sense to practice handling with an unsterile sample of the lens of the identical type before implanting the first intraocular lens. Many manufacturers provide unsterile implants for such preparations upon request without complications.
- Successful cataract surgery begins with an exact measurement of the eye. This is usually not the responsibility of the surgeon. Inexperienced handling of the ultrasound probe or incorrect operation of the IOL-Master are sources of error that must be considered. Every novice should take this very seriously to avoid systematic errors in entire patient clusters.

It is a special task for the trainer not to demotivate the student at the beginning with failures due to difficult implantation behavior, but at the same time to shape the necessary skill from the start to be successful even with more difficult lens types when the patient situation requires it.

D. Ehrich (✉)
Augenklinik, Helios Vogtland-Klinikum Plauen, Plauen, Germany
e-mail: dirk.ehrich@helios-gesundheit.de

C. F. Kreiner
KreCo, Consulting-Gesellschaft f. wiss.-techn. Projektmanagement, München, Germany

F. Wilhelm
Universitätsklinikum Halle Saale, Greifswald, Germany

F. Wilhelm (ed.), *Ophthalmic Surgery for Beginners*, https://doi.org/10.1007/978-3-662-70287-1_10

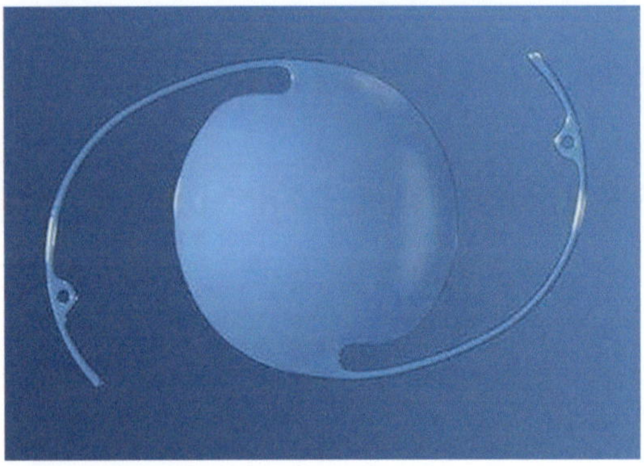

Fig. 10.1 PMMA lens with suture loops for scleral fixation

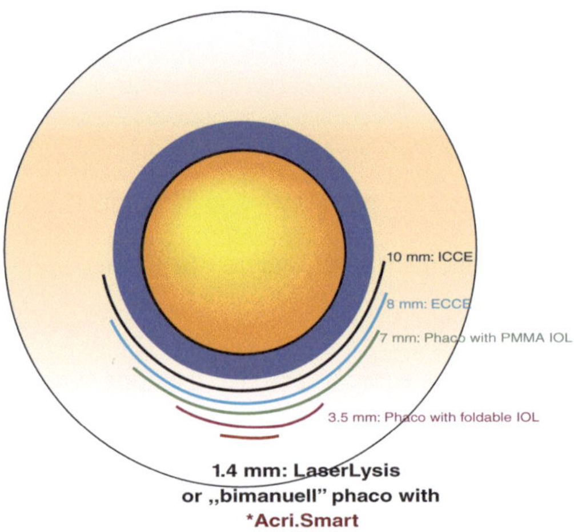

Fig. 10.2 Schematic representation of the necessary incision sizes for ICCE, ECCE, and phacoemulsification with form-stable and foldable lenses

Decisive differences exist regarding lens material and its long-term stability as well as the design of the lens, which determines a variety of properties such as implantation behavior, refractive stability, or incidence of posterior capsule opacification. Many intraocular lenses have special design features such as asphericity, spectral filters, torus, multiple foci, or special designs. Not every special lens can and should be covered in this section. The authors deliberately refrain from mentioning companies or individual lens types.

Since the first successful implantation of a rigid intraocular lens made of acrylic glass by Ridley in 1949, the implants have been continuously developed. Today, form-stable implants made of PMMA (polymethylmethacrylate) are mainly used as retropupillary iris-clipped claw lenses (Fig. 10.4) in aphakia and only sporadically as sclera-fixed secondary lenses (Fig. 10.1).

In developing countries (Sect. 21.4), however, PMMA lenses are still used more frequently due to the necessary lower costs.

▶ Every aspiring ophthalmic surgeon will quickly learn that it makes a big difference for an eye whether an 8-mm or a 2.5-mm access is required for implantation (Fig. 10.2).

Today's standard includes foldable lenses (initially made of silicone, later preferably of polymerized acrylates). This marked the birth of three-piece lenses. These consist of a lens body that can be folded to half its size like a sheet of paper without being damaged and returns to its predetermined refraction in the eye. Attached to it are two c-shaped loops made of a stiff material with high intrinsic tension to securely fix and center the artificial lens in the capsular bag (Fig. 10.3).

The decisive advantage was the possible reduction of the implantation incision, resulting in smaller, operation-induced astigmatism and reduced occurrence of incision insufficiencies with fistula formation or iris prolapse, as well as lower infection risks and irritation states. Ultimately, it was also the beginning of sutureless cataract surgery.

For a young surgeon, these lenses are not easy to implant. In the early years, there were no shooter systems, and they were implanted with a folding forceps. Especially the silicone lenses were difficult to hold in the forceps due to their higher intrinsic tension and unfolded rather abruptly in the eye. The haptics were difficult to control due to their stiffness, to avoid endothelial contact or posterior capsule ruptures. It was

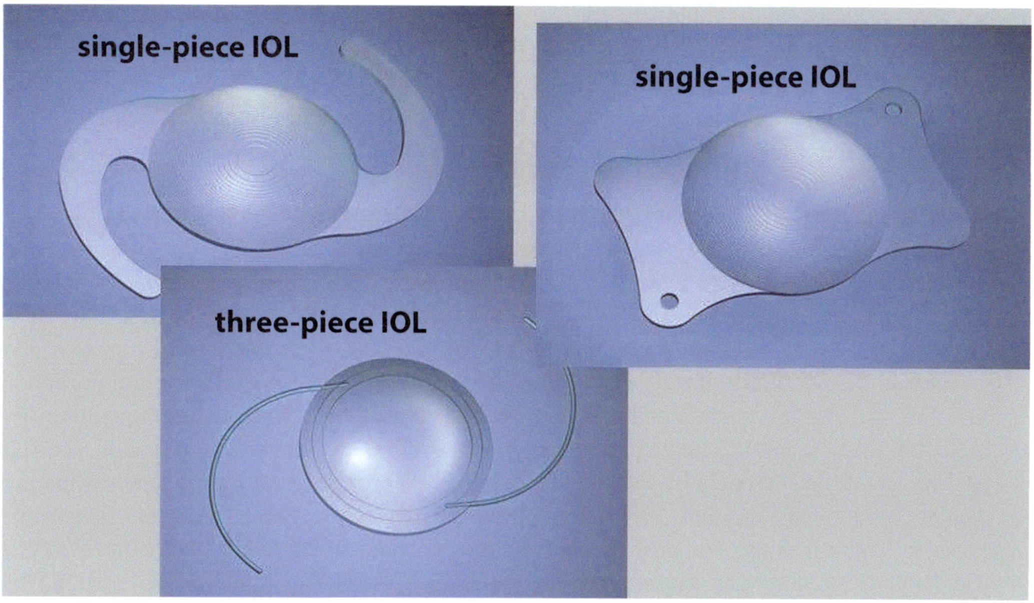

Fig. 10.3 Schematic comparison of one-piece/three-piece IOL

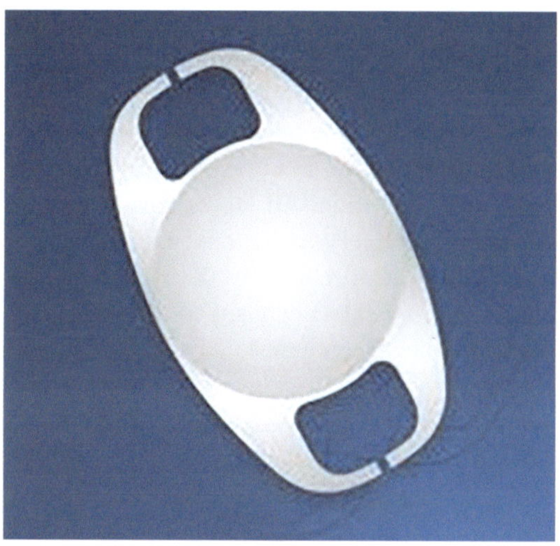

Fig. 10.4 Iris-claw lens

more straightforward to use the soon-to-be-available one-piece hydrophilic acrylic foldable lenses, which unfolded much more gently due to their soft character. Initially, however, these lenses were more problematic in the medium term with refractive changes due to capsular bag shrinkage and increased incidence of posterior capsule opacification. Experienced surgeons tended to use three-piece intraocular lenses during this time.

A significant improvement was brought by hydrophobic acrylates, angulation of the haptics, blunting of the haptic ends, sharp edges of the optics to minimize posterior capsule opacification, and the introduction of cartridge-guided shooters. The latter, in particular, significantly minimized the risk of infection, as the lens could be implanted without any contact with the eye surface. Additionally, the lens in the shooter is not only folded but rather rolled, so intraocular lenses with a 6 mm diameter usually fit through 2.2–2.5 mm incisions, depending on the system used, and in extreme cases through 1.4 mm [1].

- As with any technological advancement, there were also missteps. In the last 20 years, this applied to two quite renowned companies with implant failures due to clouding of the central lens body months to years after surgery. The polymers used were obviously not as long-term stable as hoped. Since thousands of patients had received these lenses in the meantime, a high number of explantations were required to fix the problem.

A particular form of undesirable changes in acrylic polymers is the so-called glistening (multiple tiny water droplet-like changes caused by polymer synthesis), which leads to increased glare sensitivity. Newer lens acrylates are largely free of this.

The vast majority of currently available lenses are one-piece and, in some cases, already preloaded in the shooter from the factory.

- ▶ Twist or push? This is a good example to understand the necessary operational diversity. For twisting the shooter, the surgeon needs both hands, but the implantation can be very controlled, especially with higher diopters and small incisions or difficult capsular bag situations. For pushing, only one hand is needed, and the second can fix the eyeball, which is particularly necessary with docking shooters. However, the implantation speed is more difficult to control. Many surgeons prefer one system or the other, making it impossible to agree on a standard lens in a purchasing consortium. The introduction of a preloaded lens from a renowned company, whose injector is designed to allow both twisting and pushing, was almost ingenious.

The structural properties are considered largely mature. The focus of technological development today is on improved optical properties.

There are a variety of additional features that allow for very patient-specific solutions.

10.2 Lens Types

The common lens types are briefly presented below.

10.2.1 Aspheric Lenses

The cornea is aspherically structured, so it is logical to transfer this asphericity to the lens body. Indeed, this ideally leads to improved image quality. However, a very good centering of the IOL is a basic requirement. The degree of asphericity varies depending on the manufacturer. Therefore, experience is also needed for the patient to benefit from an aspheric IOL.

10.2.2 Blue/Violet Filter Lenses

The medical community is divided regarding blue/violet filter lenses. These were introduced in 2003 due to the experimentally proven phototoxicity of the blue/violet spectrum portion on retinal physiology. Since the aging natural lens also exhibits a yellowish coloration, postoperative color perception by patients is often perceived as natural. As a result, these filter lenses have become widely used. With the increased oxidative stress from blue/violet light and the theoretically associated accelerated aging processes, one would expect a lower incidence of age-related macular degeneration in the group of patients with spectral filter lenses. So far, this evidence has not been successfully demonstrated in reliable studies, but it remains a target of scientific work. Each surgeon must position themselves on this issue. Many patients also inquire about UV protection. All lenses have this, with the majority of UV radiation being known to be already filtered corneally (keratopathia photoelectrica in welders or visits to tanning salons without protective goggles).

10.2.3 Toric Lenses

Several factors are necessary for successful astigmatism correction: It begins with an exact measurement of the eye, which is prone to errors. Relevant keywords are "sufficient contact lens abstinence," the existing "device base," "measurement inaccuracies due to reduced patient compliance or user inexperience," and the "use of the correct calculation formula." Since there are a multitude of possible combinations of sphere and torus, each lens is custom-made for the patient and thus generally represents a special lens subject to additional payment.

Even more than with aspheric lenses, a good centering with exact axis alignment is a foundation of success for toric implants. Initial problems with toric lenses regarding rotational stability or postoperative deformations "in loco" are now significantly reduced due to technological advancements. Proper suction of the viscoelastic material at the end of the operation is important. Sometimes, a post-rotation is necessary on the first postoperative day if the axis position deviates.

Capsular bag ruptures, zonular insufficiencies, or vitreous prolapse can make the insertion of a toric lens impossible. Therefore, the implantation of a toric lens belongs in experienced surgical hands.

10.2.4 Multifocal Lenses (which can also be toric)

This lens type is certainly the prototype of the premium lens. The desired goal of being glasses-free is the most perceived advertising message from an ophthalmological perspective. However, they are also the intraocular lenses with the greatest potential for conflict, as they involve a compromise of desired and undesired properties. When the incoming light is split into two or more foci, the contrast decreases. The typical ring structure leads to increased glare and halo formation at the respective transitions due to refraction and diffraction, which can be particularly disturbing when driving at night. Unlike the aforementioned IOLs, multifocal lenses also require a certain neural adaptation period, as the visual impression is created in the visual cortex, and multifocal perception is something to get used to and must be decided based on the patient's needs and abilities.

Often, the desire to be glasses-free is paramount, even when there is no significant lens opacity, as the loss of accommodation ability can turn simple or previously non-existent glasses situations into very complicated ones. With these lenses, the preselection of patients into suitable and rather unsuitable multifocal lens wearers is the real art, which requires a lot of experience.

It is also important to select the specific lens type according to the life circumstances and professional requirements, as these differ significantly in the extent of near, intermediate, and distance vision. Initially, multifocal lenses were more bifocal and either distance or near-dominant; nowadays, current models are more trifocal.

With the introduction of EDOF (Extended Depth Of Focus) IOLs in recent years, the problems of multifocal lenses are addressed by reducing halos and night glare and particularly enhancing the intermediate range, which plays a much larger role in everyday life in today's screen-dominated time than before. Even more than with toric lenses, a perfect rhexis and centering are prerequisites for success, so these patients also belong in the hands of experienced surgeons [2].

10.2.5 Add-on Lenses

These are piggyback implants on already existing artificial lenses, which are placed in the sulcus between the iris and the pseudophakos. They are available in spherical, toric, and multifocal forms, so these properties can be added later or relatively easily removed in case of lack of success or acceptance. These can be patients who initially opted for a different target refraction or against torus and multifocality, or for whom these special lenses were not yet available at the time of cataract surgery. Due to the sulcus position, the predictability of optical corrections is naturally somewhat more difficult.

10.2.6 Iris-clip lens for aphakia Correction

The phakic PMMA intraocular lens (Fig. 10.4), originally developed for anterior chamber implantation, which is fixed to the iris stroma with two claws on each side, led to the development of a surgical method in which these lenses are clipped to the iris from behind in a reversed retropupillary manner. This has made an elegant aphakia correction possible and has largely replaced the previously common scleral fixation. Due to the implantation in the posterior chamber, the corneal endothelium remains protected even in the presence of significant iridodonesis, as is often found in PEX-induced aphakia.

10.2.7 Phakic Intraocular Lenses

These are used to correct particularly higher refractive anomalies in younger people without lens opacities and with still relevant accommodation ability. In addition to the iris-fixated anterior chamber lenses made of PMMA or silicone already mentioned in Sect. 10.2.6, the intraocular contact lens (ICL) is mainly used (Fig. 10.5). This is implanted retropupillary between the back surface of the iris and the lens. In some patients, a cataract or secondary glaucoma develops due to the ICL. However, these two main complications are offset by high patient satisfaction, as high refractive anomalies up to +12 and −22 diopters can usually be corrected, for which a refractive laser procedure on the cornea would no longer be sufficient [3]

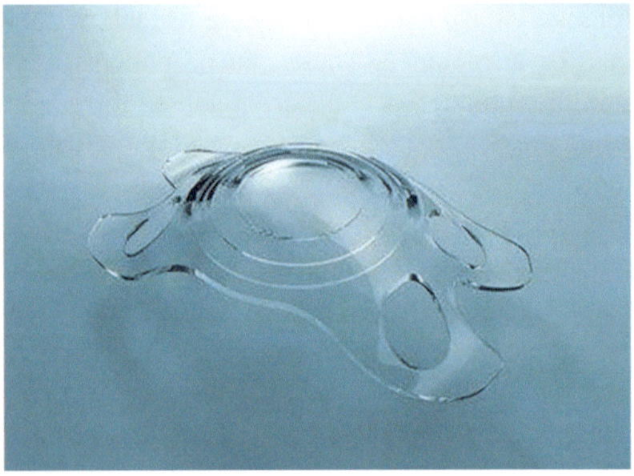

Fig. 10.5 Phakic implant

Anyone who implants artificial lenses will be confronted with the issue of dysphotopsias sooner or later. These are frustrating because they cannot be prevented either by patient selection as with multifocal lenses or by precise surgical technique. On the contrary: the typical dysphotopsia patient has a perfectly positioned lens with an ideal rhexis and full postoperative vision and is still unhappy.

Positive dysphotopsias are distinguished from negative dysphotopsias. Typical positive dysphotopsias are color distortions or blinking light reflections, while negative dysphotopsias manifest as a dark temporal crescent or prismatic perceptions.

The incidence of dysphotopsias is probably significantly higher immediately postoperatively than known, but is tolerated by many patients. Fortunately, the unpleasant perceptions usually fade over time, which is likely due to cognitive processes. However, there are still some patients who suffer so much that lens explantations have to be performed.

▶ The possible dysphotopsias must not be forgotten in patient education!

References and Further Reading

1. Burrato L, Brint S, Boccuzzi D (2014) Cataract surgery and intraocular lensens. Slack Incorporated. ISBN 9781617116049
2. Alio JL, Pikkel J (2019) Multifocal intraocular lenses. Springer. ISBN 9783319380148
3. Assia EI, Apple DJ, Kleinmann G (2014) Premium and specialized intraocular lenses. Bentham Science Publishers. ISBN 9781608058327

11 Intraocularly Administered Fluids and Medications

Peter Wölfelschneider and Christine F. Kreiner

Contents

11.1 Introductory Notes

In this chapter, substances that are available to the beginner during operations to perform individual surgical steps as gently as possible on the tissue are discussed. The selection does not claim to be complete; these examples represent groups of substances that every beginner should know. The aim is to provide an overview of the individual preparations, with particular emphasis on explaining the principles of their effects and applications.

P. Wölfelschneider (✉)
Augenzentren Rhein-Ruhr MVZ GmbH, Bochum, Germany
e-mail: dr.peter.woelfelschneider@augenzentren-rheinruhr.de

C. F. Kreiner
KreCo, Consulting-Gesellschaft f. wiss.-techn. Projektmanagement, München, Germany

11.2 Substances

This overview considers “balanced salt solution” (BSS), viscoelastics, air, dyes, drugs that affect pupil size, “recombinant tissue-type plasminogen activator” (rtPA), anesthetics, and antibiotics (see Table 11.1).

The intravitreal administration of drugs is treated separately in Chap. 18.

11.3 Volume Ratios in Intraocular Injection

Before discussing the actual handling, the volumes involved should be addressed. The volume of the anterior chamber is between 200–400 μl, it is usually 3.5 mm deep and has a diameter of

F. Wilhelm (ed.), *Ophthalmic Surgery for Beginners*, https://doi.org/10.1007/978-3-662-70287-1_11

Table 11.1 Overview of the presented substances

Substance	Application	Volume
"balanced salt solution" (BSS)	Irrigation, fluid replacement	Variable
Air	Stabilization of preformed spaces	Up to 400 µl
Viscoelastics	Stabilization of preformed spaces, gentle manipulation of tissues	Variable up to multiple fillings of the AC
Dyes	Visualization of boundary structures	Up to 400 µl
Miochol	Constricting the pupil	Up to 400 µl
Adrenaline, Mydrane	Dilating the pupil	Up to 100 µl
"recombinant tissue-type plasminogen activator" (rTPA)	Dissolving fibrin	Up to 200 µl
Anesthetics	Pain treatment	Up to 150 µl
Antibiotics	Anti-infective prophylaxis and therapy	Usually < 100 µl, (dose-dependent)

about 12.3 mm. On average, there is about 250 µl of fluid in front of the iris and another 60 µl behind it. Approximately 2–3 µl of aqueous humor is produced per minute, which has a pH of 7.2. For comparison, it should be remembered that in pharmacy, the volume of a drop of water is given as 50 µl.

Table 11.2 provides an overview of the specific requirements that fluids for intraocular use must meet.

Table 11.2 Requirements for Fluids for Intraocular Use

Osmotically compatible with ocular fluids
Without immunological potential
Free from endo- and exotoxins
Biocompatible, better: bioinert*
Optically transparent
Particle-free
No or only minimal impact on intraocular pressure
Easy to remove at the end of the surgery
Easy to use

* By *biocompatible* it is understood that there is no detectable negative impact on vital cells in the surrounding area. Among *biocompatible* materials, a distinction can be made between *bioinert* and **biotolerant**. *Bioinert* materials do not create chemical, physical, or biological interactions between tissue and implant, nor do they release toxic substances. *Biotolerant* means that a fibrous membrane forms at the interface between implant and material, which is not rejected. This is a property that, for example, is not desirable for intraocular implants!

11.4 Surgical Access

This is usually done through lamellar incisions (phaco tunnels and paracenteses) near the limbus in the corneal tissue (Chap. 13). Basically, the access should be chosen so that it is possible to operate under safe visibility during the surgery without touching vulnerable tissue outside the incision area. This also avoids additional transparency reduction due to scar formation. The incision geometry follows the principle that the length of the incision in the tissue should be about half the width to achieve a watertight wound closure for endophthalmitis prophylaxis. This can be secured by the intrastromal injection of BSS at the end of the procedure. The stromal swelling becomes visible through a localized whitening of the corneal tissue in the affected area. In some cases, a suture may be required, which is usually done with 10/0 nylon material. The planned incision width should be achieved on the first attempt. An incision that is too narrow results in increased force being required to insert the instruments during the procedure, leading to additional tissue trauma. An incision that is too wide leads to increased outflow of aqueous humor and thus to flattening of the anterior chamber. This makes intraocular manipulation during the procedure more difficult (Chap. 13). Significant pressure increases can result from the usually continuous irrigation. To prevent this, it must always be ensured intraoperatively that sufficient fluid can drain!

11.5 Handling of Syringes and Needles

The substances to be administered are contained in a syringe that is adjusted to the necessary amount of substance and the dimension of the anterior chamber. Industrially pre-filled and already drawn-up products are used, or it becomes necessary to draw up the substance into a syringe. The substance must be introduced into and/or removed from the eye with a chosen "needle".

▶ Three important questions need to be answered, for which the answer must be given before use on the eye:

1. Can the plunger of the syringe be moved without force? For this, the plunger should be moved until a drop is visible at the tip of the needle.
2. This simultaneously answers the question of the needle's patency!
3. Is the connection between the needle and the syringe secure, so that the needle does not move through the eye like a projectile during injection and cause severe injuries? The operator always keeps a fingertip on the connection between the needle and the syringe during the injection into the eye. This way, they immediately notice if the needle should come loose!

Typically, 1-, 2-, and 5-ml syringes are used. It should preferably be such that the needle can be screwed onto the syringe (for example, as a Luer-Lock connection) to prevent the needle from coming loose from the syringe. The choice of needle depends on the properties of the substance to be used. If it is viscous, the diameter must be correspondingly larger so that it can be operated safely with appropriate force and correspondingly fine movements.

11.6 Examples of Commonly Used Needles

A **"Round-end" needle** can be angled between 25 and 45°. With an inner diameter of up to 19 gauge, it is the first choice for the administration of substances with higher viscosity. Additionally, these needles are round at the opening so that no sharp edges result and the access channel can be passed as atraumatically as possible.

The **"Sautter needle"** is blunt, flattened at the tip, and slightly curved overall. It has a 27-gauge diameter to pass through a lamellar cut well and atraumatically. Therefore, it is ideal for gently and controlled dosing of low-viscosity fluids into the interior of the eye.

11.7 Balanced Salt Solution (BSS) as Irrigation Fluid for Intraocular Surgery

As early as the 1950s to 1960s, the originally used saline solutions were replaced by physiological buffered saline solutions ("balanced salt solution") due to their toxic effects. With the introduction of vitreoretinal surgery, attempts were made to better simulate the physiological composition of the vitreous body. This then led to the development of optimized BSS (e.g., commercially available as BSS plus® or Opeguard MA®), which, through the addition of bicarbonate, glucose, and the endogenous antioxidant glutathione, better corresponded to the composition of the human vitreous body and could show advantages in comparative studies [1].

BSS is also used in anterior chamber irrigation with device-controlled irrigation and aspiration (Chap. 20). Two paracenteses and a bimanual approach are common. For this, handpieces in the 23-gauge format, which are slightly curved, are mostly used. The irrigation handpiece has two lateral openings, and the aspiration handpiece has an opening near the tip, inside the convexity of the instrument. The accesses are preferably placed at 10 and 170°. This allows the surgeon to freely guide the two instruments with balanced ergonomics and a good view of the surgical field without the hands obstructing each other. Care must be taken to ensure that the cornea is not deformed during intraocular manipulation. This prevents the formation of Descemet folds as well as the gaping of the accesses and thus increased outflow of fluid from the anterior chamber. The stream of the irrigation fluid must not be directed against the endothelium, and the anterior chamber must not be collapsed by excessive aspiration (cf. Chap. 20).

11.8 Viscoelastics

In Table 11.3, the properties of the most commonly used viscoelastics are clearly summarized based on osmolarity, viscosity, elasticity, pseudoplasticity, and cohesion.

Physicochemical Properties

Osmolarity
Indicates the osmotic pressure on the tissue.
Measured in mOsm/l.
The values for fluids used in cataract surgery range from 270–340 mOsmol (isoosmotic).
If an intraocular fluid is hyperosmotic, thus above this aforementioned value, it leads to dehydration of the cornea (often mistakenly called "dehydration").
If an intraocular fluid is hypoosmotic, thus below this value, it results in swelling of the cornea and thus a stromal edema.

Viscosity
– Is the measure of the thickness of a fluid.
– Measured in mPa.s ("centistokes"; cs or centipoise (cps)).
– Changes with temperature.
The viscosity of substances used intraocularly ranges between 4000–200,000 cps.

Elasticity
This refers to the ability to restore the original shape after the application of external forces.
For intraocular use, the viscoelasticity of the substance is of essential importance, as after phacoemulsification, the viscosity and thus the protective effect must be restored.
All currently used intraocular viscoelastics possess the property of viscoelasticity.

Pseudoplasticity
This refers to the ability of a substance to transition from a gel state to less viscous states under shear forces.
Shear forces become effective in used viscoelastic fluids during:
– Manipulations with an instrument: 1–10 (1/sec),
– Irrigation: 10–100 (1/sec),
– Phacoemulsification: 100–300 (1/sec),
– Passage through the cannula: 1,000 (1/sec).

Table 11.3 Overview of viscoelastics in ophthalmic surgery

Viscoelastic substances used in ophthalmic surgery
Sodium salt of linear hyaluronic acid, originally obtained exclusively from rooster combs, now predominantly produced by biofermentation from bacterial strains (*Streptococcus equisimilis*, *Streptococcus pyogenes*, *Pasteurella multocida*) with different molecular weights
Hypromellose (hydroxypropyl methylcellulose, HPMC): Still the most commonly used variant because it is inexpensive
Chondroitin sulfate: No longer routinely used as an intraoperative fluid today, but mainly in dermatology

Cohesion

This refers to the ability of molecules to hold a substance together through true chemical bonds or intramolecular forces with mutual effects.

Long molecular chains intertwine and mix. This is characteristic of fluids with a high molecular weight.

Intraocular fluids with high cohesiveness have the advantage of being easy to aspirate intraoperatively, but they offer less protective effect for the tissue during phacoemulsification.

11.8.1 Task of Intraoperatively Used Viscoelastic Fluids

Since the endothelial cells of the cornea in adults do not have the ability to regenerate, the most important task of intraoperatively used viscoelastic fluids is to protect the cells and tissue during direct contact with instruments, the irrigation jet from the infusion or the cannula, the ultrasound energy, other noxae, and from deposits.

They coat the instruments and prevent the tissue from drying out during the surgery. The surgical area, such as the anterior chamber or the capsular bag, can be stabilized or expanded in terms of extension.

▶ Before use, the cannula should be completely free of air, as air bubbles can otherwise enter the surgical area and impair visibility intraoperatively.

Viscoelastics help in the positioning of objects such as an artificial lens. They enable the repositioning and stabilization of the vitreous body, which cannot be instrumentally grasped in the event of a capsular rupture or lens dislocation. Prolapsed iris can be gently pushed back with their help.

▶ Especially in these situations, viscoelastics prove to be the gentlest instrument!

Other applications (although much less common) include the dissolution of synechiae, stopping of bleeding, assistance in the removal of the lens nucleus or cortex, and support in keratoplasties to protect the corneal endothelium.

Viscoelastic fluids can be used pre-corneally, in the anterior and posterior chambers, as well as for coating intraocular lenses.

Dispersive fluids, i.e., those with very low cohesion and a tendency to overlay the tissue, are more difficult to remove from the eye.

▶ It is important to ensure that viscoelastic substances are removed from the eye as completely as possible, as otherwise extreme postoperative intraocular pressure spikes can result!

11.9 Storage Recommendations

Most viscoelastic, intraocularly usable substances based on hyaluronic acid must be stored cool, as prolonged storage at room temperature (more than a week) can lead to a decrease in viscosity.

▶ It is recommended to take the viscoelastic out of the refrigerator only on the day of use [2–4].

11.9.1 Air

The use of air may be necessary in various surgical steps to gently separate two tissues, such as an atonic iris from the posterior surface of the cornea. It is used to stabilize a preformed space, such as the anterior chamber, while a wound is being closed with a suture. It also serves to keep fluid away from tissue structures, such as dye from the posterior surface of the cornea.

▶ Air must be drawn through a sterile microfilter to ensure sterility and freedom from particles.

11.9.2 Dyes

Brilliant Blue G

This is a synthetic dye used as a food additive and for marking protein bands in biochemistry. It is approved for the intraoperative staining of the lens capsule and also for use in vital staining in posterior segment surgery. Almost no toxic effects have been demonstrated at moderate staining intensity [5].

Trypan Blue (TB)

The anionic diazo dye was first described by Paul Ehrlich in 1904. **Trypan Blue** is used, for example, in vitality tests ("live dead assay") because it can only penetrate the cell membrane of dead cells due to its high molecular weight. This effect is also used on ocular tissue, for example, to evaluate donor corneas. Regarding biocompatibility in living organisms, liver cell damage has been known since the 1940s (with TB 0.5%); there is also teratogenic potential. Intraocularly, TB has been used since the 1990s for staining the anterior lens capsule to make it visible in mature cataracts, and it has been used in vitreoretinal surgery for about several years. The usual clinically used concentrations in vitreoretinal surgery are normally between 0.6 mg/ml and 1.5 mg/ml. However, significant toxic effects on different retinal cells have also been demonstrated for TB, partly at clinically used concentrations. The neurosensory retina appears to be more sensitive to TB than the retinal pigment epithelium [6].

▶ Dyes should be used very carefully. Before introducing them into the anterior chamber, the endothelium should be protected by an air bubble to counteract toxic damage from a surgical perspective as well.

11.10 Medications that Affect Pupil Size

Intraoperative pharmacological influence on pupil size is often necessary in intraocular surgery.

Acetylcholine Chloride (Miochol)

For pupil constriction, it is usually sufficient to introduce a small volume of **acetylcholine** as a 1% solution into the anterior chamber. It then works by directly stimulating the M. sphincter pupillae. With appropriate local application using a fine cannula, pupil constriction can even be preferentially induced in certain sectors. However, if the cholinoceptors on the effector cells were previously blocked by anticholinergic substances (tropicamide, homatropine, scopolamine, atropine), the responsiveness to acetylcholine is reduced [7]. The solution must be freshly prepared. The medication should be dissolved in the supplied mannitol and should only be applied using the supplied filter. No more than a total of 2 ml should be used, as it can lead to sphincter atrophy. Very sensitive patients may experience bradycardia and breathing difficulties with constrictions in the bronchial system.

Adrenaline (English: Epinephrine), Mydrane® (0.2 mg tropicamide, 3.1 mg phenylephrine hydrochloride, and 10 mg lidocaine hydrochloride)

For pupil dilation in the opened eye, sympathomimetics such as **adrenaline** and **phenylephrine** (Neo-Synephrine) are considered. However, after instillation of adrenaline in the usual dilution of 1:1000, clinical permanent damage to the corneal endothelium has been observed and confirmed in animal experiments. The harmful component here appears to be the sodium disulfite added to the adrenaline as a stabilizer. Therefore, a dilution to 1:5000 is recommended, especially if endothelial "weakness" is already apparent preoperatively. The local anesthetics mixed in the case of Mydrane can also be damaging to the endothelium.

However, **endogenous substances** can also affect pupil size during a surgical procedure due to mechanical iris irritation. They can individually counteract applied sympathomimetics and parasympatholytics [7].

Very sensitive patients may develop tachycardia, cardiac arrhythmias, and hypertension.

Tissue Plasminogen Activator

The "recombinant tissue-type plasminogen activator" (rTPA) is used intraocularly for the treatment of persistent fibrin membranes with good tolerance. In the anterior segment of the eye, 25 µg rTPA (Actilyse) is introduced into the anterior chamber. A reduction in fibrin is sometimes only gradual. Postoperatively, manageable minor bleeding may occur, and very rarely, localized corneal opacities.

Anesthetics

Procedures in the anterior chamber of the eye can very often be performed using a combination of drop anesthesia and intraocularly applied local anesthetic. The use of 0.15 ml lidocaine 1% has proven to be uncritical in terms of endothelial damage and effective in terms of pain relief, even in cataract surgery. The aforementioned Mydrane has also proven effective.

▶ Any manipulation of the iris should be avoided, as this form of anesthesia often does not provide sufficient pain relief.

Antibiotics

Before administration, the user should be clear about the indication or the antibiogram and the corresponding indication. Concentration and volumes must be strictly defined, as significant tissue damage, particularly to the corneal endothelium, can otherwise occur. It should be noted once again that a required volume can only be left after the corresponding removal of an equivalent amount (Chap. 18).

References and Further Reading

1. Thaler S, Haritoglou C, Schuettauf F (2013) Neuroprotektive Ansätze. Ophthalmologe 110:941–947
2. Auffarth GU (2001) Viskoelastische Substanzen in der Opthalmochirurgie. Uni-med, Bremen-London-Boston
3. Kuhn F (2016) Vitreoretinal surgery, strategies and tactics. Springer, Bremen-London-Boston
4. Meyer-Schwickerath G (1984) Viskochirurgie des Auges. Enke, Bremen-London-Boston
5. Gerding H (2009) [Aktueller Stand der Entwicklung und Anwendung von Farb- und Markierungsstoffen für die vitreoretinale Chirurgie]. Klin Monatsbl Augenheilkd 226:220–223
6. Thaler S, Schüttauf F, Haritoglou C (2009) Biokompatibilität von Farbstoffen für die vitreoretinale Chirurgie. Ophthalmologe 106:11–15
7. Mackensen G, Neubauer H (1988) Augenarztliche Operationen. Springer, Bremen-London-Boston

Basics of Suturing and Knotting in Ophthalmic Surgery

12

Frank Wilhelm, Erik Chankiewitz and Uwe Wilhelm

Contents

With the introduction of clear cornea phacoemulsification, corneal suturing became unnecessary. In refractive surgical procedures and intravitreal operative drug administrations (IVOM), suturing is required only in exceptional cases. Even with the new techniques of lamellar keratoplasty and trocar-guided pars plana vitrectomy, sutures are hardly necessary anymore. Fortunately, the number of eyeball injuries requiring corneal sutures has steadily decreased over the past decades. Consequently, despite the increase in surgical procedures in ophthalmology in recent decades, the proportion of operations requiring sutures under the microscope has decreased.

Due to this development, there are few opportunities for the aspiring ophthalmic surgeon to gain experience in suturing under the microscope in clinical routine. Nevertheless, he must strive to learn this skill. Possessing it is particularly important in the rare but often complicated situations!

- ▶ Correct suturing and knotting are prerequisites for secure wound closure

This article presents basic rules and provides tips on how to perform suturing in ophthalmic surgical procedures.

- ▶ Every step of a procedure requires careful planning!

In preparing for each operation, the surgeon must first develop a plan of what needs to be done.

- ▶ The basic rule always applies that "as much as necessary and as little as possible". Often, the best procedure is the one that does not need to be performed at all!

F. Wilhelm (✉)
Universitätsklinikum Halle Saale, Greifswald, Germany

E. Chankiewitz
Augenklinik, Städtisches Klinikum Braunschweig gGmbH, Braunschweig, Germany
e-mail: erik@chankiewitz.de

U. Wilhelm
MVZ Roswitha und Daniel Krause, Dortmund, Germany

F. Wilhelm (ed.), *Ophthalmic Surgery for Beginners*, https://doi.org/10.1007/978-3-662-70287-1_12

For example, in the case of a corneal wound with a lamellar configuration, suturing can often be avoided by using a contact lens. This prevents scar formation with additional fibrosis in the suture area.

In addition to surgical textbooks that explain the various procedures in detail but contain little about suture techniques and the possible problems, courses and wet labs are offered for aspiring ophthalmic surgeons to practice these (Sect. 7.2). In the operating room, tips and tricks are often conveyed by the mentoring surgeon depending on the situation.

▶ Tips from an experienced surgical nurse on handling suture material and instruments should not be neglected!

Even though the surgical assistant usually hands the needle holder to the surgeon already loaded with the needle, the surgeon must be able to remove the needle with the thread intact from the packaging. It is necessary for every surgeon to familiarize themselves with the range of suture materials and available instruments in the clinic before a procedure (Chaps. 5 and 6).

12.1 Suitable Suture Material

Various suture material manufacturers recommend specific threads and needles for each indication (see Chap. 6). However, it has been shown that implementation can vary significantly depending on the experiences of individual surgeons, including their preferred instruments, the chosen surgical technique, and the tissue to be sutured [10].

12.1.1 Skin, Conjunctiva, and Tenon

In well-vascularized tissues such as skin and conjunctiva, the healing process is completed after a few days. When suturing the conjunctiva, special care must be taken to ensure that the cut edges, which often roll in due to their inherent elasticity, are brought out with the teeth of the fine forceps and accurately aligned by the sutures. For beginners, single button sutures are recommended here [11]. To prevent postoperative disturbances from prominent knots, the knot should be tried to submerge. This means the first stitch is made from bottom to top in the loose part and then from top to bottom in the firm part. The connective tissue Tenon beneath the conjunctiva should be carefully considered during wound adaptation. With skillful needle guidance, it can often be grasped simultaneously with the conjunctival suture and sewn without gaps.

12.1.2 Cornea

In the avascular cornea, wound healing proceeds differently and more slowly. Corneal wounds primarily adhere through fibrin, provided the wound edges are cleanly adapted. If the wound closure is not performed correctly, complications such as fistulas, infections, and epithelial implantation may occur due to wound dehiscence [3].

12.2 Suturing

The following provides important tips regarding the correct suture technique.

12.2.1 Practice the Hand Knot and the Instrument Knot

In the operating room, the ophthalmologist must be able to quickly and securely tie a knot in any situation. Therefore, it is advisable for beginners to practice the individual steps with a piece of string before performing the first suture on a patient. While the surgical knot involves tying with the fingertips, which can also be done semi-instrumentally if necessary, the instrument knot using needle holders and/or tying forceps has become established under the operating microscope due to the limited visibility.

- Due to the limited surgical field that the surgeon sees through the microscope, it is absolutely necessary to ensure a secure grip of the needle in the needle holder to achieve a safe guidance for gentle suturing with the lowest possible penetration force.

12.2.2 Needle Holder and Needle

Suturing begins with the selection of the needle holder and the clamping of the needle. For corneal and conjunctival sutures, needle holders without a lock have become established in ophthalmology. Many surgeons prefer curved needle holders. In this case, the needle must be grasped so that the convex curvature of the needle holder and the needle tip point in the same direction and the needle forms a right angle with the curve of the needle holder. This allows the needle to be guided precisely and securely during tissue penetration.

In special situations, it may be necessary to clamp the needle at an angle (Fig. 12.1). In these cases, the needle can only be securely grasped for suturing with a straight needle holder.

If the needle is accidentally grasped at the tip area during clamping, it results in damage to the tip, making it blunt and hindering gentle tissue penetration.

- In case of improper handling, for example, after touching or bumping the needle tip, bead-like thickening can be observed under the operating microscope (Fig. 12.2). In this case, it is strongly advised to replace the damaged needle!

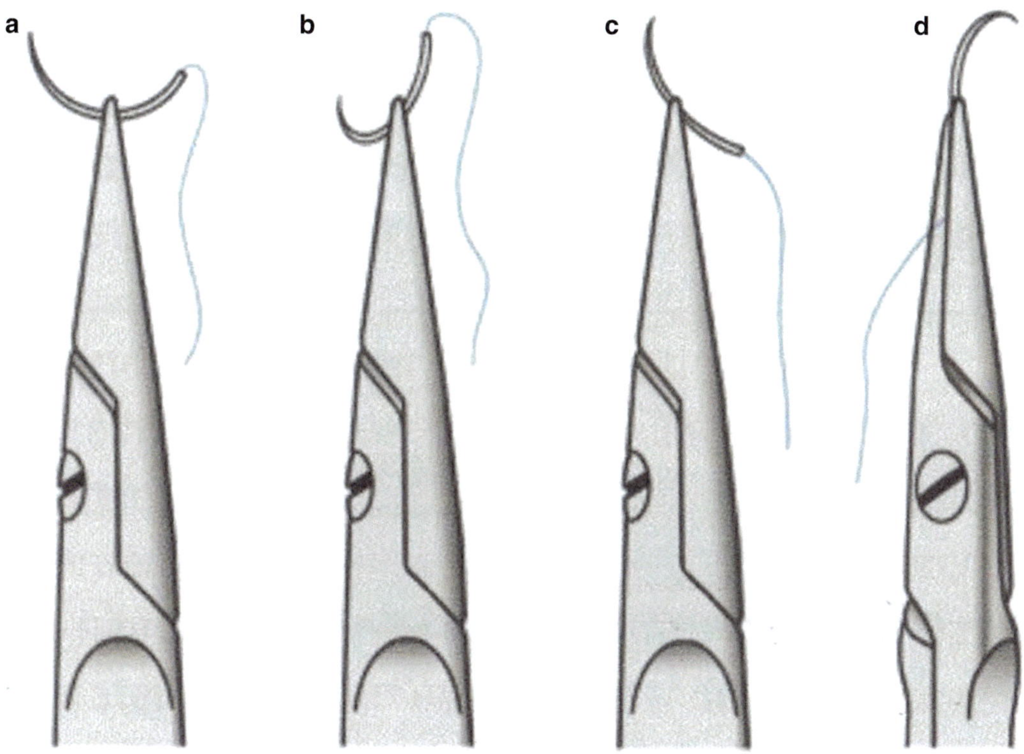

Fig. 12.1 The needle must form a right angle with the guiding line of the needle holder (**a**) to guide the needle precisely and securely during tissue penetration. In special situations, it may be necessary to clamp the needle at an angle (**b–d**). (Mod. after 2)

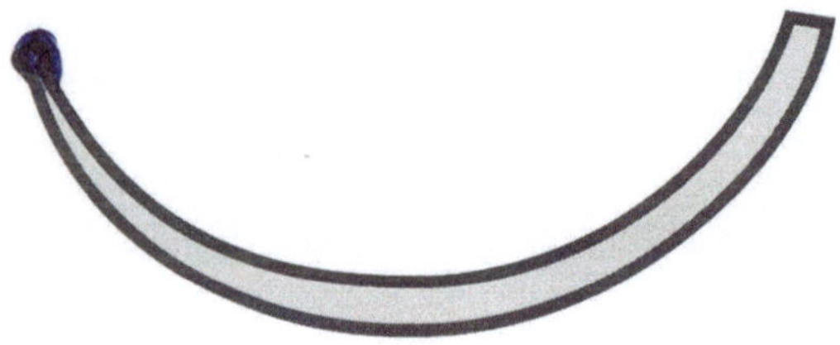

Fig. 12.2 Bead-like thickening results from damage to the needle tip

Grasping the needle too far at the proximal, round end leads to twisting and can cause bending or even breaking during the suturing process. It is recommended to clamp it at the transition to the rear third (Fig. 12.3), but the optimal point for grasping the needle also depends on the curvature, bending and breaking strength, and the consistency of the tissue to be sutured.

- The firmer the consistency of the tissue to be sutured, the closer to the middle the needle must be clamped.

12.2.3 Fundamentals of Microsurgical Suturing

During the suturing process, the penetration is dictated by the curvature of the needle. Since suturing is generally done "towards oneself," the needle is held in the "forehand" position. It is distinguished whether the surgeon is suturing with the left or right hand. The supination of the surgeon's hand results in an arched movement that follows the curvature of the needle, allowing the tissue to be penetrated gently with minimal pressure and without significant deformation (Fig. 12.4).

In selected situations, it may be necessary to suture "away from oneself." For this, the needle is held in the backhand position, and the arched movement is performed through the pronation of the hand. (This approach is necessary, for example, when suturing corneal transplants.)

- Care must be taken to pierce perpendicular to the wound edge to avoid shifting the wound surfaces and distorting the tissue when tightening the knot.

It has proven effective to first pierce the needle through only one edge of the wound and then release the needle so that the needle tip indicates the direction in which the thread must be guided through the second wound lip to achieve an exact adaptation of the opposing fixation points (Fig. 12.5).

Then, the needle is grasped again behind the tip and precisely pierced through the second wound lip in the predetermined direction. This approach is generally recommended for beginners and for experienced surgeons in difficult initial situations with swollen corneal stroma, as it results in a secure and precise wound closure and minimizes the extent of suture-induced astigmatism.

An exception is the double continuous diagonal suture in penetrating keratoplasty according

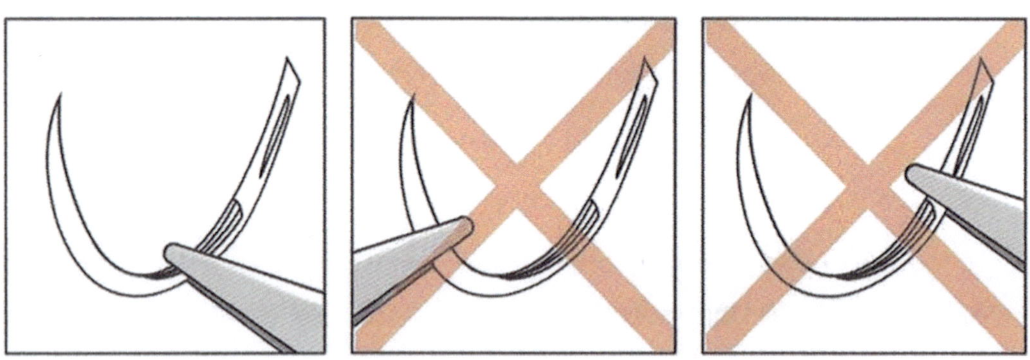

Fig. 12.3 It is recommended to grasp the needle between the middle and rear third of the curve

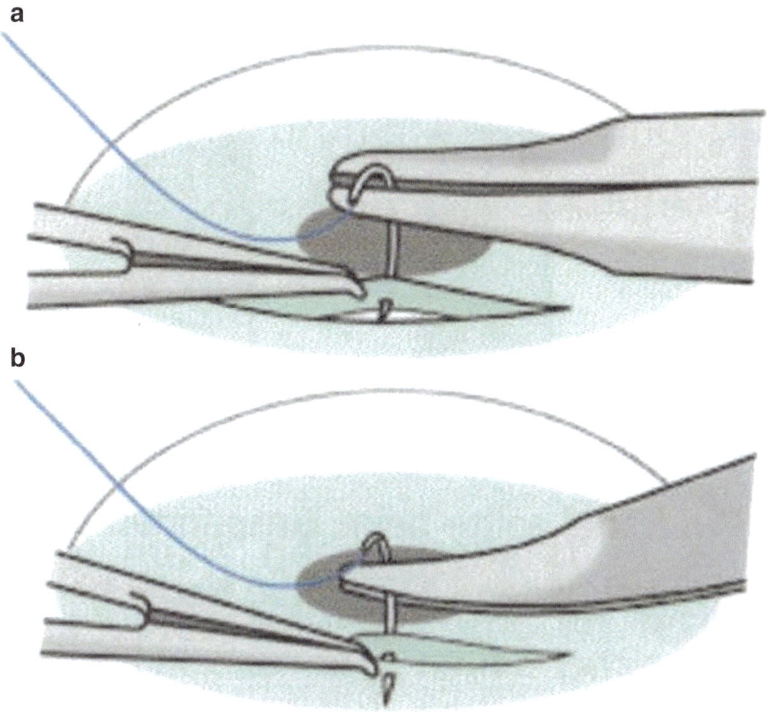

Fig. 12.4 The suturing movement follows the needle curvature: (**a**) vertical insertion of the needle tip, (**b**) gentle penetration of the tissue through the arched supination movement of the surgeon with the needle

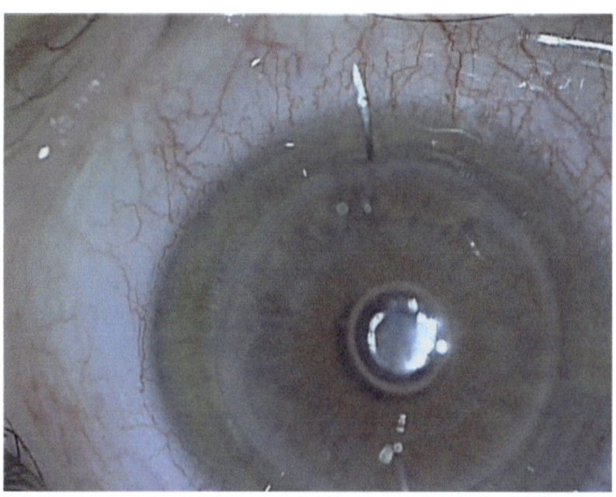

Fig. 12.5 The needle is pierced through the first wound lip and then released by the needle holder to indicate the direction in which the suture must be guided through the second wound lip, ensuring that there is no shifting of the wound edges against each other after the knot is tied

to Hoffmann [7]. In this case, the needle is pierced in and out at an angle to the wound edge. The guidance of the two sutures, one running superficially and the other deep, results in a clean adaptation without gaping.

For individual sutures on the cornea, it is important that the wound edges are adapted at the same depth with the opposite side (Fig. 12.6). The extent of the inner wound gap depends on the depth of the suture guidance.

For this purpose, the surgeon can enlarge the image under the operating microscope as needed so that the boundary between the stroma and the Descemet's membrane is clearly visible in depth. The needle can then be controlled to pierce in and out closely in front of it, achieving a secure wound closure over the entire corneal thickness.

- Since gaping wounds on the eye surface are filled with granulation tissue and often colonized by bacteria, incomplete adaptation results in fistulas and step formations, which can cause a foreign body sensation with subsequent

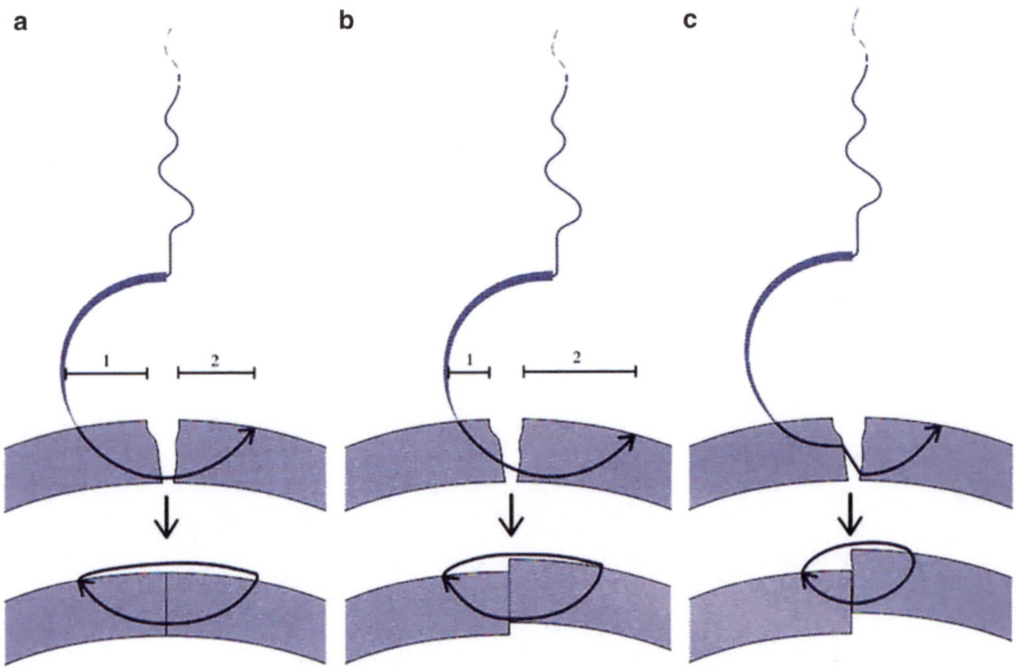

Fig. 12.6 Exact adaptation of opposing wound edges deep lamellar before the DM (**a**) ensures a tight wound closure, which is not the case with different stitch distances (**b**) or penetration depths (**c**). (Mod. after 9)

vascularization in the patient and induce higher astigmatism!

12.2.4 The limbus suture is started first!

Before closing any wound, it must be clarified at which point the suturing will begin. In the case of a cornea-sclera wound due to an injury, the first suture must always be the limbus suture [12]. After that, it can be decided how many sutures will likely be needed. These should be distributed successively according to the wound course to arrange the distances between the individual sutures in such a way that no tissue overlap results [4]. Distortions and folds of the wound edges, which mainly affect the cosmetic result on the skin, cause significant astigmatism on the cornea.

Beginners in ophthalmic surgery should definitely opt for single button sutures again: interrupted on the cornea, the conjunctiva and on the skin.

- It is important to arrange the stitches in such a way that a secure wound closure is achieved with as few sutures as possible (Fig. 12.7).

- With increasing experience, the single button sutures can then be replaced by continuous

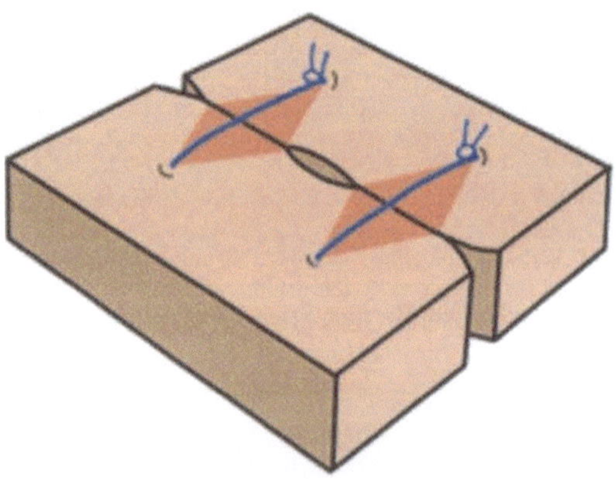

Fig. 12.7 When adapted by EKN, the wound edges are sealed only in the area compressed by the suture. Leaks can result in between! (Mod. after 4)

or cross sutures. In the case of swollen and jagged wound edges, it may be necessary to temporarily place individual sutures as "assembly aids" or situational sutures to better place the final adaptation threads afterward. Subsequently, the situational sutures should be removed again. Especially when placing several single button sutures with the same direction of pull, loosening of previously placed threads can occur after the corneal stroma has de-swollen. In this case, it must be decided which suture needs to be replaced.

12.3 Knots

When tying a knot, some basic rules must be observed. The thread ends must be sufficiently long to form the knot at all. The length of the longer thread end required to execute the knot and grasp the short end depends on the number of planned turns (Fig. 12.8).

The second thread end should, if possible, not be too long, as loops can form when pulling through, which can tighten and may not be easily loosened. The short thread end is grasped with the needle holder, then the long end is wound around the instrument, and the short thread end is pulled through the loop resulting from the winding [6]. To practice the movement sequence for the instrument knot, dry exercises on suitable models are recommended (Fig. 12.9).

- The needle itself must not be used to tie the knot! It should be placed within the microscope field so that it does not need to be searched for after cutting.

- When tying with instruments, special care must be taken to ensure that the edges of the needle holder and forceps are smooth, as otherwise the vulnerable thread can easily be damaged. This is especially important

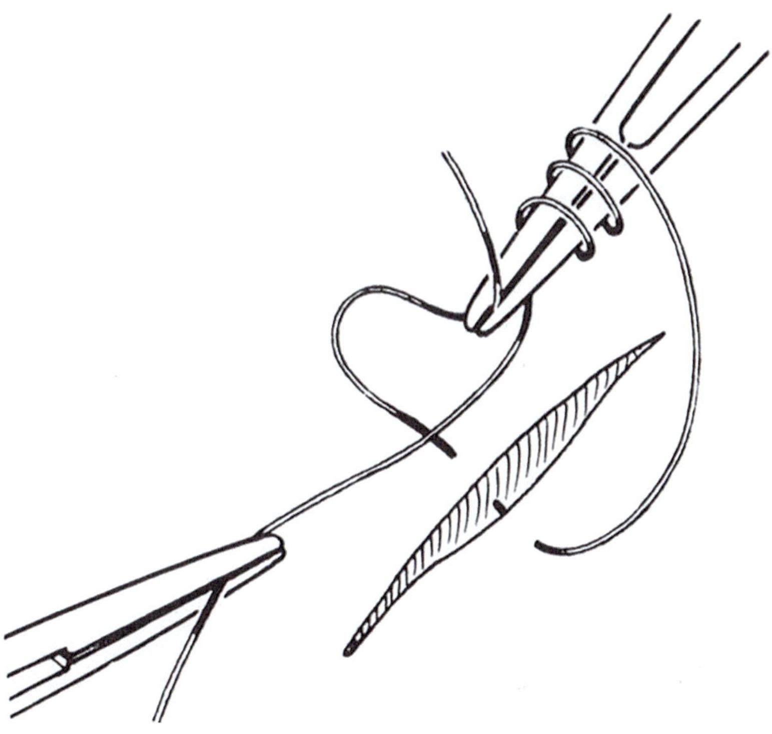

Fig. 12.8 When tying with instruments, the thread ends must be sufficiently long to form the knot at all!

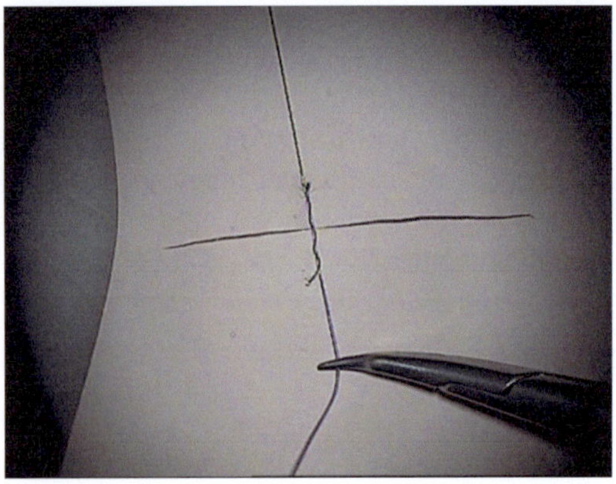

Fig. 12.9 The movement sequence for the instrument knot can be practiced on the model in the dry lab

when very thin monofilament suture material is used. Monofilament threads should never be stretched too much, as they can twist and possibly break.

Depending on the direction in which the thread is looped during the execution of the second winding, a "granny knot" or a "reef knot" is formed [1]. While the reef knot usually adapts the wound edges very stably through two individual loops, the granny knot leaves the possibility open that it can be tightened even more after forming the second throw (Fig. 12.10). The reef knot is also known from sailing as a square knot [5], in which the two overlapping thread windings lock each other.

12.3.1 The First Knot

The first knot should be placed exactly as a surgical knot in a double winding to increase the friction between the thread loops and thus counteract the separation of the wound edges due to tissue tension. This knot must always be tightened in the "running direction" of the loop. Then it must be checked whether the tension is sufficient or whether the wound edges distance themselves from each other again due to tissue tension.

- If the wound edges gape apart, one end of the thread can be passed under the opposing thread again to achieve an additional winding. This is gentler than reopening and relooping the knot.

At this point, the question arises as to how many windings are necessary for the knot at all.

12.3.2 Number of Windings

The number of windings depends on both the type of suture material and the tension of the tissue to be sutured. With high tissue tension and monofilament material, more windings are necessary for a tight wound adaptation.

In principle, a knot should be tied with the smallest possible number of windings to make

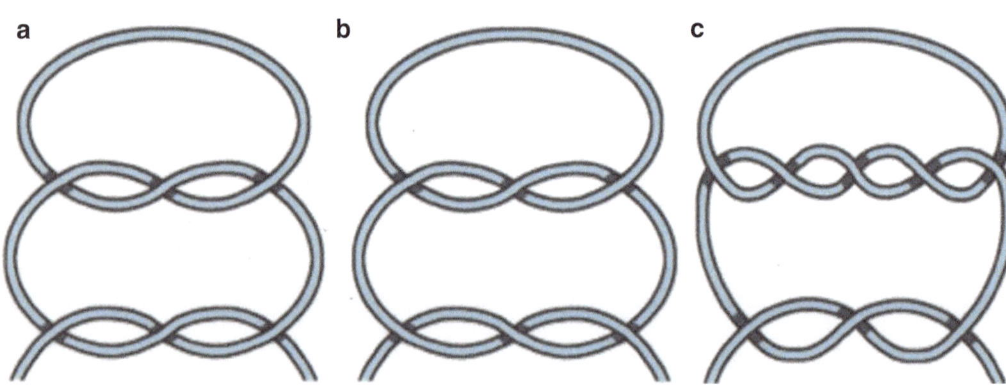

Fig. 12.10 **a**,**b** **a** Granny knot. **b** Square knot. **c** Surgical knot. (Mod. after 1)

it overall smaller. This is not significant for skin sutures that are removed early. However, large knots on the conjunctiva and cornea lead to pain and blepharospasm due to the foreign body irritation and are often not tolerated by patients.

12.3.3 Smooth or Overhand Knot

When forming the knot, a distinction is made between a smooth knot and an overhand knot in the first winding (Fig. 12.11). If the threads are not tightened in the running direction, the knot overhands and slides on the second thread end (Fig. 12.12).

▶ In principle, the two consecutive loops of a knot should differ by only one winding (Fig. 12.10), otherwise it overhands when tightened and does not hold. However, the knot becomes bulkier due to the increased use of suture material, which is why it is also recommended to deviate from this rule for corneal sutures if necessary [8].

12.3.4 Burying the Knot

Corneal threads should be buried. Therefore, it is necessary to design the knot particularly carefully here, to tighten it securely, and to cut the thread ends as short as possible. This is best achieved by cutting the tightly held monofilament thread close to the knot. It is broken over the edge of a microscalpel (Fig. 12.13). In doing so, the surgeon can precisely determine the distance to the knot, whereas when using scissors, the knot may be obscured by the branches of this instrument, making it difficult to accurately estimate the length of the thread ends at the knot.

▶ This approach is recommended exclusively for monofilament sutures to shorten the ends with a single, controlled action.

When using multifilament suture material on the skin and conjunctiva, this makes little sense, as the thread would otherwise split into its individual fibers. Here, a suitable pair of scissors should be preferred (Fig. 12.14).

When sinking the knots into the corneal tissue, care should be taken to ensure that the threads can be removed as gently as possible later. Therefore, after the knot has been rotated into the deeper stroma, it is then rotated back up to just below the surface. This aligns the thread ends in the direction of pull, whereas if this retraction is omitted, they act like small barbs that, after fibrosis has formed around the knot, make it difficult to remove the threads at a later time (Fig. 12.15).

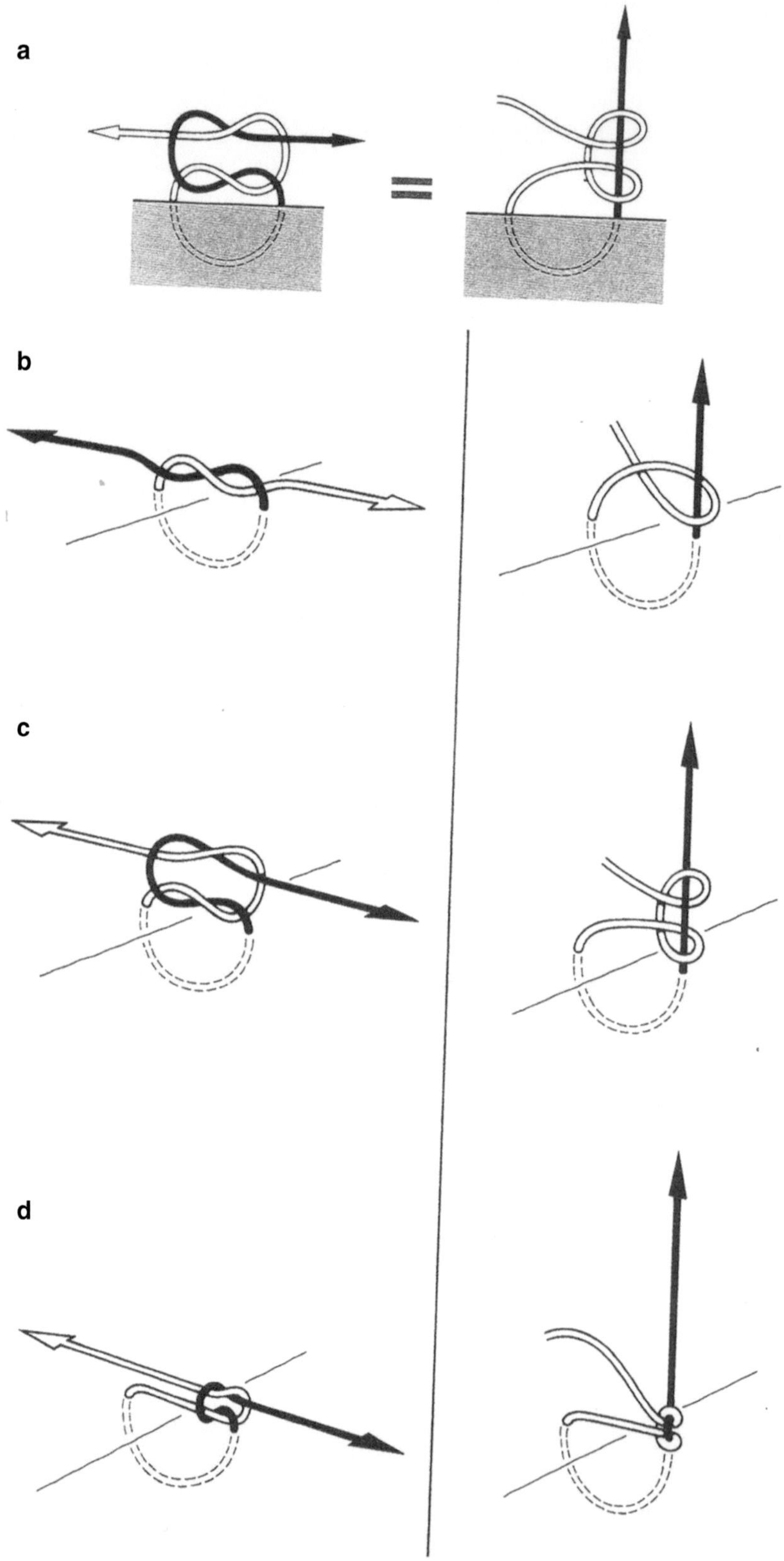

Fig. 12.11 (**a**–**d**) left side smooth/square knot, right side overhand knot. (Mod. after 4)

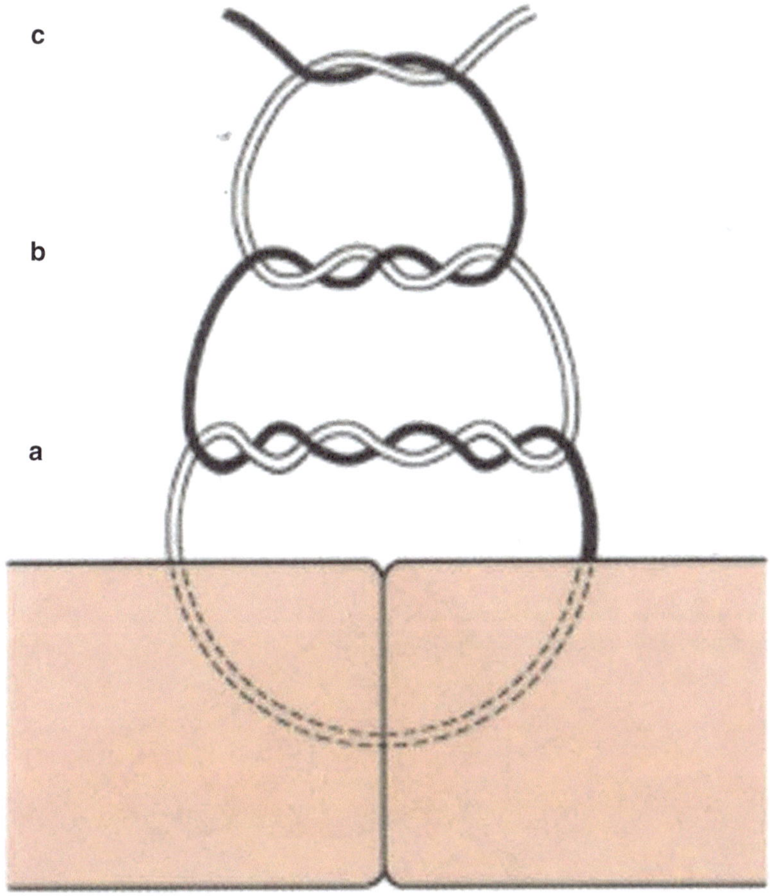

Fig. 12.12 **a–c** With monofilament suture material, an additional securing loop **c** follows the adaptation knot **a** and the securing loop **b**. (Mod. after 4)

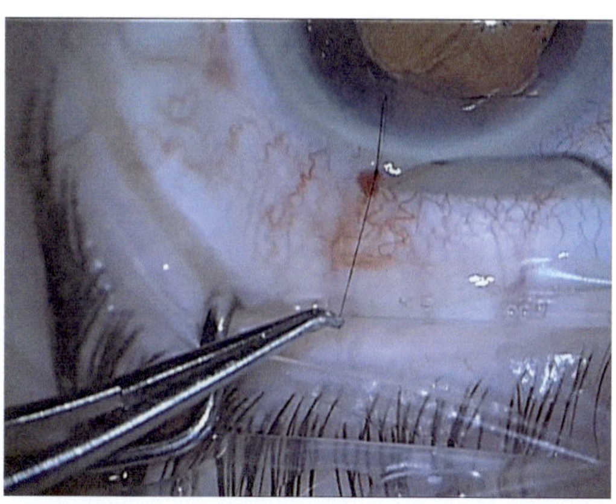

Fig. 12.13 To break the monofilament suture close to the knot over the edge of the microscalpel, the thread must be held tightly!

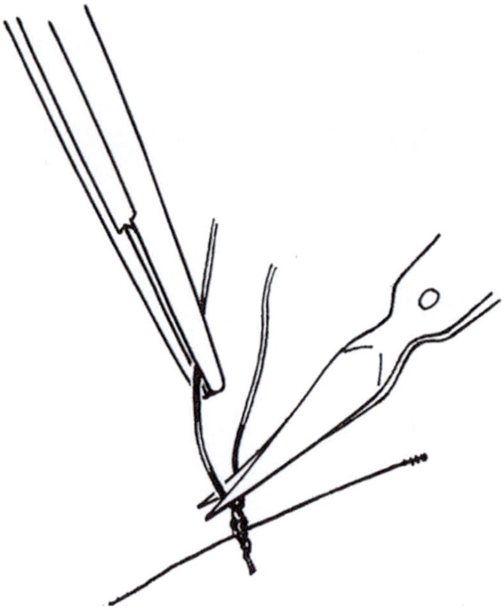

Fig. 12.14 The shortening of the thread ends to the appropriate length is done with scissors for skin and conjunctival sutures

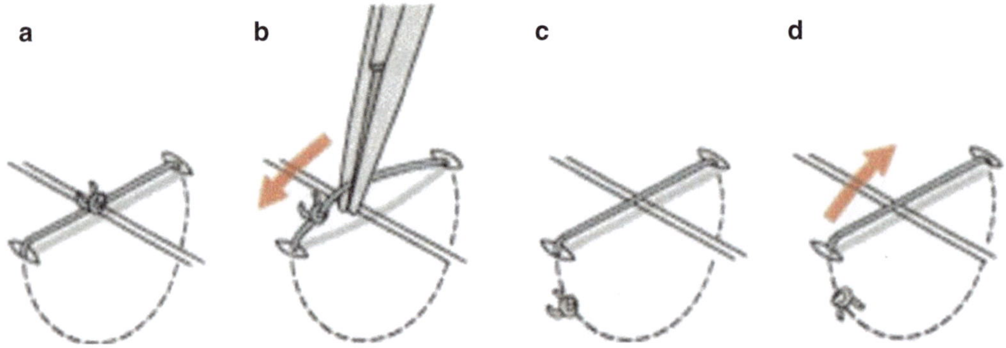

Fig. 12.15 **a–c** After tying, the knot is tightened **a** and rotated into the corneal stroma **b**. This aligns the thread ends so that they act like barbs **c**, which, particularly due to fibrosis after remodeling processes during wound healing, makes it difficult to remove the knots. Therefore, the knots are rotated back up to just below the corneal surface by pulling the thread in the opposite direction, aligning the ends in such a way (**d**) that the thread along with the knot can be more easily removed

References and Further Reading

1. Becker T (1989) Kurzgefasster Operationskurs. Johann Ambrosius Barth Leipzig. 315 S
2. Castroviejo R (1968) Keratoplastik. Thieme, Stuttgart, p 453 S
3. Domarus v D et al (1996) Trauma, Operationen und Wundheilung des Auges. In: Naumann GOH (Eds) Pathologie des Auges, Band I, pp 301–377. Springer, Berlin
4. Eisner G (1978) Augenchirurgie. Einführung in die operative Technik. Springer, Berlin
5. Friedrichsen W (1986) Das Segelhandbuch. Hoffmann und Campe, Hamburg

6. Harms H, Mackensen G (1966) Augenoperationen unter dem Mikroskop. Thieme, Stuttgart
7. Hoffmann F (1976) Nahttechnik bei perforierender Keratoplastik. Klin Monatsbl Augenheilkd 169:584–590
8. Kuhn F (2008) Ocular Traumatology. Springer, Berlin
9. Rohrbach M, et al. (2002) „Ophthalmologische Traumatologie". Textbuch und Atlas. Schattauer Stuttgart – New York. 434 S
10. Schargus M (2017) Einführung in die Ophthalmochirurgie, Teil 1: Nahtmaterial und Instrumentarium – was nehme ich wozu? Ophthalmo-Chirurgie 29:127–138
11. Sundmacher R et al (1988) Chirurgie der Konjunktiva und Sklera. In: Mackensen G, Neubauer H (Eds) Augenärztliche Operationen Teil 1, Springer, Berlin, pp 333–382
12. Viestenz A et al (2018) Einführung in die Ophthalmochirurgie, Teil 9: Verletzungen des Auges – was ist zu tun bei der Erstversorgung? Ophthalmo-Chirurgie 30:317–324

Incision Techniques in Ophthalmic Surgery

13

Jens Heichel and Thomas Hammer

Contents

In order to operate on the surface of the eye (conjunctiva) as well as intraocularly, the most precise planning possible is required. What is the goal of the procedure, and what interventions might still be necessary subsequently? These questions must be asked before every operation, but especially when operating on the surface of the eye (Chap. 15).

Through various incisions, the surgeon can gain access to the anterior segment of the eye (anterior chamber). For this, it is also absolutely necessary to have a thorough thought process about the course of the operation in advance, with a clear definition of the objective of the surgical intervention.

Modern cataract surgery is increasingly seamless and shows a clear trend towards minimally invasive procedures. Accordingly, the smallest possible incisions in the corneal area are preferred, whereas older access techniques with scleral preparation techniques have somewhat unjustly fallen into oblivion. The aim is to achieve sufficient wound closure and induce the lowest possible postoperative astigmatism while still ensuring convenient surgical handling.

13.1 Incision Techniques in the Conjunctiva

The main indications for surgery in the conjunctival area are tumor excisions, wound closures after trauma, and pterygium removals. Larger operations, such as reconstruction in cases of symblepharon, are to be excluded here (Chap. 15).

J. Heichel (✉)
Klinik und Poliklinik für Augenheilkunde, Universitätsklinikum Halle/Saale, Halle/Saale, Germany
e-mail: jens.heichel@uk-halle.de

T. Hammer
Klinik und Poliklinik für Augenheilkunde, Universitätsklinikum Halle/Saale, Martin-Luther-Universität Halle-Wittenberg, Halle/Saale, Germany

Augenarztpraxis, Augenzentrum "Frohe Zukunft", Halle/Saale, Germany
e-mail: thomas.hammer@uk-halle.de

F. Wilhelm (ed.), *Ophthalmic Surgery for Beginners*, https://doi.org/10.1007/978-3-662-70287-1_13

▶ In advance, the surgical area must be examined using a slit lamp microscope to detect changes in the conjunctiva. This includes postoperative conditions (Cave: bleb after glaucoma surgery) as well as pathological changes in the context of infectious or inflammatory pathologies (Cave: pemphigoid).

In principle, the conjunctiva has good wound healing properties. Reasons for this include its rich vascularization and regenerative epithelium. Nevertheless, the tissue of the conjunctiva is limited, so tissue-sparing and careful surgery is essential. The preparation is done with scissors (e.g., Westcott or Vanas), as vessel compressions for hemostasis can already be achieved during the incision proces (Chaps. 2, 5 and 15).

The good mobility and elastic connection to the surface of the eyeball via the Tenon's capsule can be helpful. Thus, the subconjunctival injection of anesthetics significantly facilitates the preparation and also provides an option for postoperative pain prophylaxis.

Fine surgical forceps can be used for preparation. In some cases, the use of swabs is sufficient and ensures better protection of the mucosa. An eyelid speculum allows the surgical field to be held open. If preparation near the conjunctival fornices is necessary, temporary sutures can be used to rotate the eyeball.

13.1.1 Incision Technique

The conjunctiva does not have classic tension lines. Nevertheless, radial wound courses in the lid fissure area are favorable, as they are compressed by blinking and are less exposed to shear forces during horizontal eye movements.

By gently lifting with surgical forceps and forming a conjunctival fold, the incision can be made with scissors. Subsequently, the small access is suitable for blunt dissection to facilitate further wound opening. The small scissors can be used to enter the pocket thus created to continue the incision.

13.2 Access Routes to the Anterior Segment of the Eye

Operations in the anterior segment of the eye are considered common interventions in ophthalmic surgery. Not only in the context of cataract surgery, but also for acute pressure relief, medication administration, or diagnostic aqueous humor sampling, paracenteses are necessary. Other frequently performed interventions in this area include DMEK (Descemet Membrane Endothelial Keratoplasty), ab interno canaloplasty, glaucoma stent implantation, or refractive procedures (Chap. 20).

A selection of various microsurgical scalpels, which are used in anterior segment surgery, is shown in Fig. 13.1. Table 13.1 provides an overview of the characteristics of corneal and sclerocorneal incisions (Figs. 13.2 and 13.3).

▶ Before performing a procedure in the anterior chamber of the eye, knowledge of the existing corneal architecture, including thickness ratios and anterior chamber depth, is essential.

13.2.1 Localization of the Incision

In advance, it must be clear what the access will ultimately be used for. If it is merely for medication administration or a puncture of the anterior chamber of the eye for sample collection, the simple preference of the surgeon regarding their handedness can also be considered.

▶ Fixation with a surgical forceps (Kolibri) when entering the eyeball should be done exactly oppositely (from the opposite side) to avoid rotation of the eyeball.

Furthermore, the surgeon must be clear about where the most indeal location for entering the AC is. If tissue or a foreign body is to be retrieved from the anterior chamber, it is often necessary to choose the access from the opposite

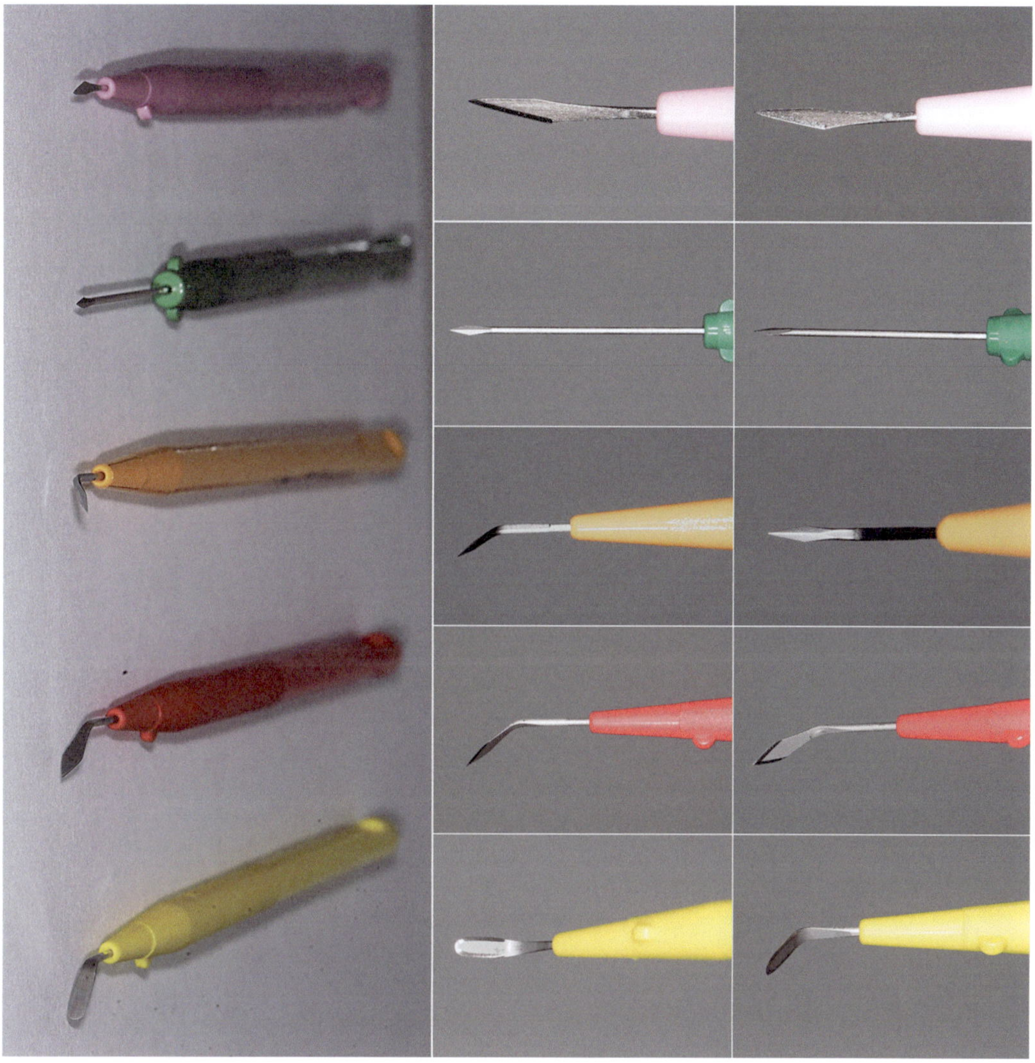

Fig. 13.1 Microsurgical blades for anterior segment surgery (overview on the left; detailed images at different angles). **Pink:**15° paracentesis knife. **Green:**20-gauge lance in a straight design (for vitreoretinal infusion openings or paracentesis incisions in the cornea with a cut width of 1.18 mm). **Orange:** 20-gauge lance in an angled design. **Red:**Phaco lance with a 45° bend and a cut width of 2.4 mm. **Yellow:**Tunnel knife with a 45° bend and a width of 2.0 mm for lamellar preparations

side or at a right angle. The same consideration applies if two entry sites are to be created, which are ultimately to be used via a bimanual system (irrigation/aspiration). Here, it is usually sensible to choose the distance between both incisions to be approximately 150 to 180 degrees apart (e.g., 3 o'clock/9 o'clock position).

As a basic rule, it is advisable to incise as peripherally as possible. The border to the vascularized limbus region to the clear cornea is suitable. Some bleeding may occur. The advantage of this peripheral approach is that the optical axis is less affected. Additionally, the access is largely astigmatism-neutral and, due to the vascularization, promises more secure wound healing.

Finally, the surface tissue of the eye must also be considered. If there is already a significant thinning of the corneal stroma, e.g., due to a scar or another substance defect, or if a dry

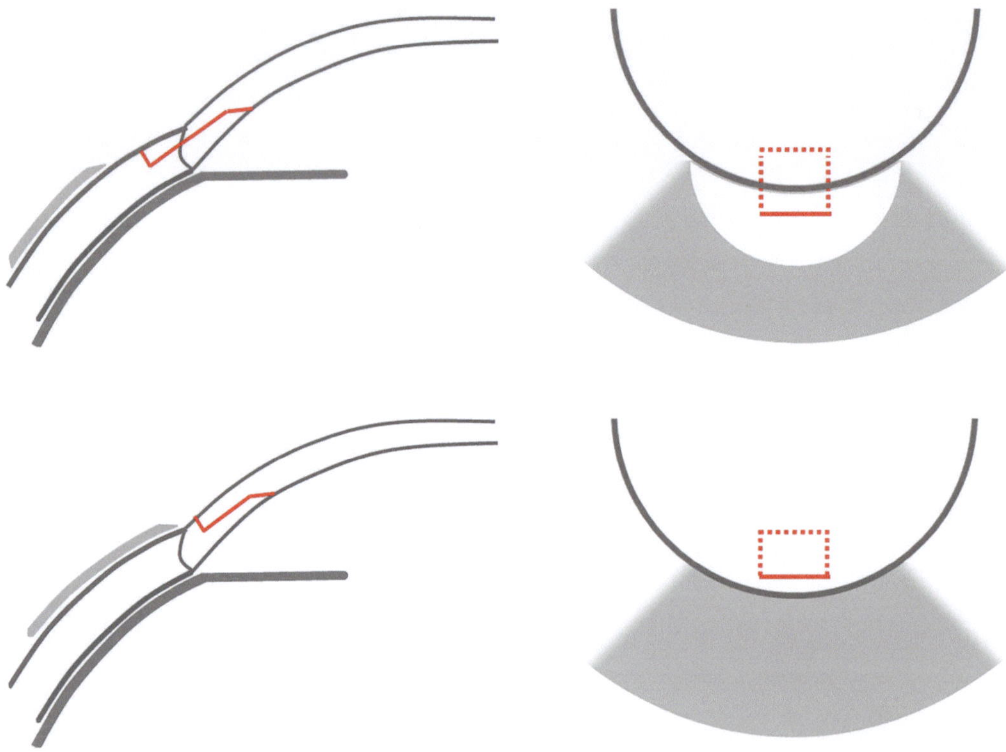

Fig. 13.2 Scleral and corneal incision (schematic representation). Upper row: Scleral incision with preceding conjunctival preparation (left in cross-section, right from the 12 o'clock position). Lower row: Corneal incision (left in cross-section, right from the 12 o'clock position)

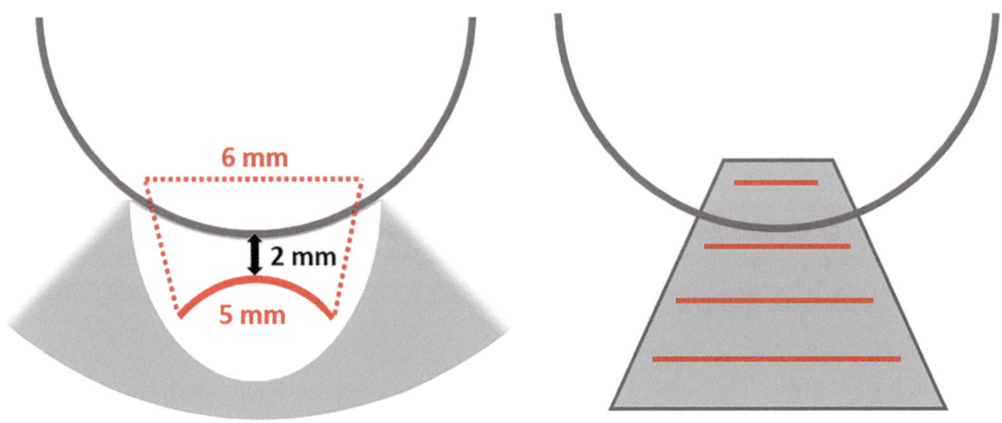

Fig. 13.3 "Frown-Incision" (left) and "Incisional Funnel" (right, schematic representations from the 12 o'clock position). Through an intrascleral arcuate tunnel preparation (arc length: 5 mm; at least 2 mm distance from the limbus), an opening of the anterior chamber over 6 mm (depending on the preparation technique even 8 to 10 mm) can be achieved. The "Incisional Funnel" describes the relationship of equal astigmatic effects depending on the incision width and location in relation to the cornea

Table 13.1 Comparison of corneal and sclerocorneal incisions

	Corneal	Sclerocorneal
Indications	– Findings after fistulating glaucoma surgery – Anterior synechiae – Limbal conjunctival scars	– In cataract surgery with nucleus extraction – Large, non-foldable or only limited foldable IOL
Advantage	– Low tendency to bleed – Preservation of the trabecular meshwork – Postoperative deep anterior chamber, largely self-sealing watertight wound closure by stromal swelling – Hardly any relevant scarring	– Sufficient wound closure through blood supply and conjunctival coverage – No corneal involvement
Disadvantage	– Small inner wound lip – More corneal edema – Slow scarring and thus longer susceptibility to ruptures – Risk of descemetolysis	– Bloody access – Essential damage to the trabecular meshwork – Greater preparatory effort
Contraindication	– Microcornea – Corneal thinning in the context of dystrophies and degenerations	– Scleromalacia
Complication	– Insufficiency – Need for additional suturing, e.g., in high myopia	– Scleral perforation with ciliary body injury
Influence on refraction	The influence on induced astigmatism increases from scleral to corneal. Thus, a 3.5 mm scleral incision induces less astigmatism than an equally long corneal incision (see Fig. 13.3)	

eye is expected in the relevant region, e.g., due to a conjunctival prominence, the area should not be chosen for access. Only a sufficiently large stromal thickness allows for self-sealing corneal incisions (Chap. 20).

▶ The location of the incision can be used to mitigate corneal astigmatism (alignment with the steep meridian).

13.2.2 Size of the Incision

The size of the incision is determined by the size of the instrument/implant with which one intends to penetrate the eye, or by the structure in the eye that one wants to remove through the access. The rule is that the opening should be kept as small as possible. For a simple anterior chamber irrigation with medication administration or for sample collection, it is important to keep the incision as small as possible to avoid inducing unnecessary pressure drop and to achieve good wound closure. If only a puncture is required, the paracentesis opening can be just large enough for the hub of the blunt cannula to penetrate and the access to be sealed later by the wound lips. This can prevent unnecessary loss of anterior chamber fluid due to displacement in the x–y axis.

▶ An intraoperatively stable anterior chamber can avoid numerous complications and should be aimed for through good access preparation. Postoperatively, this can minimize wound leaks.

In addition to the instruments, possible implants must also be included in size planning. For certain intraocular lenses (IOL), it is necessary to choose the smallest possible diameter as the incision size (e.g., 6 mm large IOL optic). This full incision width should be created only just before the actual use, otherwise an unnecessarily unstable anterior chamber due to fluid loss may result.

▶ Too small a wound carries the risk of blunt tissue trauma such as tears of the corneal stroma or Descemetolyses. The most gentle insertion of the instruments into the anterior chamber must be ensured by an appropriate incision size.

13.2.3 Direction of the Incision

The incision technique can be performed from the outside inwards, but also from the inside outwards. The incision technique starting from the outside is easier to learn and more widespread. Penetrating the eye and performing the incision from the inside outwards requires greater surgeon experience and is partly necessary for creating larger accesses (v. Graefe incision). The surgeon cuts "on the way back" when withdrawing the knife after insertion.

When choosing the direction, the angle of penetration into the cornea must also be considered. The incision technique can be performed perpendicular to the surface (short wound tunnel) or almost surface-parallel tangential (long wound tunnel). The longer the stromal wound gap, the easier it is to close the wound through stromal hydration or suturing. It is important to know the anatomy of the eye. Shallow anterior chambers predispose to iris incarceration in the paracentesis (Caution: intraoperative floppy iris syndrome [IFIS] with alpha-1 antagonists) (Chap. 2, 20).

The following incision positions are differentiated (see Fig. 13.2)

1. Scleral incision (scleral tunnel)
2. Sclerocorneal incisions
   - posterior incision over the scleral spur and trabecular meshwork
   - middle incision over the Schwalbe's line
   - anterior incision over the end of the Bowman's layer
3. Clear-cornea incision (in front of the conjunctival insertion)

▶ Despite their size, scleral tunnels can often remain sutureless. However, there is a slightly increased risk of intra- and postoperative bleeding (Caution: preparation through vascularized tissue). Wound closure after completion of wound healing is more sufficient due to a stronger fibrin reaction than, for example, the clear-cornea access.

References and Further Reading

1. Anders N, Pham DT, Antoni HJ, Wollensak J (1997) Postoperative astigmatism and relative strength of tunnel incisions: a prospective clinical trial. J Cataract Refract Surg 23:332–336
2. Ernest PH, Neuhann T (1996) Posterior limbal incision. J Cataract Refract Surg 22:78–84
3. Ernest PH (1994) Cataract incision architecture. Int Ophthalmol Clin 34:31–57
4. Kohnen T, Lambert RJ, Koch DD (1997) Incision sizes for foldable intraocular lenses. Ophthalmology 104:1277–1286
5. Rainer G, Menapace R, Vass C, Annen D, Findl O, Schmetterer K (1999) Corneal shape changes after temporal and superolateral 3.0 mm clear corneal incisions. J Cataract Refract Surg 25:1121–1126
6. Rainer G, Vass C, Menapace R, Papapanos P, Strenn K, Findl O (1998) Long-term course of surgically induced astigmatism after a 5.0 mm sclerocorneal valve incision. J Cataract Refract Surg 24:1642–1646
7. Singer JA (1991) Frown incision for minimizing induced astigmatism after small incision cataract surgery with rigid optic intraocular lens implantation. J Cataract Refract Surg 17(Suppl):677–688

Minor Eyelid and Lacrimal Duct Surgery

14

Jens Heichel, Christoph Schmidt and Anke Steinmann

Contents

The eyelids serve to protect the eye by warding off foreign bodies and UV radiation. They participate in tear production and distribute the tear fluid. Thus, they significantly contribute to maintaining the surface homeostasis (preservation of optical properties, protection against drying out) of the eye. As a functional unit with the lacrimal drainage system, the eyelids are also responsible for tear drainage.

Oculoplastic procedures on the eyelids and the lacrimal drainage system present a special situation for patients and practitioners. On the one hand, diseases in these areas lead to significant distress, as they are characterized by severe functional disorders (e.g., watery eye, so-called epiphora). On the other hand, the structures are located in the central midface, thus directly accessible to visual perception and thereby shaping the aesthetic appearance of the person.

Eyelid surgery includes the removal of tumors, the correction of eyelid malpositions, and the improvement of aesthetics. In every oculoplastic intervention, the goal must be to achieve the best possible restoration of function with appropriate aesthetic rehabilitation, in addition to healing. These goals and perceptions can vary significantly between patients and doctors, which is why a good preoperative evaluation of the possibilities and limitations, as well as the definition of treatment goals, is indispensable before any oculoplastic procedure.

Two main symptoms characterize the lacrimal drainage system: increased tearing (epiphora) and a—not always coexistent—mucopurulent secretion. The treatment of a tear

J. Heichel (✉)
Klinik und Poliklinik für Augenheilkunde, Universitätsklinikum Halle/Saale, Halle/Saale, Germany
e-mail: jens.heichel@uk-halle.de

C. Schmidt
Augenärztliche Gemeinschaftspraxis "Augen im Zentrum", Greifswald, Germany
e-mail: c.schmidt@augen-im-zentrum.de

A. Steinmann
Coesfeld, Germany

F. Wilhelm (ed.), *Ophthalmic Surgery for Beginners*, https://doi.org/10.1007/978-3-662-70287-1_14

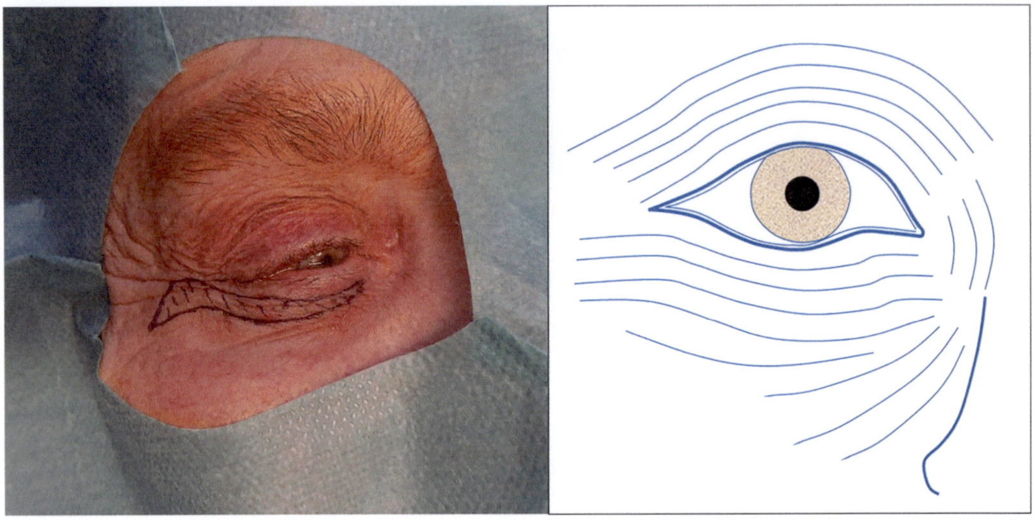

Fig. 14.1 Physiological tension lines of the skin, as considered in the example shown here during a lower eyelid blepharoplasty

drainage disorder includes surgical rehabilitation of the lacrimal drainage system. This must be preceded by targeted diagnostics.

▶ The physiological tension lines of the skin must be considered in periocular surgery (Fig. 14.1). Eyelids and tear drainage pathways also form a functional unit (Chap. 2).

14.1 General Preliminary Considerations

Good preparation is essential before a surgical procedure on the eyelids. This includes not only an exact determination of the indication but also extensive patient education, in which the patient's wishes as well as the medical goals, limitations, and possibilities must be precisely defined. Since these are usually elective surgeries, this should not be overlooked. In case of doubt, the patient should be given more time to consider.

14.1.1 Examination of the Eyelids

Numerous pathological changes can occur on the eyelids. This is partly due to the enormous variety of tissues found in this small area. In addition to inflammatory changes (e.g., blepharitis), numerous tumors and degenerative processes can occur.

Through a careful examination, the planned surgical procedure must and can be simulated and thus tested for its suitability. The horizontal tension relationships (snap-back test, horizontal traction test, distraction test) must be evaluated. This can be assessed during a forced eyelid closure. Furthermore, tumors and scars should be looked for to exclude a secondary mechanical component. The physiological protective reflexes should also be evaluated (Bell's phenomenon, corneal reflex) (Chap. 2).

▶ In the snap-back test, the lower eyelid is pulled down with the finger and released. Normally, the eyelid margin immediately reattaches to the surface of the eyeball. The time to return to the starting position is measured in seconds (s) (Grade I = 2–3 s; Grade II = 4–5 s; Grade III = > 5 s; Grade IV = lower eyelid remains in ectropion position).

▶ Through horizontal traction, the tear punctum can normally be displaced laterally by a maximum of 1 mm (horizontal traction test).

▶ The lifting of the eyelid should not be possible more than 5 to 6 mm from the eyeball (distraction test).

For ptosis surgery, measuring the eyelid fissure height in the primary position as well as in upward and downward gaze is essential. The position of the eyelid can be quantified with the MRD (margin-reflex distance 1 for the upper eyelid and 2 for the lower eyelid). Furthermore, the levator function must be measured, excluding the involvement of the M. frontalis. The examinations are explained in Sect. 14.3.2.

▶ Photodocumentation should always be sought in oculoplastic issues.

14.1.2 Operating Table

Planning the operation in advance allows for precise preparation of instruments and consumables. This starts with the type of disinfection and analgesia and ends with the dressing material. Possible allergies and medications that prolong bleeding time must be considered. What suture material and which implants (e.g., lid-loading) are needed?

Generally, the instruments for oculoplastic procedures are linited. (Fig. 14.2). Nevertheless, one should be prepared for certain situations (e.g., increased bleeding → cauterization; increased sensitivity to glare or reduced compliance → bulb protection cap) (Chap. 5).

14.1.3 Patient Management During the Operation

Communication with the patient is a very important factor. The patient's ability to speak and understand language, as well as their hearing ability, are essential. If applied incorrectly, communication can also become a disadvantage. Therefore, a sense for the situation must be developed, as not every patient wants to be informed about the procedures immediately during the operation in the same way. Generally, patients want a rough idea of what is happening and how long the procedure is expected to last.

In any case, patients should be prepared for potentially unpleasant situations in advance during the consultation (e.g., pain). The statement that it might "hurt soon" but will "pass quickly" creates an appropriate expectation and allows for coping strategies. Statements like "It's bleeding a lot today." or "I've never seen anything like

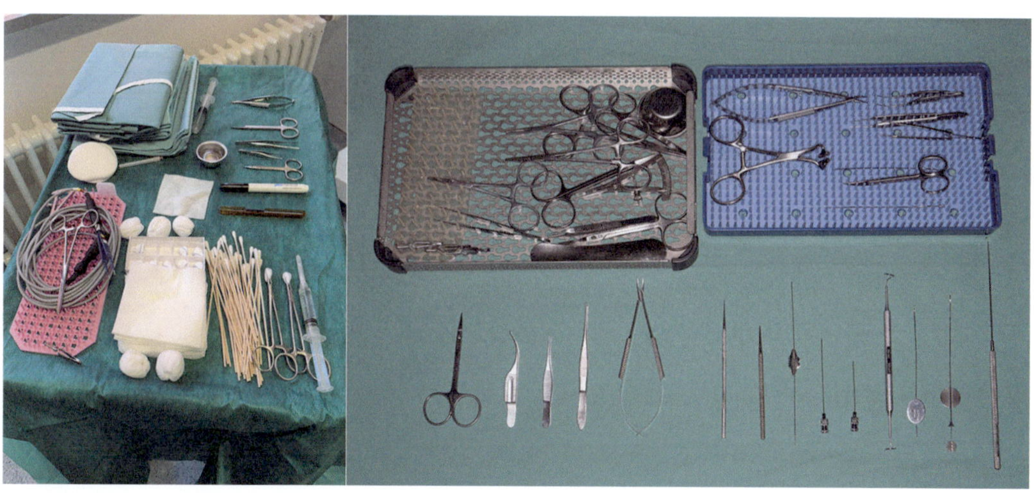

Fig. 14.2 Operating table for minor eyelid and lacrimal surgery

this before." or "The blood pressure keeps going up." should be avoided at all costs.

If it is possible to guide the patients through the unpleasant situation of the operation with a calm and factual manner, one will encounter great gratitude and cooperation.

▶ During an operation under local anesthesia, the doctor, the surgical assistant, and the patient form a team.

14.2 Eyelid Malpositions

The eyelid malpositions to be discussed here are the entropion and the ectropion of the lower eyelid as well as the ptosis. Due to space constraints, only the most common causes, namely the involutional forms, can be examined here.

14.2.1 Involutional Entropion

Due to reduced tension of the eyelid support apparatus, there is an inward tilting of the eyelid margin with consequent eyelash rubbing (trichiasis). The consequences are, in addition to a strong foreign body sensation, increased tearing (due to reflex secretion) and microlesions in the area of the conjunctival and corneal epithelium. Furthermore, ulcerations (on the eyelid margin, conjunctiva, and cornea) can occur. The reduced tolerance of the senile ocular surface to this permanent mechanical stress is of particular importance.

Temporary Measures

If a major surgical correction is not possible in the near future, the following measures can be used for temporary stabilization:

- Bandage contact lens,
- Tape traction,
- Injection of botulinum toxin A into the preseptal orbicularis muscle,
- everting sutures ([22]; Fig. 14.3).

Wies Procedure

At approximately 5 mm from the eyelid margin (tarsal height at the lower eyelid approximately 4 mm), a full-thickness, eyelid-margin-parallel incision is made across nearly the entire width of the eyelid. Three U-sutures are then placed, which, starting from the conjunctiva and the lower eyelid retractors in the area of the inferior wound edge, are brought out to the superior wound edge ventral to the tarsus and 2 mm subciliary. The distance between the U-legs is approximately 3 mm. This achieves an outward tilting. Furthermore, postoperative muscle fibrosis prevents the overriding of preseptal orbicularis muscle parts. The remaining wound closure is performed continuously in the skin-muscle layer (Fig. 14.4). For the U-sutures, absorbable

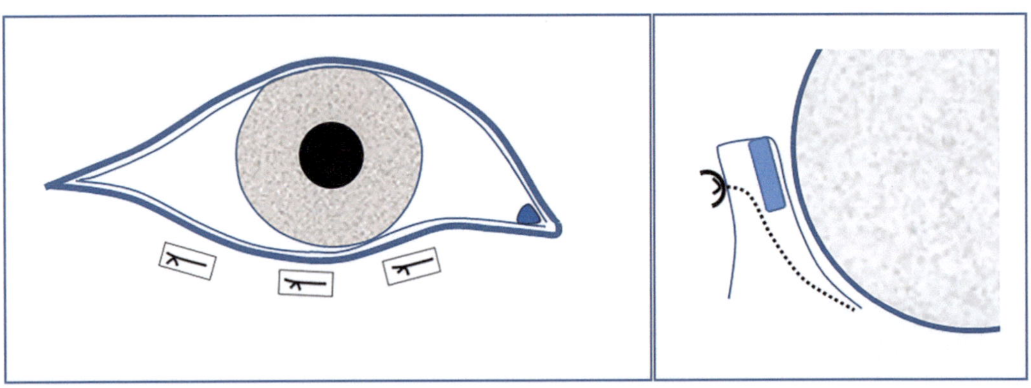

Fig. 14.3 Everting sutures. The U-sutures are passed from the lower fornix approximately 2 mm below the lash line anterior to the tarsus and tied over silicone bolsters. (Suture material used: 4-0 to 5-0, absorbable or non-absorbable)

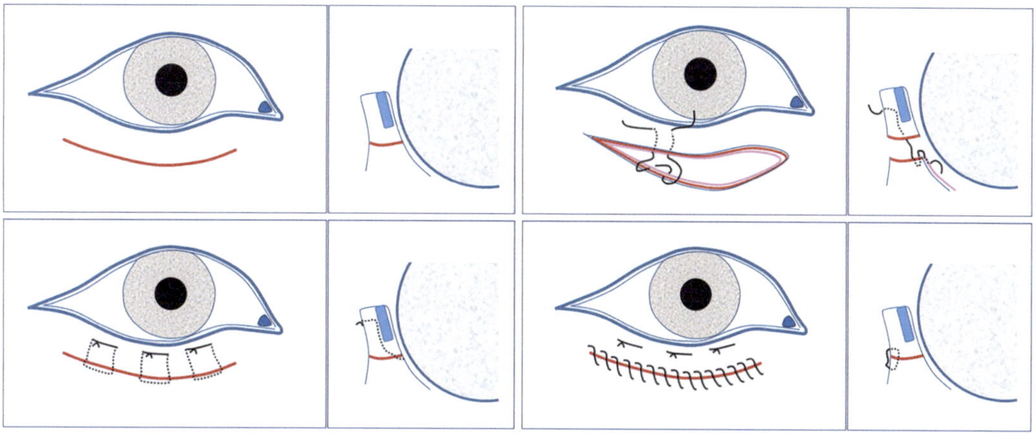

Fig. 14.4 Procedure according to Wies. (From top left to bottom right)

or non-absorbable suture materials of size (4-0), 5-0, or 6-0 can be used. The skin-muscle closure is performed with absorbable or non-absorbable suture materials of size 6-0 or 7-0.

▶ An immediate postoperative overcorrection (ectropion) is indeed desired in the Wies procedure. If this persists for more than five days, individual U-sutures can be removed prematurely.

Wies-Quickert Procedure

If, in addition to the overriding of the orbicularis muscle, there is reduced horizontal tension of the eyelid, the Wies technique can be extended by a horizontal shortening. For this, a corresponding eyelid block including the eyelid margin is excised (Fig. 14.5). The eyelid margin suture is performed according to the options listed below (Sect. 14.4.3).

Jones Procedure

In this modification, the lower eyelid retractors are tightened. The eyelid-margin-parallel incision below the tarsus of the lower eyelid is not full-thickness but only up to the lower eyelid retractors. Through a special suturing technique, the retractor layer is folded and thus tightened. This modification can be well combined with a lateral tarsal strip procedure or a resection of parts of the preseptal orbicularis muscle (Fig. 14.6).

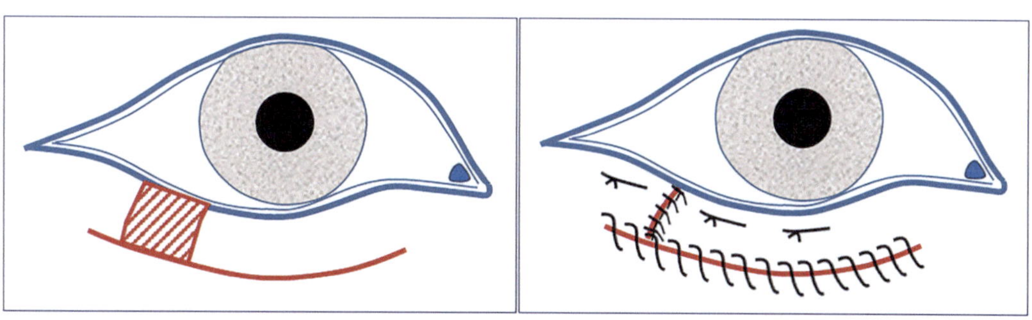

Fig. 14.5 Procedure according to Wies-Quickert

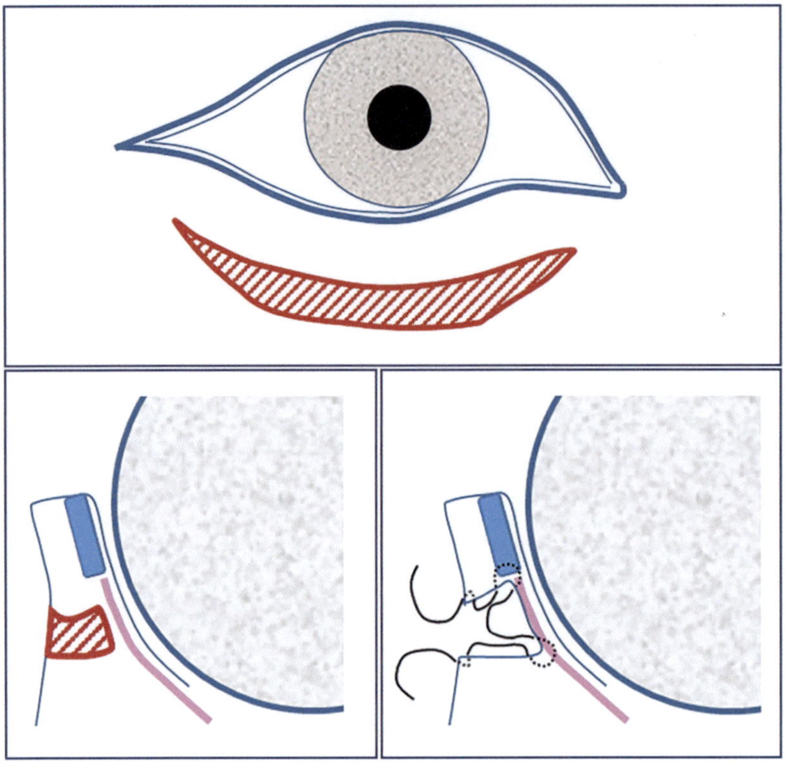

Fig. 14.6 Procedure according to Jones (retractor folding). The red hatched area shows the removal of a skin-muscle strip (containing preseptal orbicularis parts). The retractors are shown in pink. For the retractor folding, Vicryl 6-0 or 7-0 can be used

14.2.2 Senile Ectropion

The correction of involutional ectropion is usually somewhat more complex compared to entropion. The horizontal tension is reduced and must be increased through appropriate measures. Sometimes the fold of the conjunctiva is significantly widened, and there is an ectatic conjunctival sac. Secondarily, severe blepharitis can occur.

Lateral Tarsal Strip Procedure

This procedure is also called tarsal strip procedure. Through a horizontal skin incision starting from the lateral canthus, the tarsus is dissected over the desired distance (usually 5 to 8 mm). All tissues covering the tarsus are removed. The resulting tarsal strip is shortened according to the tension conditions and then fixed to the periosteum of the temporal orbital rim with a U-suture (suture material: non-absorbable or absorbable, polyfilament, size 4-0 to 5-0). The procedure can be well combined with a skin-muscle tightening and is suitable for the correction of both ectropion and entropion (Chap. 2) (Fig. 14.7).

- The tarsal strip must be fixed as far dorsally as possible to the periosteum to avoid the lid margin from standing away from the eyeball. A temporal-superior traction effect is desirable. The effect can be simulated during the surgery by applying traction with forceps.

Inverting Sutures

The course of the inverting sutures is exactly opposite to that of entropion correction. Inverting sutures can be used in any ectropion surgery (Fig. 14.8).

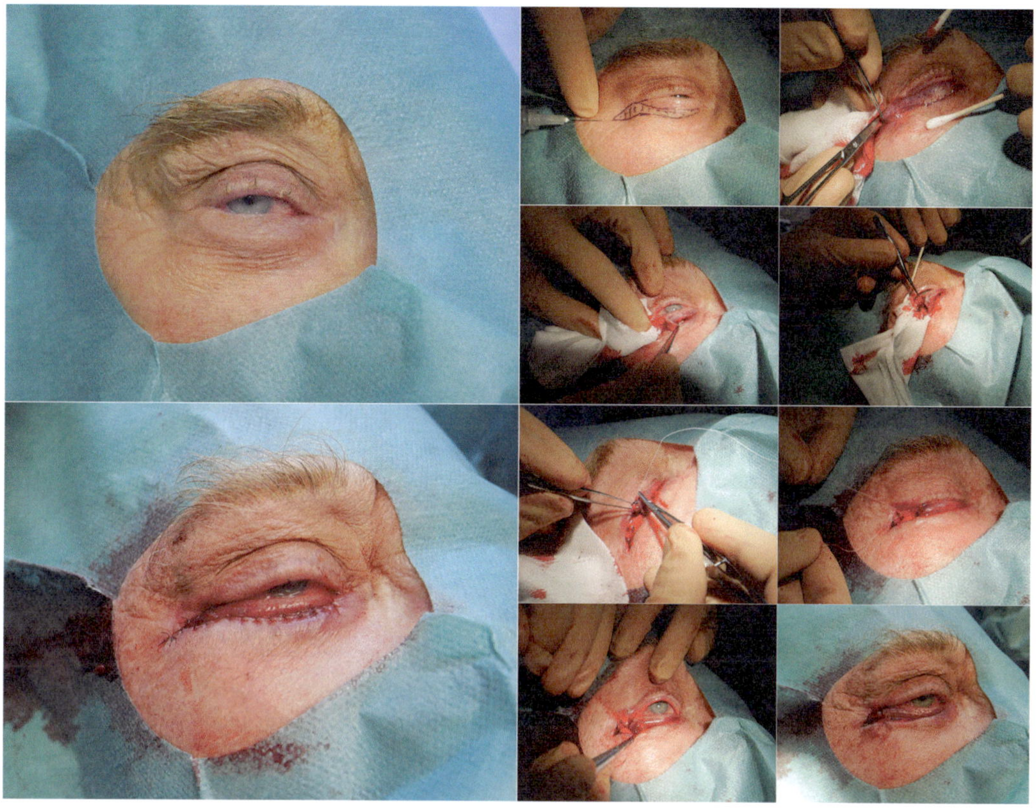

Fig. 14.7 Lateral tarsal strip procedure with partial resection of preseptal orbicularis muscle

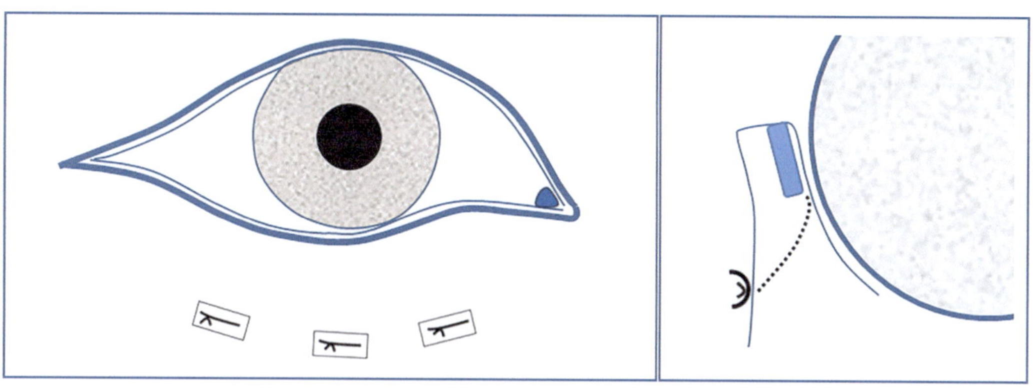

Fig. 14.8 Inverting sutures

14.2.3 Paralytic Ectropion

Paralytic ectropion due to facial nerve damage is a common issue. Due to exposure keratopathy, quick action is sometimes required. Here, a lateral tarsal strip procedure can be combined with a tarsorrhaphy.

Temporary Tarsorrhaphy

A simple way to temporarily improve eyelid closure is the temporary tarsorrhaphy. Here, the upper and lower lid tarsus are adapted with U-sutures, which are tied over bolsters (Fig. 14.9). No lid margin tissue is removed.

Permanent Tarsorrhaphy

If the lid margins are to remain permanently connected, a permanent tarsorrhaphy can be performed. Various techniques have been described for this. A simple modification is derived from the temporary tarsorrhaphy and involves additional freshening of the lid margins by removing the skin on the lid margin (so-called permanent marginal tarsorrhaphy). The tarsus adaptation is also done using intratarsal U-sutures and silicone bolsters. However, the anterior lamella is additionally adapted with individual knotted sutures (e.g., 6-0, absorbable or non-absorbable).

14.3 Aesthetic Eyelid Surgery

Improving the aesthetics of the eyelids must be subordinate to any functional aspects. Therefore, eyelid margin position, mobility, and complete eyelid closure must never be endangered by aesthetic surgery (Chap. 2).

▶ In aesthetic eyelid surgery, the function of the eyelids and thus the eye must not be endangered.

14.3.1 Upper Eyelid Blepharoplasty

A dermatochalasis of the upper eyelid potentially leads to functional and aesthetic limitations (visual field). The excess can be eliminated through an upper eyelid blepharoplasty. In addition to symmetry with the opposite side, the correct dosage must be observed (Caution: overcorrection). Preoperatively, traction of the skin can be performed by lifting it with the fingers to simulate the possible removal. As an intraoperative guideline, approximately 2 cm of skin should remain between the lower edge of the brow and the upper eyelid margin. However, there are often significant interindividual

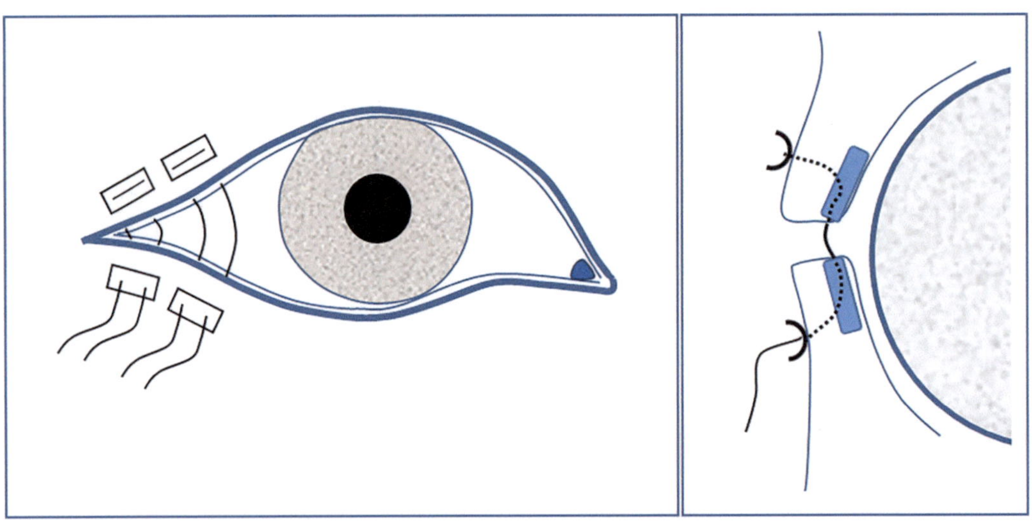

Fig. 14.9 Temporary tarsorrhaphy

differences. An example of an upper eyelid blepharoplasty is shown in Fig. 14.10.

- Local anesthesia creates a subcutaneous support, which significantly facilitates the incision. The incision should be made along each wound edge in one go as much as possible to create a homogeneous and step-free wound edge.

- All markings must be applied before local anesthesia.

14.3.2 Levator Folding

To correct a senile ptosis, folding of the levator muscle (M. levator palpebrae superioris) can be performed. A prerequisite for levator surgery is a largely well-preserved function of the muscle. Therefore, the levator function must be assessed beforehand by manually excluding the cooperation of the M. frontalis. The physiological levator function is > 14 mm and should be at least 9 mm for levator folding.

- The assessment of levator function is performed starting from the downward gaze, excluding brow elevation via the M. frontalis by manually fixing the brow by the examiner. A millimeter scale is placed at the upper eyelid margin and marks the zero point. The patient is then asked to look up. The position of the upper eyelid margin now reached is projected onto the millimeter scale and marks the levator function in mm.

The incision is made along the upper eyelid crease and should be marked. Typically, this is shifted superiorly in the context of involutional ptosis and may need to be corrected slightly downward (8 to 10 mm). After local anesthesia and cutting through the skin and orbicularis muscle, the orbital septum is exposed and opened under vertical tension. The preaponeurotic fat pad can now be visualized. The levator aponeurosis

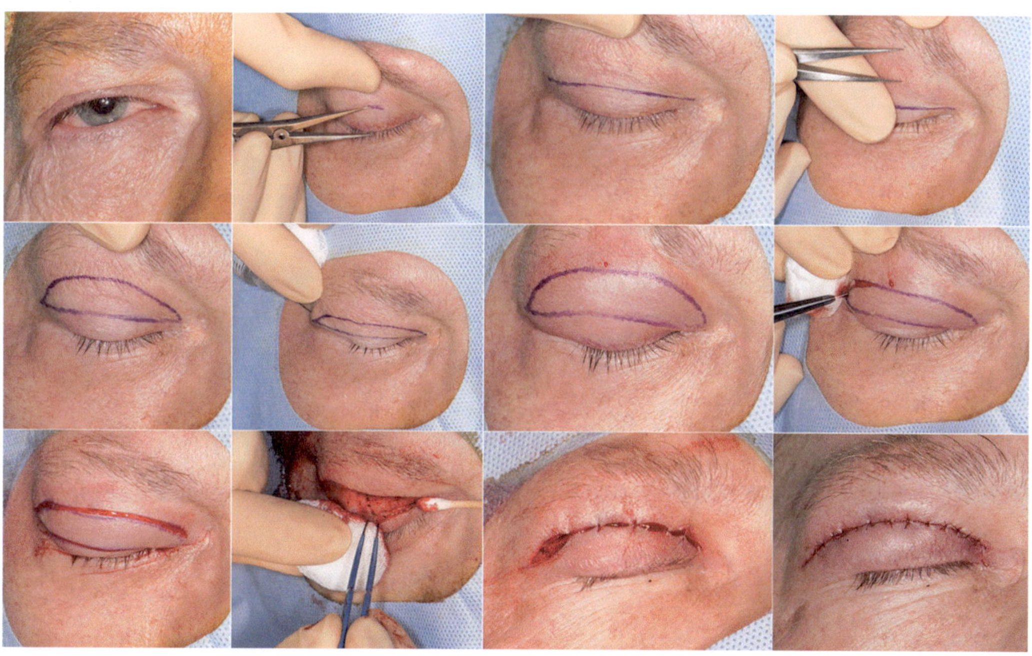

Fig. 14.10 Upper eyelid blepharoplasty (suture material: 6-0 or 7-0, mono- or polyfilament, absorbable or non-absorbable). Considering a distance of 10 mm each from the upper eyelid margin and to the brow, 12 mm of excess skin could be excised. (Caution: The patient also has a concurrent brow ptosis)

lying dorsally to it is exposed up to the transverse superior ligament (Whitnall). Subsequently, three folding sutures (non-absorbable suture material of strength 6-0 to 7-0) are placed in the aponeurosis and led inferiorly through the tarsus. The suture path must be placed intratarsally to avoid perforation towards the conjunctiva tarsi. Initially tying the folding sutures in loops, a simulation of the eyelid lift can be performed. Only when a good eyelid lift with good eyelid closure and satisfactory eyelid curvature is achieved, the final knotting of the sutures is done. The remanining wound closure includes closing the orbital septum with continuous suture (7-0, absorbable) and a skin-muscle suture (6-0 or 7-0, absorbable or non-absorbable), which can be performed in single-knot or continuous technique (Chap. 2 and 6) (Fig. 14.11).

▶ Ptosis surgery is contraindicated in severe dry eye syndrome or limbal stem cell deficiency. Furthermore, myogenic and neurogenic causes of ptosis must be excluded before any surgical ptosis correction.

14.4 Minor Tumor Surgery

Tumors of the eyelid are common. The distinction between benign and malignant forms is essential. This cannot always be determined based on clinical aspects, although ulceration, loss of eyelashes (madarosis), infiltration, neovascularization, and size progression are classic signs of malignancy. Photodocumentation should always be sought. Only a histopathological examination provides certainty.

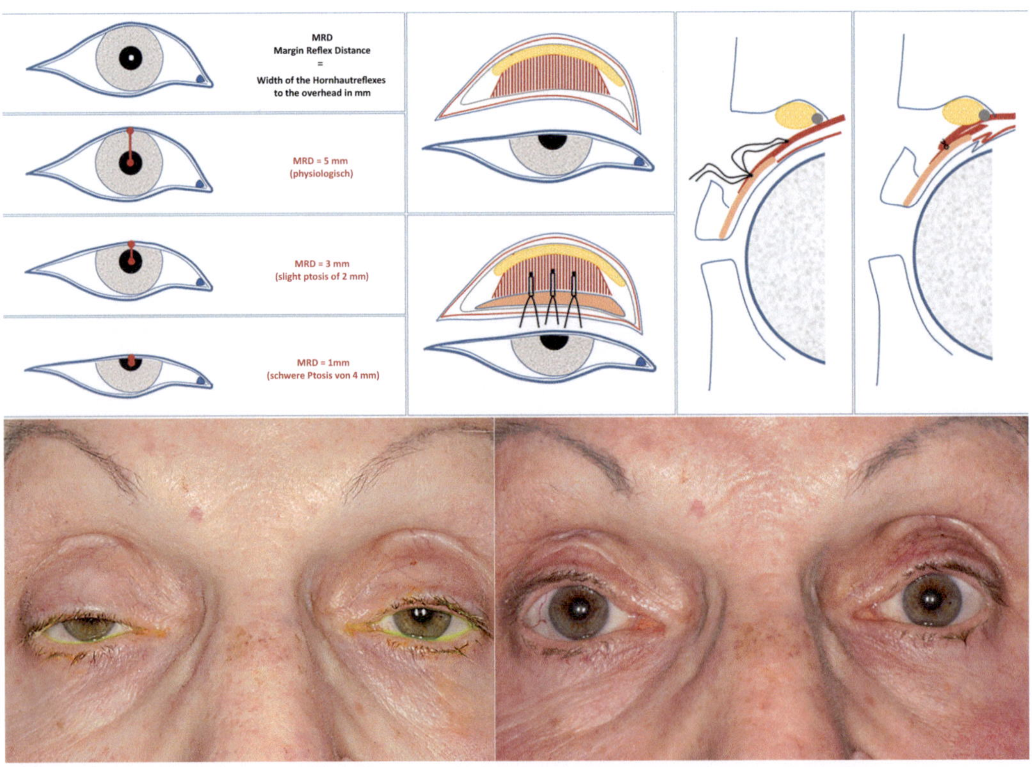

Fig. 14.11 Grading of ptosis using MRD 1 (Margin Reflex Distance) and levator folding. Three folding sutures are led from the levator aponeurosis to the tarsus. The levator aponeurosis is to be exposed up to the transverse superior ligament (marked in gray in the graphic). The preaponeurotic fat tissue is shown in yellow, the tarsus in orange. Below are images of a patient with involutional ptosis before (left) and after (right) bilateral levator folding

▶ The care of patients with malignant tumors should be placed in experienced hands. The question of safety margins and subsequent complex reconstruction techniques requires a high level of experience. Sometimes these patients need to be managed interdisciplinarily.

14.4.1 Excision of Chalazia

A chalazion is an encapsulated (fibrous pseudocapsule) chronic inflammatory process that originates from a sebaceous gland of the eyelid. The process can bulge towards the tarsal conjunctiva or towards the epidermis and is accessible to surgical remediation through these routes. If an external (epidermal) approach is chosen, the incision should be made parallel to the eyelid margin, and a suture is required for wound closure. With an internal (conjunctiva tarsi) approach, the incision is made vertically to the eyelid margin. Wound closure can usually be omitted (Chap. 2) (Fig. 14.12).

▶ In any case, a partial resection of the fibrous capsule structures with subsequent histological examination should be performed to rule out rare differential diagnoses (e.g., sebaceous gland carcinoma, metastasis, etc.).

14.4.2 Local Flap Transpositions

If the position of the eyelid margin is endangered by direct wound closure (Caution: Ectropion), a flap transposition must be applied to change the force vectors. Direct wound closure is often possible with corresponding excess skin on the upper eyelid (Fig. 14.13).

▶ In a flap transposition, vertical tensile forces towards the eyelid margin must be avoided. However, an increase in horizontal tension is possible. This is especially important to note on the lower eyelid (greater tendency for ectropion due to narrower tarsus).

Limberg Flap

The Limberg flap is a local flap transposition. By extending the incision from one of the vertical wound poles, a corresponding skin flap can be swung into the defect (Fig. 14.14).

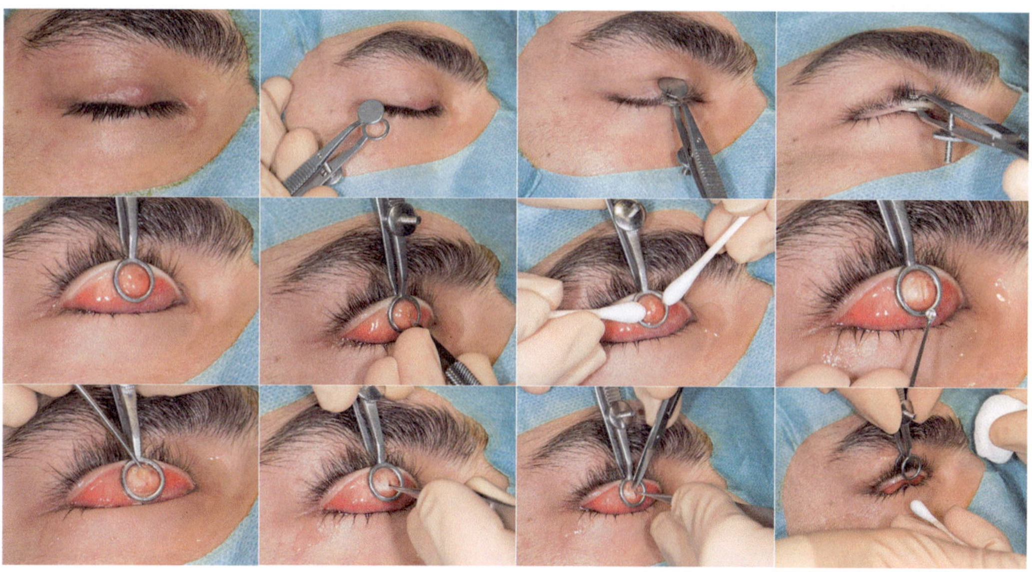

Fig. 14.12 Procedure of a chalazion surgery on the upper eyelid. (Conjunctival approach)

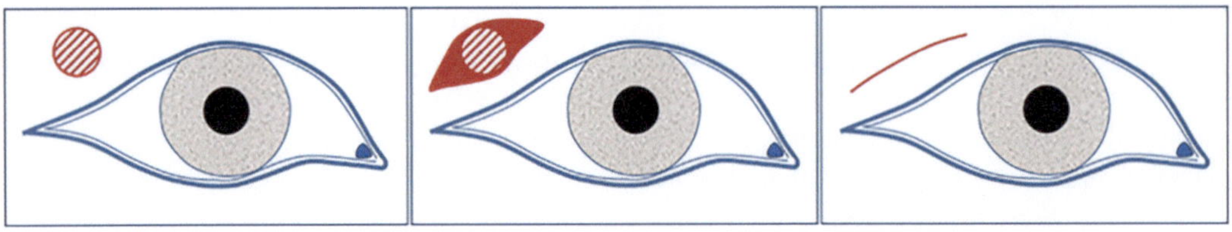

Fig. 14.13 Direct wound closure with existing excess skin

Horizontal Flap Transposition

After mobilizing a larger horizontal skin area, it is relocated so that the defect area can be covered without tension. At the base of the skin flap to be transposed, small compensatory triangles (Burow) must be removed (Fig. 14.15).

Skin Flap from the Upper Eyelid or Cheek

Larger defects may sometimes not be reconstructed by simple skin transpositions. Here, it may be necessary to use excess skin from the upper eyelid or cheek. It is important that the used skin is sufficiently mobilized to avoid traction and consequent eyelid malpositions (Fig. 14.16).

14.4.3 Excision of Tumors of the Eyelid Margin and Primary Eyelid Margin Suture

Tumors of the eyelid margins sometimes require a block excision of the affected area. Accordingly, a eyelid margin suture is necessary, which must adapt both eyelid layers (anterior and posterior eyelid layer) separately. Reduced horizontal eyelid tension is advantageous. The technique of an eyelid margin suture is shown in Fig. 14.17 (Chap. 2).

14.4.4 Displacement of the Eyelid Margin by Canthotomy and Cantholysis

If the horizontal tension is too great, there is a risk of postoperative dehiscence. To avoid this, a canthotomy (**horizontal** splitting of the lateral canthus) and, if necessary, additionally a cantholysis (**vertical** severing of the lateral canthal tendon) can be performed. This can usually bridge 5 mm of the defect (Chap. 2) (Fig. 14.18).

▶ Canthotomy and cantholysis are also suitable for acute decompression of the orbit.

14.4.5 Semicircle Flap Technique

The arc transposition in the area of the lateral canthus is attributed, among others, to Tenzel. Through an arc-shaped incision, the skin can be swung into the defect. A cantholysis is also necessary here, as otherwise no displacement of the eyelid margin is possible. In the area of the new eyelid margin, a suture adaptation of

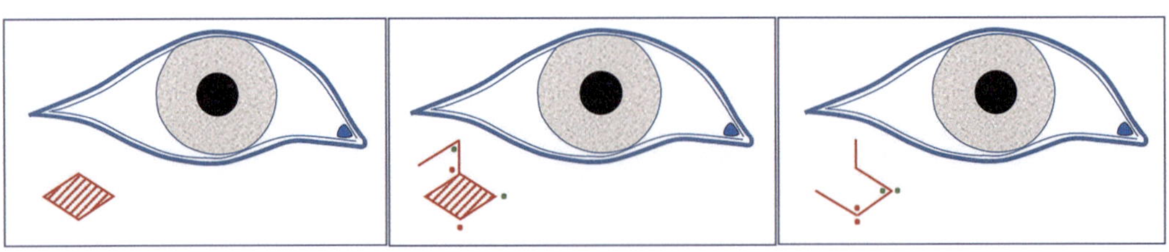

Fig. 14.14 Limberg flap. (Red and green dots added for didactic reasons)

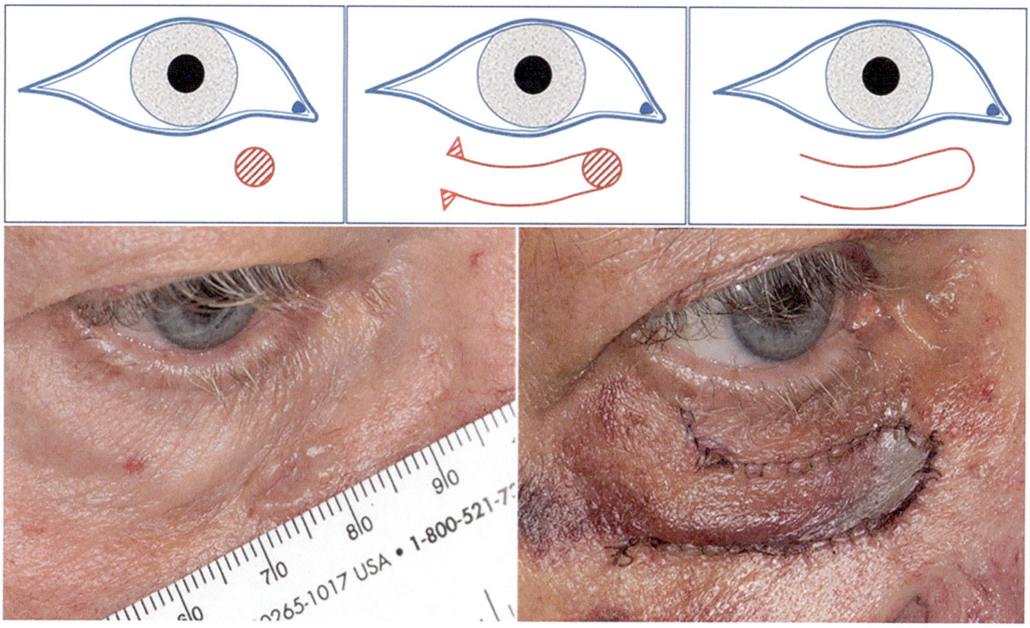

Fig. 14.15 Horizontal flap transposition using Burow's compensatory triangles in schematic representation and patient example with basal cell carcinoma on the medial lower eyelid. (Note the preserved attachment of the lower eyelid to the eyeball surface)

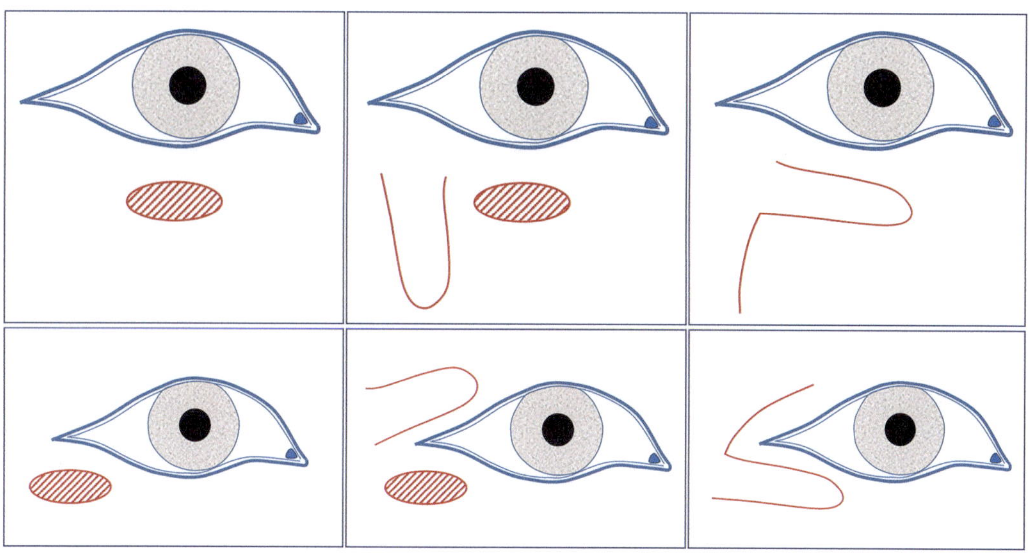

Fig. 14.16 Skin flap from the cheek (upper row) and from the upper eyelid (lower row)

the conjunctiva with the skin is performed using U-sutures (e.g., 7-0, polyfilament, absorbable). The closure of the eyelid margin is carried out according to the principles of eyelid margin suturing (Fig. 14.17 and 14.19).

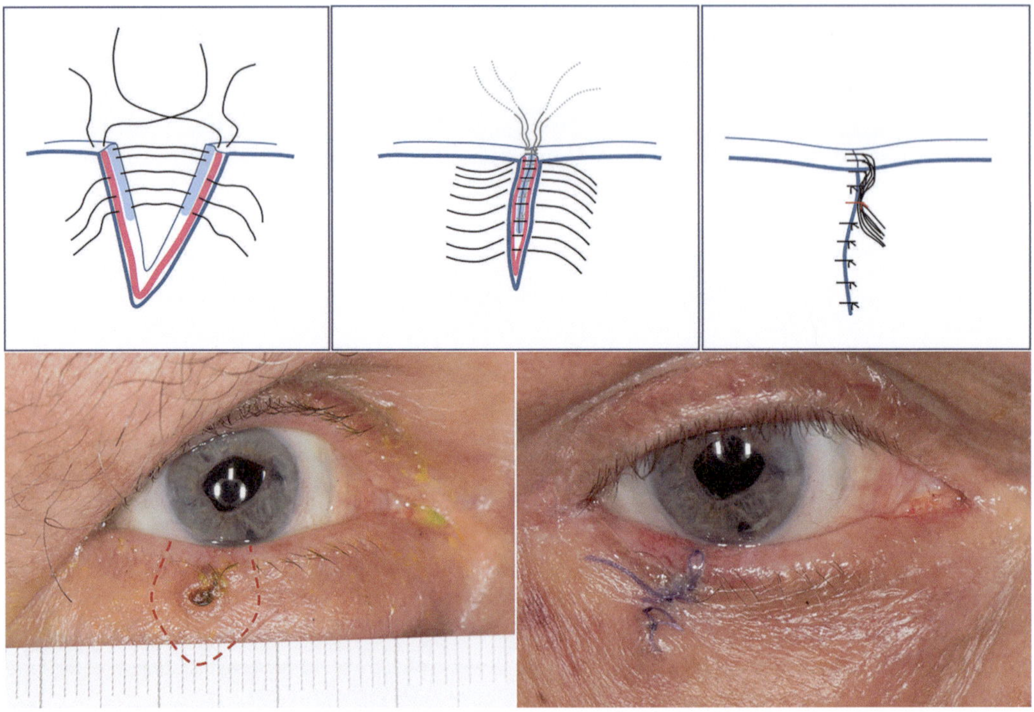

Fig. 14.17 Eyelid margin suture in schematic representation and patient example. (Blue: posterior eyelid layer; pink: anterior eyelid layer; red suture fixes the intermarginal sutures)

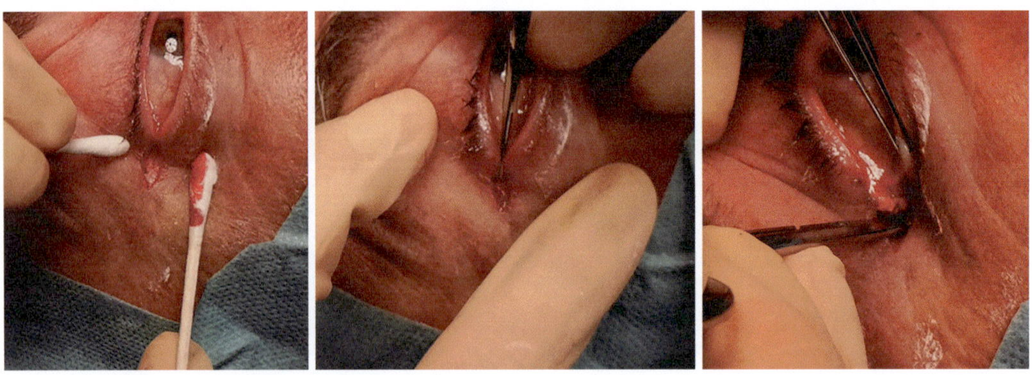

Fig. 14.18 Canthotomy and Cantholysis

14.5 Minor Lacrimal Surgery

The goal of lacrimal surgery is to improve tear drainage and to treat chronic inflammations. It is generally very complex and can only be partially presented here.

Before treating a disease of the lacrimal drainage system, a thorough medical history and clinical examination must be conducted. The latter includes special test procedures and also involves a diagnostic irrigation of the lacrimal drainage system. The goal is to classify the tear

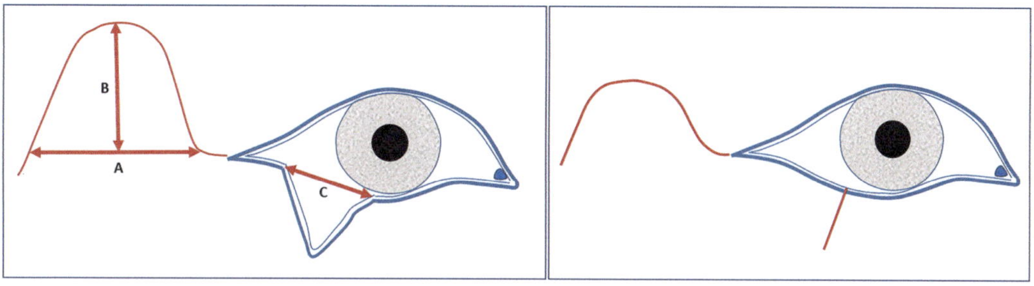

Fig. 14.19 Semicircle Flap Technique (A = 2 x C; B ≥ A)

Tab. 14.1 Classification of lacrimal duct stenosis

Criterion	Classification
Degree of stenosis	Absolute
	Relative
Type of stenosis	Mechanical
	Functional
Localization of stenosis	Presaccal
	Intrasaccal
	Postsaccal
Time of manifestation	Congenital
	Acquired - primary (PANDO) - secondary (SALDO)

PANDO - primary acquired nasolacrimal duct obstruction
SALDO - secondary acquired lacrimal drainage obstruction

drainage disorder as accurately as possible (Tab. 14.1).

The basic diagnostics in the area of the lacrimal drainage system include the inspection and palpation of the eyelids and the lacrimal sac region, the examination of eyelid tension, the conjunctival dye test, the manual compression of the lacrimal sac, and the diagnostic irrigation of the lacrimal drainage system. To rule out reflex hypersecretion, a Schirmer test and the determination of the tear film break-up time should be performed. If a mechanical tear drainage disorder can be detected, an Ear Nose Throat (ENT) consultation must be initiated to exclude a possible causative pathology in this region.

14.5.1 Correction of the Position of the Lacrimal Punctum

An outward tilting of the lacrimal punctum prevents adequate immersion in the tear lake. This results in a functional disorder. Through a diamond-shaped excision in the area of the inner eyelid below the lacrimal punctum, an Eversio puncti lacrimalis can usually be very effectively corrected (Fig. 14.20). The highest point should be at least 3 mm away from the eyelid margin to avoid injury to the lacrimal punctum ampulla.

14.5.2 Therapeutic Irrigation of the Lacrimal Ducts

A classic indication for therapeutic lacrimal duct irrigation is congenital dacryostenosis with persistence of the Hasner membrane. Within the first year of life, the intervention can be performed under local anesthesia (anesthetic eye drops; 40% glucose solution orally) on the changing table. The child is wrapped in a cloth ("swaddling") and held by an assistant. This allows approximately 90% of children to be successfully treated.

The therapeutic lacrimal duct irrigation involves the following steps (Fig. 14.21):

- Dilation of the upper lacrimal punctum (alternatively, the lower one can also be used, although the angle of entry into the lacrimal sac is less favorable);

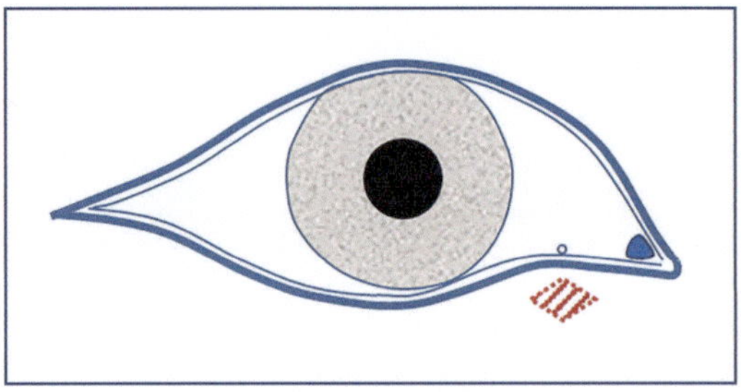

Fig. 14.20 Oval or diamond-shaped excision below the lacrimal punctum. The excision is performed only on the inner eyelid

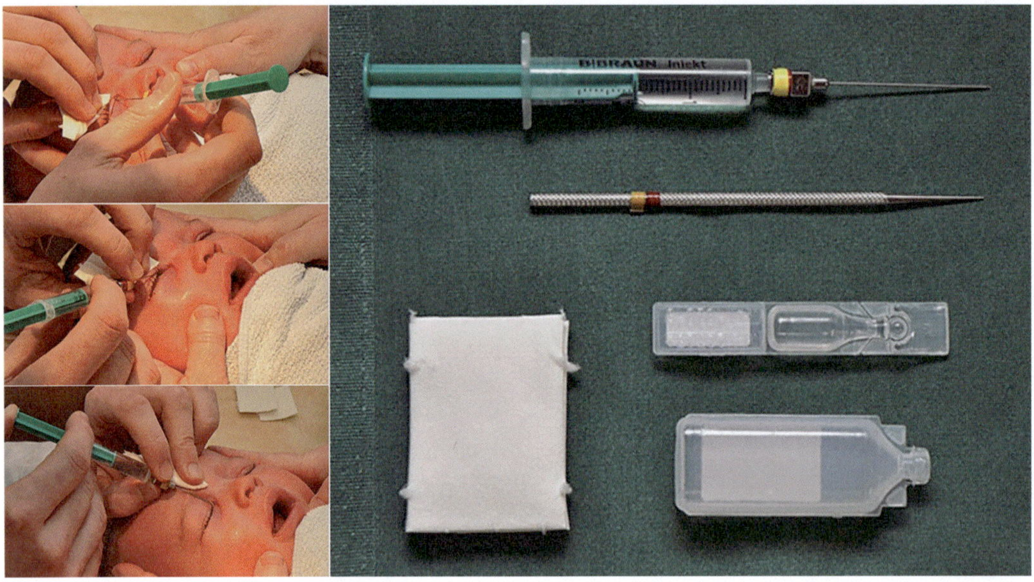

Fig. 14.21 Therapeutic lacrimal duct irrigation in childhood and required instruments. (Bangerter cannula and conical probe, 2-ml syringe, physiological saline solution, anesthetic eye drops, swabs)

- Horizontal probing up to the periosteal stop (hard stop);
- Positioning of the lacrimal duct irrigation cannula and further probing towards the nose under slight irrigation pressure.

▶ Therapeutic lacrimal duct irrigation in childhood under local anesthesia requires experience. Lacrimal duct irrigation purely for diagnostic purposes is contraindicated in young children, as it can lead to injuries and iatrogenic lacrimal duct stenosis.

14.5.3 Relief of a Lacrimal Sac Empyema

As a result of a postsaccal lacrimal duct stenosis, there is a retention of secretions in the lacrimal sac. This usually leads to chronic, often mild, dacryocystitis. However, during acute exacerbations, the full picture of acute dacryocystitis can develop, characterized by severe pain and swelling in the lacrimal sac region. In addition to systemic intravenous antibiotic therapy, incision of the lacrimal sac is an effective means to manage this life-threatening situation (caution: sinus vein thrombosis). The procedure for a stab incision of the lacrimal sac is shown in Fig. 14.22.

▶ Acute dacryocystitis with abscess is an ophthalmological emergency. Patients must be admitted for inpatient treatment. In the course

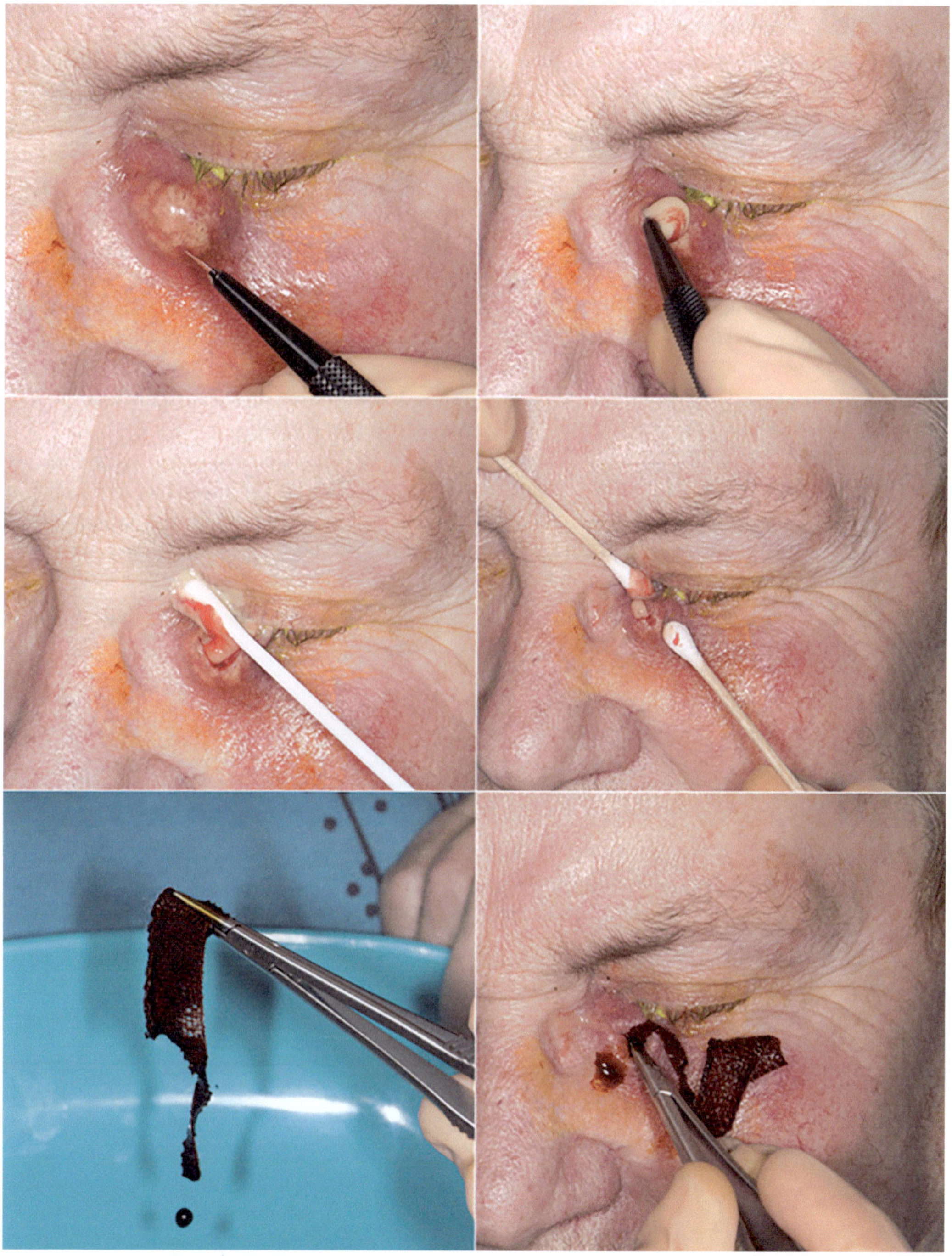

Fig. 14.22 Stab incision of the lacrimal sac, swab collection, and loop drainage (povidone-iodine 7.5%) in acute dacryocystitis

of treatment, almost always a restoration of the lacrimal ducts through dacryocystorhinostomy is necessary.

14.5.4 Intubation of the Lacrimal Ducts

The temporary splinting of the lacrimal drainage system aims to bridge the opened passageway and thus keep it open during wound healing, ultimately increasing the success rate of the surgery. Indications for lacrimal drainage system intubation include trauma, lid and tumor surgery affecting the lacrimal drainage system, as well as stenosis recurrences or situations associated with a high recurrence rate for lacrimal drainage system stenoses (e.g., narrow anatomical conditions, previous surgeries, ENT pathologies, etc.). The variety of possible intubation techniques for the lacrimal drainage system is very large (Table 14.2). The ring intubation according to Murube del Castillo and the technique according to Ritleng will be discussed in more detail here.

Ring Intubation according to Murube del Castillo

The splinting of the tear ducts is primarily used for stabilization after tear duct injuries. After retrograde probing of the injured canaliculus stump using a special probe (e.g., pigtail probe according to Worst), a guide thread (Polypropylene 6-0) is inserted. Over this, a silicone tube can now be threaded and pulled into the TNW. After shortening the tube, the thread is tied, forming a ring (Fig. 14.23). The intubation is usually left in the TNW for three months (Chap. 2).

▶ The primary reconstruction of a tear duct injury requires intubation of the efferent tear ducts to bridge the injured mucosal portion.

Monocanalicular Nasal Intubation according to Ritleng

As a very versatile intubation technique, the monocanalicular nasal procedure according to Ritleng can be applied. Using a special probe, which has a lateral slit, a TNW probing is performed starting from the tear duct, through the lacrimal sac to the nasolacrimal duct or the

Tab. 14.2 Intubation techniques for splinting the lacrimal drainage system. (Selection)

Location of the stenosis	monocanalicular/monocanaliculonasal	bicanalicular/ bicanaliculonasal
Canaliculi	Minimonoka® (Fayet & Bernard)	Ring intubation (Murube del Castillo)
	Lacrijet® for tear duct injuries	Ring intubation set ("Erlangen model")
		bicanalicular self-stabilizing set®
Lacrimal sac and/or	Monoka® (Ritleng)	bicanaliculonasal intubation (Jünemann)
Nasolacrimal duct	Masterka®	BIKA intubation set®
	Lacrijet®	Intubation set Ritleng+®
		Nunchaku®
Osteotomy as part of	Minimonoka® (Fayet & Bernard)	bicanaliculonasal intubation (Crawford, O'Donoghue)
a DCR	Monoka® (Ritleng)	Nunchaku®
	Mono-Crawford®	
Conjunctiva/nose as part of	Lester-Jones tube (StopLoss™ tube)	
a conjunctivorhinostomy	Tube de Metaireau®	

DCR dacryocystorhinostomy
®FCI, Paris, France

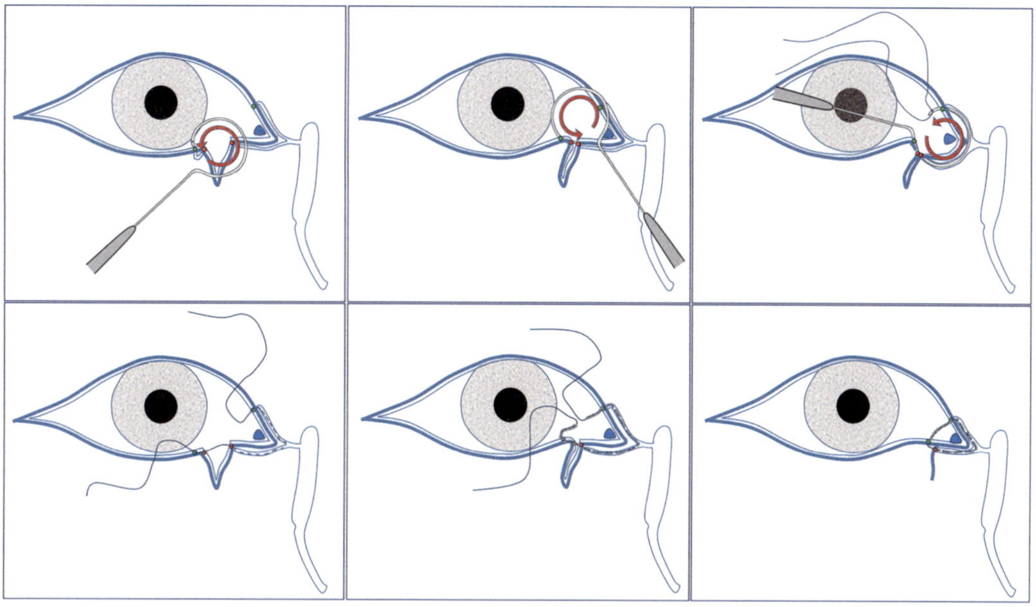

Fig. 14.23 Ring intubation of the TNW according to Murube del Castillo

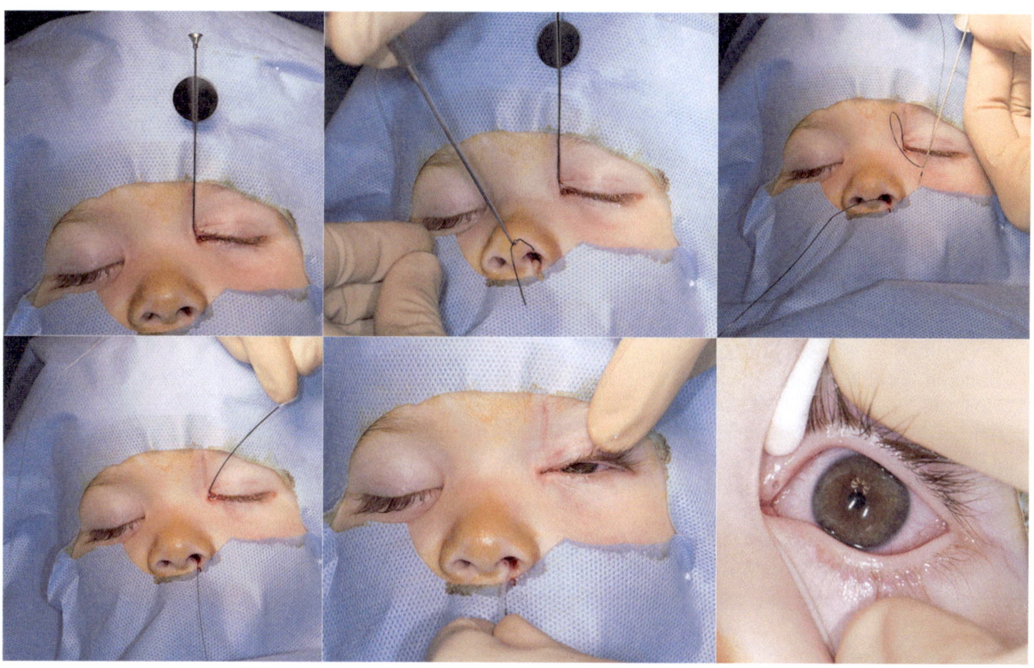

Fig. 14.24 Lacrimal duct intubation using Ritleng technique in an 18-month-old child with congenital dacryostenosis. (Left eye)

lower nasal passage. Subsequently, a guide thread is inserted at the end of which the silicone part is already attached. The guide thread rolls up in the nasal cavity and can now be extracted from the nostril with a hook. Since the guide thread tapers after about 30 cm, this thin part allows for lateral separation from the lacrimal drainage system probe through the slit. The silicone part is then pulled in over the thread remaining in the lacrimal drainage system until it snaps into place with its shoe in the lacrimal punctum. The excess part of the intubation can be shortened through the nostril (Chap. 2) (Fig. 14.24).

References and Further Reading

1. Anderson R, Dixon R (1979) Aponeurotic ptosis surgery. Arch Ophthalmol 97:1123–1128
2. Anderson R, Gordy D (1979) The tarsal strip procedure. Arch Ophthalmol 97:2192–2196
3. Blaskovics L v, Kettesy A (1970) In: Vörösmarthy D (Hrsg) Eingriffe am Auge. 4. Aufl. Enke, Stuttgart, p 176
4. Collin JRO, Rathbun JE (1978) Involutional entropion: a review with evaluation of a procedure. Arch Ophthalmol 96:1058–1064
5. Frueh BR, Schoengarth LD (1982) Evaluation and treatment of the patient with ectropion. Ophthalmology 89:1049–1054
6. Heichel J (2017) Stufenkonzept zur Therapie der konnatalen Dakryostenose. Klin Monatsbl Augenheilkd 234:1250–1258
7. Heichel J, Reich W, Stadie V, Viestenz A, Eckert A (2020 Jan) Interdisziplinäres Management von Tumoren der Lid- und Periorbitalregion. Klin Monatsbl Augenheilkd 237(1):46–56
8. Heichel J, Struck HG, Viestenz A, Glien A, Plontke S (2020) Erkrankungen des Tränenapparats, Teil 1: Anatomie. Physiol Diagn Laryngorhinootol 99:112–125
9. Heichel J, Struck HG, Viestenz A, Glien A, Plontke S (2020) Erkrankungen des Tränenapparats, Teil 2: Grundlagen der Therapie. Laryngorhinootologie 99:247–261
10. Jindal K, Sarcia M, Codner MA (2014) Functional Considerations in Aesthetic Eyelid Surgery. Plast Reconstr Surg 134:1154–1170
11. Jones LT, Reeh MJ, Wobig JL (1972) Senile Entropion: A New Concept for Correction. Am J Ophthalmol 74:327–329
12. Klingenstein A, Hintschich C (2018) Update Oberlidblepharoplastik. Ophthalmologe 115:266–274
13. Lee OS (1951) Operation for correction of everted lacrimal puncta. Am J Ophthalmol 34:575
14. Lew HR (1995) Suture repair of involutional entropion. Aus New Zealand J Ophthalmol 23:247–248
15. Müllner K (1998) Ritleng-Intubationsset zur Schienung verletzter Tränenwege. Klin Monatsbl Augenheilkd 213:238–240
16. Olver JM (1998) Surgical tips on the lateral tarsal strip. Eye (Lond) 12:1007–1012
17. Pitz S (2010) Stellenwert der horizontalen Lidspaltung nach Wies in der Entropiumchirurgie. Klin Monatsbl Augenheilkd 227:26–28
18. Riedel KG, Beyer-Machule CK (1991) Die temporale Tarsalzungenplastik zur Korrektur von Unterlidfehlstellungen. Forstchr Ophthalmol 88:569–573
19. Rokohl AC, Guo Y, Mor JM, Loreck N, Koch KR, Heindl LM (2020) Intubationssysteme in der Tränenwegchirurgie – eine aktuelle Übersicht. Klin Monatsbl Augenheilkd 237:20–28
20. Rokohl AC, Kopecky A, Guo Y, Kakkassery V, Mor JM, Loreck N, Koch KR, Heindl LM (2020) Chirurgische Resektion mit ophthalmoplastischer Rekonstruktion. Goldstandard beim periokulären Basalzellkarzinom Ophthalmologe 117:95–105
21. Schaudig U, Heidari P, Schumacher S (2012) Ektropium und Entropium des Unterlids. Ophthalmologe 109:443–449
22. Schöpfer O (1949) Über einen einfachen Eingriff zur Behandlung des Entropiums. Klin Monatsbl Augenheilkd 115:40–42
23. Sommer F (2010) Operative Ektropium- und Entropiumkorrektur. Ophthalmologe 107:897–904
24. Struck HG (2009) Tränenwegsverletzungen und ihre chirurgische Versorgung. Ophthalmologe 106:223–228
25. Wabbels B (2019) Botulinumtoxin in der Augenheil kunde. Klin Monatsbl Augenheilkd 236:825–836

Procedures on Conjunctiva and Cornea

15

Martin Miertsch, Frank Wilhelm, Christoph Schmidt, Anja Viestenz and Erik Chankiewitz

Contents

Practicing operations on the conjunctiva and cornea is of particular value for beginners in ophthalmic surgery. These are usually performed exclusively extraocularly and involve suturing and knotting.

M. Miertsch (✉)
Greifswald, Germany

C. Schmidt
Augenärztliche Gemeinschaftspraxis „Augen im Zentrum", Greifswald, Germany
e-mail: c.schmidt@augen-im-zentrum.de

A. Viestenz
Klinik und Poliklinik für Augenheilkunde, Universitätsklinikum Halle/Saale, Halle/Saale, Germany
e-mail: sekretariat.augenklinik@uk-halle.de

E. Chankiewitz
Augenklinik, Städtisches Klinikum Braunschweig gGmbH, Braunschweig, Germany
e-mail: erik@chankiewitz.de

F. Wilhelm
Universitätsklinikum Halle Saale, Greifswald, Germany

15.1 Cornea

The most common procedures on the cornea involve placing and removing sutures, which will be exemplarily addressed here.

Corneal sutures are necessary after injuries to the eyeball and in the context of intraocular procedures. Individual sutures, such as those placed as tunnel sutures or for the treatment of small perforating injuries of the cornea, are particularly suitable for beginners, as the risk of anterior chamber flattening or tissue prolapse during manipulation is low in these cases.

- There are rules that make it easier for beginners in ophthalmic surgery to perform single button sutures. It should be ensured that:
- An operating microscope is used in principle,
- non-absorbable suture material Nylon 10-0 is used (see Fig. 15.1),
- The needle is inserted perpendicular to the wound edge,

F. Wilhelm (ed.), *Ophthalmic Surgery for Beginners*, https://doi.org/10.1007/978-3-662-70287-1_15

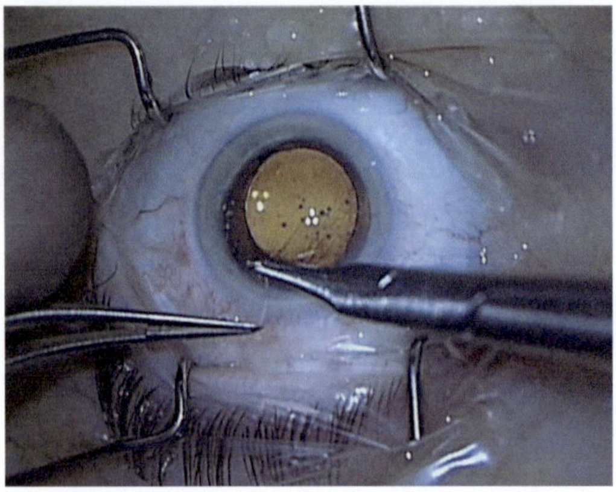

Fig. 15.1 Performing a single button suture on a corneal tunnel after cataract surgery (Technical details are discussed in detail in Chap. 12.)

- Opposite wound edges are precisely apposed (deep lamellar),
- The suture movement follows the curvature of the needle,
- The monofilament suture is cut close to the knot,
- The knot is tightened and rotated into the corneal stroma,
- The induced astigmatism is considered when aligning and adjusting the suture tension.

The removal of individual corneal sutures is possible for the experienced surgeon at the slit lamp. If there are multiple single button sutures after the treatment of extensive corneal wounds or continuous sutures, for example, in the context of a corneal transplant, removal in the operating room under the microscope is advisable. In addition to a suitable lid speculum for pulling the threads, a suture forceps or a fine needle holder is required as instrumentation. A micro knife (Chap. 13) can be used for cutting. A fine needle is also possible and more cost-effective. Just like with the blade of the micro knife, the suture can be cut with the lateral edge of the needle. The flat part of the instrument is then used to lift the suture end over the epithelium, which can then be grasped with the forceps.

- It is important to ensure that:
  the suture is cut in such a way that the end in the direction to be pulled is left as long as possible to securely grasp it with the forceps or fine needle holder,
- The pull is directed towards the adapted wound so that the opening of the wound is not provoked and the wound edges do not gape apart.

After suture removal, it is recommended to check the condition at the slit lamp. Depending on the extent of the primary wound, the number of removed sutures, and the epithelial lesions caused by the procedure, the use of topical antibiotics and epithelializing eye ointments should be considered.

15.2 Conjunctiva

The removal of a pterygium is the most common procedure on the conjunctiva and is therefore often assigned to beginners. This operation will be exemplarily presented here, as the approach in many individual steps is comparable to other procedures on the conjunctiva, such as the treatment of wounds or the removal of small tumors.

15.2.1 Operative Procedure

After skin disinfection, taping the eyelid margins with incision foil, and inserting the lid speculum, local sub-conjunctival infiltration anesthesia with Xylocaine follows. The body of the pterygium is undermined with a probe, and the head is partially bluntly detached and partially sharply separated from the cornea with a 30° knife. The base of the excision site is cleaned and smoothed with the hockey knife and, if necessary, with small scissors. Then, the triangular excision of the pterygium is performed depending on the extent up to the plica semilunaris. Hemostasis is achieved using diathermy if needed. The use of antimetabolites such as Mitomycin C to reduce the recurrence rate should be handled restrictively, as the data on this is inconsistent [6].

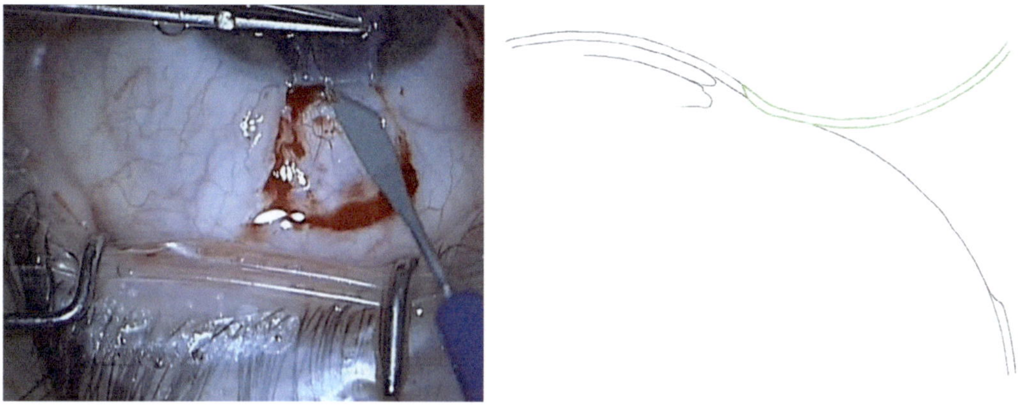

Fig. 15.2 Inclusion of deeply located limbal stem cells at the excision site

A conjunctival flap of appropriate size with limbal stem cells is obtained from the upper temporal area.

▶ Since the limbal stem cells are not found superficially at the limbus but several hundred micrometers deep, the conjunctival flap should not be prepared too thinly at the limbus!

As shown in Fig. 15.2, an appropriate micro knife (here a 30° knife) is used to include the deeply corneal limbal stem cells.

Additionally, the orientation of the conjunctival graft must be clear to the surgeon at all times during the procedure. A spontaneous movement of the patient or strong squeezing of the eyelids can lead to displacement of the free graft. Also, during this phase of the operation, dabbing should generally be avoided (or done only by the surgeon) as the graft may otherwise adhere to it. If the conjunctival graft were to be implanted in the wrong orientation, i.e., not with the limbal stem cells at the corneal edge, the likelihood of recurrence is very high.

The authors therefore recommend leaving the conjunctival graft fixed at the limbus in an area of about ½ hour during preparation. A correspondingly long 10–0 nylon suture is anchored intrasklerally at the limbus at the lower corner of the excision site and led to the corresponding limbal edge of the conjunctival graft. The suture ends are left long (Fig. 15.3). Only then is the final severing of the remaining bridge at the upper limbus performed (Figs. 15.4 and 15.5).

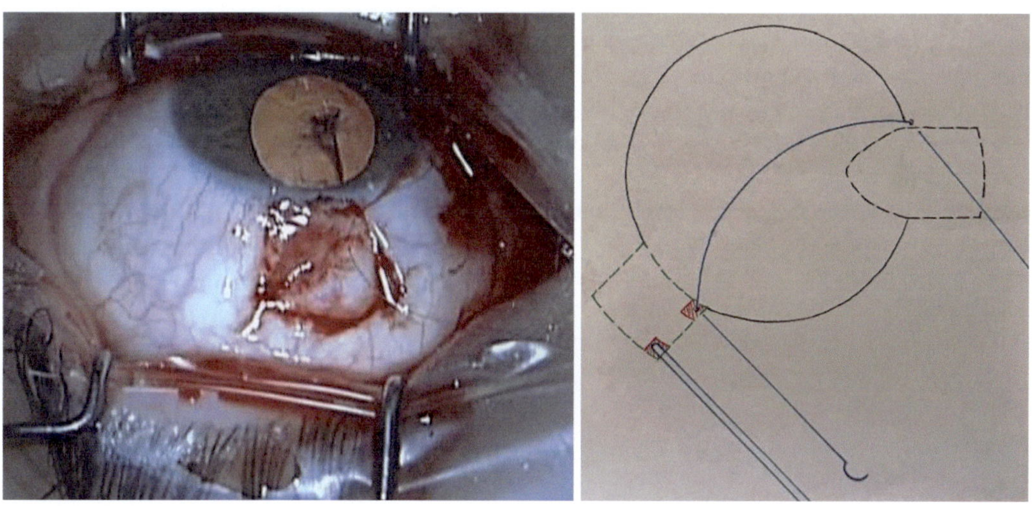

Fig. 15.3 Placing a long suture from the excision site to the graft corner

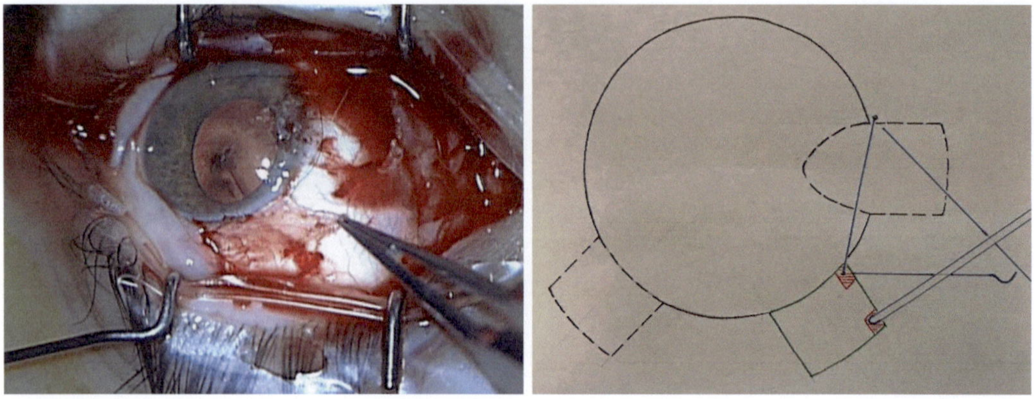

Fig. 15.4 With the help of the pre-placed long 10-0 nylon suture, the graft is simultaneously controlled and safely swung into the excision site in a limbus-to-limbus position by pulling at two graft corners and fixed with 10-0 nylon single button sutures

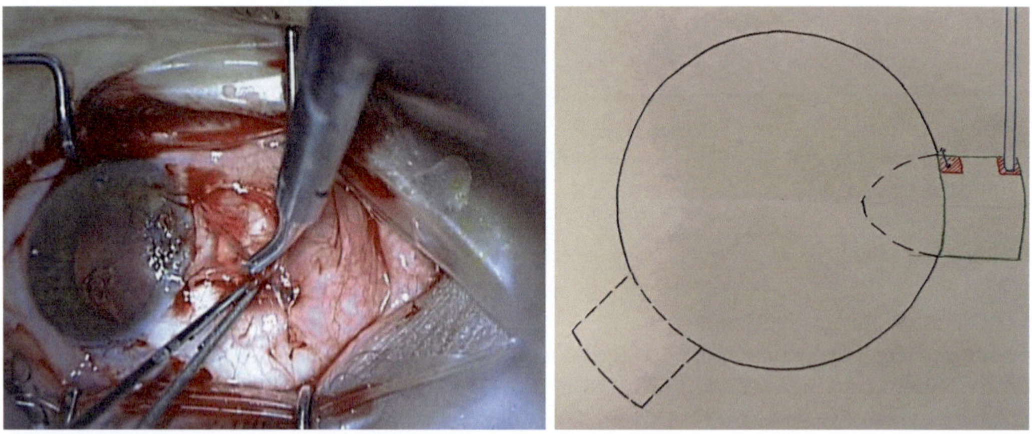

Fig. 15.5 The graft is apposed tension-free with 10-0 nylon single button sutures

At the excision site of the conjunctival graft, suturing is also performed with 10-0 nylon single button sutures. It is important to ensure that the conjunctiva to be adapted lies directly and without a gap at the "excision limbus" to avoid provoking a pterygium recurrence at the excision site. The suture ends should be left long as they can be removed more easily later.

When using a limbus-overlapping therapeutic contact lens (e.g., 20 or 22 mm diameter) at the end of the procedure, the patient does not experience any significant foreign body sensation postoperatively due to the long sutures.

▶ The routine histological examination of every excised pterygium is mandatory [4, 5, 8].

15.2.2 Postoperative Therapy

To reduce the recurrence risk after pterygium surgery, both corticosteroids (topical or subconjunctival) and cyclosporine A can be used postoperatively [7]. Depending on the findings, these should be applied over several weeks to months under control (e.g., preservative-free cortisone eye drops).

▶ Postoperative monitoring of intraocular pressure is necessary to identify steroid responders!

Considering the underlying condition, the lubricating therapy should be continued regularly (preferably with preservative-free preparations) for life.

15.3 Amniotic Membrane Transplantation

The transplantation of an amniotic membrane (AM) is suitable for many indications [9]. In the eye, it is primarily used for chronic or acute surface problems of the cornea and conjunctiva. Here, the basic technique, which is easy to perform, will be presented. In cases of deep corneal ulcers, AM layers are used to fill deep stromal defects, known as the inlay technique [10]. Erosions are treated using the onlay technique.

The amniotic membrane itself is a bioproduct that is semi-transparent, anti-inflammatory, non-immunogenic, anti-fibrotic, promotes epithelial growth, and is self-epithelializing. It is the fetal side of the placenta, the amniotic epithelium with a thin stromal layer underneath. It is obtained from placentas of cesarean deliveries. The selection of donors is based on the criteria for corneal donation, including serological and microbiological controls. Processing is done under cleanroom conditions. The placenta is thoroughly rinsed, the AM is peeled off, and placed on a suitable carrier. It is then cut into squares (usually 2 × 2 cm for ophthalmology). Through cryopreservation (at least −80 °C), the preparations are usable for one year [11]. With other forms of preservation, such as peracetic acid and ethanol, lyophilization, the advantage of longer shelf life at room temperature is offset by the disadvantage of the loss of biological properties [12].

15.3.1 Operative Procedure

The procedure can be performed under local drop anesthesia with an additional subconjunctival injection of a local anesthetic.

The cryopreserved amniotic membrane is delivered frozen from a cornea bank and should be thawed before use (at least 30 minutes) after checking the packaging. The thickness of the AM itself can vary greatly depending on the extraction site on the placenta. At the attachment of the umbilical cord, the amniotic membrane is particularly thick.

- ▶ The suturing of an amniotic transplant should only be performed if the ocular surface and wound (after sufficient topical antibiotic pretreatment) are germ-free.

The ulcer base is cleaned using a hockey knife and the size is determined with the help of a compass. Then, one or, depending on the depth, several AM transplants are prepared either using a trephine or simply with Wescott scissors in the appropriate size. The use of fibrin glue for fixation can be helpful but is only necessary in exceptional cases.

- ▶ With a dried ulcer base (if necessary, additionally dabbed), the applied transplants hardly shift.

Another trick is to fix a larger covering membrane with 10-0 or 11-0 sutures and carefully pull the smaller AM pieces underneath into the resulting pocket to fill the ulcer.

The last, top layer of the amniotic membrane is fixed radially with 10 or 11-0 nylon sutures with the epithelial side facing up, as already mentioned (Fig. 15.6a).

- ▶ The length of the suture ends at the knots should be chosen so that they are easy to grasp and do not injure the young, vulnerable epithelium again when removed (Sect. 15.2)!

Overlaps with the host epithelium should be avoided. The more fitting and smoother it lies, the better the corneal epithelium can grow over it. The membranes can be fully integrated into the cornea, keratocytes migrate in, and the cornea becomes increasingly transparent after a few months [13].

Finally, as with only shallow defects (erosions), an amniotic membrane can be placed over it in the onlay technique, which is not integrated and is mainly used as protection

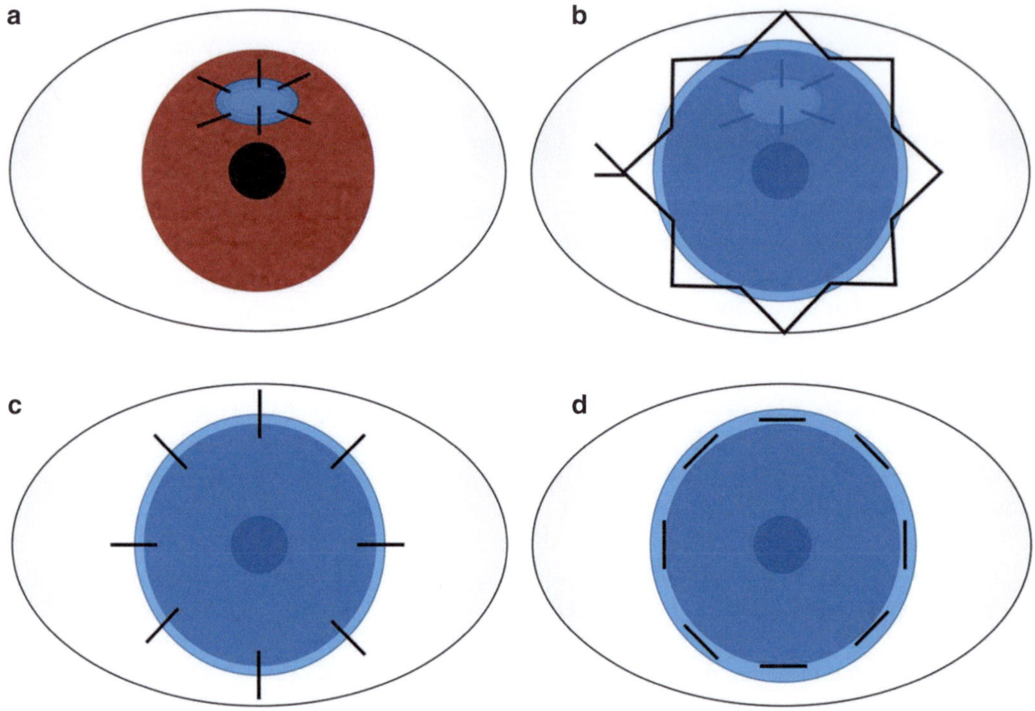

Fig. 15.6 **a–d** Common methods for fixing an amniotic membrane with sutures on the cornea. **a** Inlay technique. **b** Inlay technique in combination with onlay technique and continuous star suture. **c** Onlay technique with radial single button sutures and **d** Onlay technique with circular sutures, possible as single button or continuous sutures

and a growth stimulus. There are many variations here, and almost every surgeon modifies the technique slightly. However, it is generally advisable to choose the size of the AM transplant so that it overlaps the limbus edge, i.e., to trephine it with a diameter greater than 13 mm or cut it with Wescott scissors. When covering freshly burned eyes after a peritomy, the amniotic membrane is made even larger and spread flat under the opened bulbar conjunctiva-Tenon layer and fixed in this way. The epithelial side of the amniotic membrane should face downwards! It is advisable to pause the surface rinsing at this stage to avoid displacing the amniotic membrane. The easiest way to fix the membrane is with a monofilament suture and a semicircular needle, ideally with the suture for corneal sutures (see above). The suture can be placed either with eight to ten radial single button sutures fixed directly at the limbus or limbus-near scleral area (Fig. 15.6c). Alternatively, a continuous star suture with about six to eight stitches in the amniotic membrane and exits in the free conjunctival area can be performed (Fig. 15.6b). A circular suture with entry and exit in the amniotic membrane as a continuous or single button suture can also securely and stably fix the transplant (Fig. 15.6d).

Occasionally, the hyperemic conjunctiva bleeds heavily when pierced with the needle. However, this is not necessarily a disadvantage, as the limbal stem cells are additionally stimulated by blood or serum, and the natural fibrin glue provides additional fixation.

15.3.2 Postoperative Therapy

Finally, a contact lens should be used for protection, and in cases of burns, an Illig shell should also be used. The local antibiotic therapy must be continued. After about a week, the release of growth factors from the amniotic membrane is exhausted, and it only serves as a wound cover, similar to a bandage. It has proven effective to leave the amniotic membrane in place as long as the structure of the membrane is clearly recognizable, giving the surface enough time to heal. Repeating the procedure is possible at any time if needed.

15.4 EDTA Abrasion for Band Keratopathy

The EDTA abrasion is a relatively simple therapy for the removal of superficial epithelial corneal changes with calcification, such as band keratopathy. Band-shaped corneal degenerations can occur in the context of rheumatic underlying diseases, after intraocular inflammations, after injuries, after repeated intraocular procedures, or more rarely, hereditary. Regularly, the changes begin in the area of the palpebral fissure nasally or temporally and increase over time until the optical axis is reached. The calcifications can sometimes increase so much over time that the deposits can also detach in the form of plaques. An indication for treatment exists in the case of a reduction in visual acuity or significant photophobia.

The listed instruments and materials are needed for the EDTA abrasion:

- sterile cotton swabs,
- sterile absorbent swab material,
- funnel-shaped plastic eye cup with a diameter at the attachment of 12–22 mm (corresponding to the plastic eye cup for ultrasound biomicroscopy),
- hockey knife if needed,
- eyelid speculum,
- drape with hole or drape with integrated incision foil,
- diluted EDTA solution (1.5–3% ethylenediaminetetraacetic acid or ethylenediaminetetraacetate),
- 0.9% NaCl rinsing solution,
- one 5 ml or 10 ml disposable syringe each for the EDTA and NaCl rinsing solution,
- simple bandage lens or sclera-supported bandage lens,
- magnifying glasses or operating microscope.

15.4.1 Operational Procedure

After performing surface disinfection, topical anesthesia is administered (Chap. 9). The surgical area is covered sterilely, and an eyelid speculum is inserted. Then the plastic funnel can be inserted. This must fit tightly with the eye surface to prevent the EDTA solution from flowing away. Any superficial larger calcium plaques can be carefully removed with a hockey scalpel. With a cotton swab soaked in the EDTA solution, the corneal surface is massaged in a circular motion to dissolve the calcium deposits. EDTA is a chelating agent and forms a chelate complex with calcium during these manipulations. Simultaneously, the pathologically altered epithelium is mechanically removed by the manipulations with the swab. These fragments, along with excess EDTA, can be removed from the eye cup by rinsing with 0.9% NaCl solution and absorbent swabs. The treatment with a new cotton swab soaked in EDTA solution alternated with NaCl rinsing is repeated as needed until the plaque-like corneal changes are removed. If delicate residual changes remain in the peripheral corneal area despite multiple passes, they can also be left. It should be noted that in patients with limbal stem cell insufficiency of the cornea, this manipulation further reduces the number of functional stem cells!

▶ To reduce postoperative pain, the use of a bandage lens is necessary due to the large corneal erosion!

15.4.2 Aftercare

As local therapy, preservative-free antibiotic and lubricating eye drops are applied. Usually, after one to two weeks, the cornea is sufficiently epithelialized so that the bandage lens can be dispensed with. In the case of limbal stem cell insufficiency, this can be significantly delayed. If epithelial closure does not occur, additional measures, such as sewing on an amniotic membrane, may be indicated.

The patient should be informed in advance that it may be necessary to repeat the treatment due to a recurrence even after years.

References and Further Reading

1. Jack J Kanski, Brad Bowling (2012) Klinische Ophthalmologie. 7. Aufl. Urban & Fischer in Elsevier (Verlag). 978-3-437-23473-6 (ISBN)
2. Bradley JC, Yang W, Bradley RH, Reid TW, Schwab IR (2010) The science of pterygia. Br J Ophthalmol 94(7):815–820. https://doi.org/10.1136/bjo.2008.151852. Epub 2009 Jun 9. PMID: 19515643
3. Chui J, Di Girolamo N, Wakefield D, Coroneo MT (2008) The pathogenesis of pterygium: current concepts and their therapeutic implications. Ocul Surf 6(1):24–43. https://doi.org/10.1016/s1542-0124(12)70103-9. PMID: 18264653
4. Cursiefen C, Kruse FE, Naumann GOH (2008) Conjunctiva and limbus corneae. In: Naumann GOH, Holbach L, Kruse FE (Hrsg) Applied pathology for ophthalmic microsurgeons. Springer, Berlin, Heidelberg, S 67–75
5. Kruse FE, Völcker HE, Naumann GOH (1997) Konjunktiva. In: Naumann GOH (Hrsg) Pathologie des Auges. Springer, Berlin, Heidelberg, S 379–506
6. Eisenmann K, Zeman F, Helbig H, Gamulescu MA, Barth T (2020) Ergebnisse der Pterygiumchirurgie nach verschiedenen Operationstechniken – Ist die Exzision mit einfachem Bindehautverschluss noch lege artis? [Outcome of pterygium excision after various surgical techniques-is excision with simple conjunctival closure still lege artis?]. Ophthalmologe 117(4):359–365. https://doi.org/10.1007/s00347-019-00968-8. PMID: 31520116
7. Heindl LM, Cursiefen C (2010) Pterygium. Ätiologie, Klinik und neue adjuvante Therapien [Pterygium. Etiology, clinical aspects and novel adjuvant therapies]. Ophthalmologe 107(6):517–520., 522–524. PMID: 20393732. https://doi.org/10.1007/s00347-009-2100-4
8. Hirst LW, Axelsen RA, Schwab I (2009) Pterygium and associated ocular surface squamous neoplasia. Arch Ophthalmol 127(1):31–32. https://doi.org/10.1001/archophthalmol.2008.531. PMID: 19139334
9. Schmiedova I et al (2021) Using of amniotic membrane derivatives for the treatment of chronic wounds. Membranes (Basel) 11(12):941
10. Lee SH, Tseng SC (1997) Amniotic membrane transplantation for persistent epithelial defects with ulceration. Am J Ophthalmol 123(3):303–312
11. Thomasen H et al (2018) [Good practice procedures for acquisition and preparation of cryopreserved human amniotic membranes from donor placentas]. Ophthalmologe 115(10): p. 855–867
12. Thomasen H et al (2009) Comparison of cryopreserved and air-dried human amniotic membrane for ophthalmologic applications. Graefes Arch Clin Exp Ophthalmol 247(12):1691–1700
13. Seitz B et al (2006) Histopathology and ultrastructure of human corneas after amniotic membrane transplantation. Arch Ophthalmol 124(10):1487–1490

16 Enucleation

Jens Heichel and Arne Viestenz

Contents

The removal of the eyeball (Enucleatio bulbi, Enucleation) involves the surgical extraction of the bulbus oculi from the orbital tissue complex. According to anatomical descriptions, the essential connections to the external eye muscles, the Tenon capsule (Vagina bulbi), the conjunctiva, and the optic nerve fix our visual organ in the orbit (Chap. 2).

Enucleation is often delegated to less experienced surgeons. It should be critically noted here that, depending on the indication, the constitution of the eyeball, and the general condition of the patient, some difficulties may arise. Furthermore, it is a final ophthalmic surgical procedure, often preceded by numerous operations and thus a long period of suffering. This must be taken into account in patient management and the implementation of surgical measures. Severely disconfigured eyes are generally difficult to dissect during enucleation, making these cases unsuitable for beginners, as the possibility of scleral perforation is very high—a situation that must be avoided at all costs (Caution: intraocular malignancies; sympathetic ophthalmia)!

Another aspect is the removal of donor eyes, which should only be mentioned here. This procedure must be carried out with no less care. The procurement of donor tissue plays a very significant role in ophthalmology and should therefore be learned and performed by young colleagues. Enucleation for the procurement of

J. Heichel (✉) · A. Viestenz
Klinik und Poliklinik für Augenheilkunde, Universitätsklinikum Halle/Saale, Halle/Saale, Germany
e-mail: jens.heichel@uk-halle.de
e-mail: sekretariat.augenklinik@uk-halle.de

F. Wilhelm (ed.), *Ophthalmic Surgery for Beginners*, https://doi.org/10.1007/978-3-662-70287-1_16

donor eyes provides an excellent opportunity for every aspiring ophthalmic surgeon to practice the enucleation operation under guidance and to gain a sense of the procedures, the tissue, and the anatomical conditions. The careful preparation of the eye muscles can also help to achieve the required numbers in the context of specialist training.

16.1 Distinction Between Evisceration of the Eyeball and Orbital Exenteration

The rarely used Evisceratio bulbi (syn. Exenteratio bulbi) involves the evisceration of the eye's interior while leaving the scleral shell in situ. Thus, the anterior segment of the eye is removed, and the retina and choroid are removed by curettage. A placeholder can then be inserted into the scleral shell. The procedure can be performed under local anesthesia and is associated with a lower tendency to bleed. However, compared to enucleation, slightly higher rates of prosthesis extrusion are to be expected. Evisceratio bulbi is contraindicated in cases of intraocular malignancy and advanced endophthalmitis (Caution: scleral and optic nerve involvement).

The Orbital Exenteration (syn. Exenteratio orbitae) involves the removal of the contents of the orbital socket up to the periorbita, where the anterior layers of the eyelids can be left in place depending on the indication, to fold them into the orbit and incorporate them into the plastic reconstruction. The procedure is usually performed by colleagues from other head and neck surgical specialties.

▶ For enucleation, the eyelids, conjunctiva, and lacrimal apparatus must be free from significant pathological processes (Caution: tumor infiltration!).

16.2 Planning the Procedure

First, a clear indication must be established to define the goal and necessity of enucleation. This must be discussed with the patient in an appropriate manner and requires time, empathy, and professional competence. The procedure is typically performed under general anesthesia. Classic risk factors such as bleeding tendency and arterial hypertension should be taken care of or addressed in advance of the elective surgery. Additionally, questions regarding a bradycardic heart rhythm disorder (oculocardiac reflex) and sufficient postoperative compliance must be addressed. Bleeding tendencies, non-compliance, and complex anatomical conditions (e.g., enucleation in a child) are absolutely unsuitable for novice ophthalmic surgeons!

16.3 Classic Indications

A typical indication is the painful amaurotic eye. This situation is often the result of chronic uveitis, severe trauma, or secondary angle-closure glaucoma. Another reason is severe therapy-resistant endophthalmitis. However, enucleation is still indicated for tumors at a certain stage. This latter indication is particularly important because a possible transscleral break-through and optic nerve infiltration must be ruled out in advance. This must be urgently considered during preparation, as the optic nerve stump remaining on the eyeball must be significantly longer (at least 5 mm or longer, depending on the findings).

16.4 Possibilities of Volume Replacement

The eye socket has a volume of approximately 30 ml. The eyeball occupies about ¼ of this space. Removing the eyeball without volume replacement would therefore lead to a significant excess space in the orbit. A ptosis with a deep lid crease and the appearance of a pseudoenophthalmos would be the result (Chap. 2).

In principle, autologous and alloplastic techniques can be distinguished in orbital volume replacement. They can be classified as follows:

Overview of Autologous and Alloplastic Techniques

- Autologous Transplants
  - Pedicled: Temporalis muscle via lateral orbitotomy
  - Free: (e.g., gluteal) dermis-fat transplant
- Alloplastic Implants
  - Porous: Hydroxyapatite (biological/synthetic)
    Bioceramic
    Polypropylene
    Acrylic
  - Non-porous: Silicone plug
    Glass
    Polymethylmethacrylate
    Acrylic
  - Combined: Hydroxyapatite-silicone implant (e.g., according to Guthoff; Fig. 16.1)
- Mixed volume replacement (allogeneic-alloplastic)
  - Alloplastic implants encased by sclera

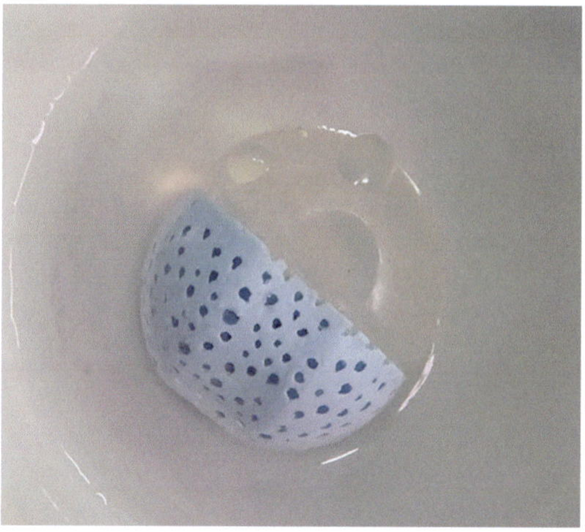

Fig. 16.1 Guthoff implant

16.5 Goals of a Proper Eye Removal

The following goals are pursued from a functional and aesthetic perspective, in addition to eliminating pathological changes:

- Movable orbital implant with good biocompatibility;
- extensive symmetry to the opposite side;
- comfortable and sufficient fit of the later prosthesis (intact fornices, adequate lid tension).

Therefore, reduced horizontal lid tension or a volume deficit (Phthisis bulbi) should be identified before enucleation. The goal is also to place the orbital implant in the intraconal space (Tenon's capsule). Due to the expected atrophy of the orbital soft tissue, the primary volume replacement should be as large as possible (Chap. 2).

▶ To achieve good prosthesis mobility, a connection between the external eye muscles and the orbital volume replacement must be established. Furthermore, a large orbital implant and intact conjunctival fornices are advantageous for this purpose (Caution: symblephara).

16.6 Procedure of an Enucleation

The following is an example of a possible enucleation procedure. It should be noted that there are numerous modifications for performing this procedure, which will not be discussed in detail here.

Before an enucleation, the indication and the side of the operation should be rechecked or confirmed by the surgeon immediately before the start of the operation. For this purpose, fundoscopy and, if necessary, sonography should be performed intraoperatively.

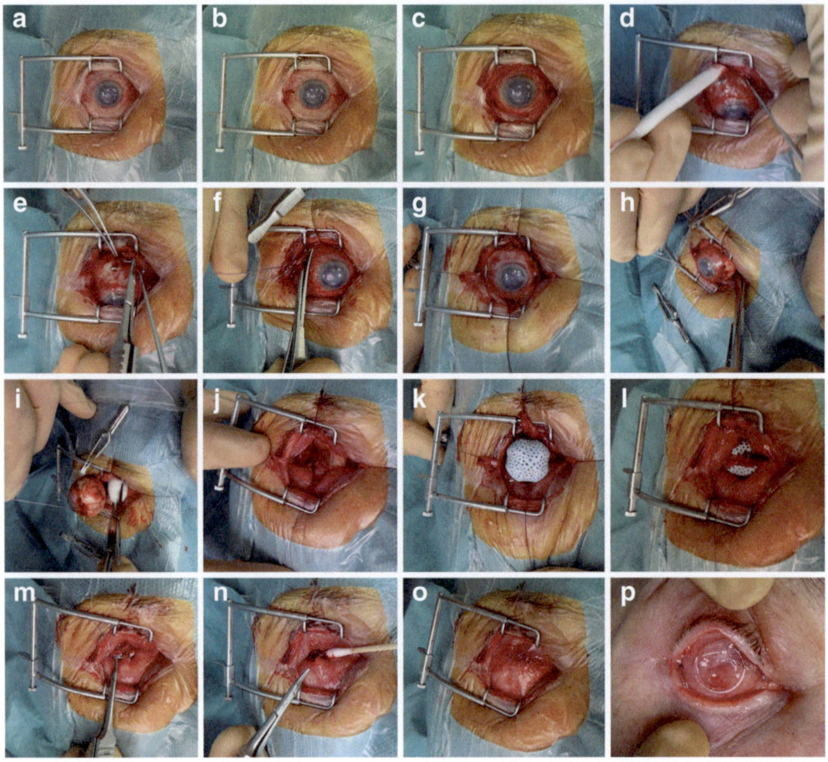

Fig. 16.2 a–p Procedure of an enucleation with implantation of an 18-mm Guthoff implant. (From top left to bottom right, explanations in the text). **a** Situs after completed disinfection and draping as well as insertion of the lid speculum. **b** Opening of the conjunctiva at the 3 and 9 o'clock positions. **c** Completion of the 360° peritomy. **d** Hooking of the straight external eye muscles (here, M. rectus superior). **e** Weaving through the muscle. **f** Severing of the muscle. **g** Situs after looping all four straight external eye muscles. **h** Insertion of the slightly opened enucleation scissors into the Tenon's capsule from the nasal side. **i** Compression of the orbital apex after severing the optic nerve. **j** Situs after removal of the eyeball. **k** Insertion of an alloplastic volume replacement into the Tenon's capsule. **l** Crossing and bringing together the horizontal muscles over the orbital implant using absorbable sutures. **m** Crossing the vertical muscles and forming a muscle cross with the horizontal muscles, fixation with absorbable suture material. **n** Tight suturing of the Tenon's capsule. **o** Suturing of the conjunctiva. **p** Insertion of a placeholder (here: Illig shell)

Procedure of an Enucleation

The procedure of an enucleation can be summarized as follows (Fig. 16.2):

1. Disinfection of skin and conjunctiva; sterile draping of the surgical field. Optionally, a parabulbar injection of adrenaline 1:200,000 can be administered (Fig. 16.2a).
2. Insertion of the lid speculum and circular paralimbal opening of the conjunctiva (if necessary, marking to better distinguish the conjunctiva from Tenon's capsule, Fig. 16.2b, c).
3. Exposure of the sclera while preserving Tenon's capsule, visualization of the four rectus muscles (Fig. 16.2d).

4. Hooking of the four rectus muscles with a strabismus hook, looping with a resorbable polyphilic 6-0 suture (weaving twice at a distance of about 2 to 3 mm from the muscle insertion) and severing of the muscle; leaving the detachment stump of the medial rectus muscle slightly longer to allow secure grasping of the eyeball (Fig. 16.2e, f, g).
5. Hooking the oblique muscles with the strabismus hook and severing it; if necessary, looping (some surgeons prefer attaching the oblique muscles to the prosthesis to improve motility).
6. Maximum abduction of the eyeball by pulling on the medial muscle insertion (alternatively, a traction suture can be used) and entering the orbit with the enucleation scissors from the medial side towards the optic nerve; the optic nerve can be felt by slightly opening the scissors (Fig. 16.2h).
7. Detachment of the optic nerve at the desired distance from the globe (aiming for 5 mm) and immediate compression of the orbital funnel with a plum-shaped swab clamped in a forceps (compression duration 3 to 5 minutes, Fig. 16.2i).
8. If necessary, sequential hemostasis by cauterization.
9. Insertion of the orbital implant into Tenon's capsule and gradual overlapping of the rectus muscles (isolated knotting of the horizontal and vertical motors respectively, and final purse-string-like weaving of the entire muscle cross with the pre-placed resorbable polyphilic 6-0 sutures of the muscle loops, Fig. 16.2j, k, l, m).
10. Tight closure of Tenon's capsule with several resorbable polyphilic 6-0 sutures (single knot technique, Fig. 16.2n).
11. Continuous suture of the conjunctiva, e.g., with resorbable polyphilic 7-0 suture (Fig. 16.2o).
12. Insertion of an Illig shell, ointment pressure bandage (Fig. 16.2p).

16.7 Aftercare

Depending on the course of the operation and the expected tendency to bleed, the bandage can initially be left in place for 48 hours. Subsequently, further daily pressure bandages are applied. As a rule, these are not required for more than five days. Antibiotic-anti-inflammatory ointments should be used under the bandages. The Illig shell should also continue to be used to prevent early shrinkage of the fornices. If no more bandages are needed, eye drops can be used instead. The central opening in the Illig shell allows wound secretion to drain. After about four weeks, fitting of a glass or acrylic prosthetic epithesis is possible. This is done by an ocularist.

References and Further Reading

1. Baino F, Perero S, Ferraris S, Miola M, Balagna C, Verné E, Vitale-Brovarone C, Coggiola A, Dolcino D, Ferraris M (2014) Biomaterials for orbital implants and ocular prostheses: overview and future prospects. Acta Biomater 10:1064–1087
2. Cleres B, Meyer-Rüsenberg HW (2014) Poröse Orbitaimplantate. Ophthalmologe 111:572–576
3. Hintschich C (2017) Dermis-Fett-Transplantation. Ophthalmologe 114(8):755–758
4. Klett A, Guthoff R (2003) Wie lässt sich die Prothesenmotilität verbessern? Ophthalmologe 100:445–448
5. Langer C (2002) Enukleation des Bulbus. In: Wilhelm FW, Duncker GIW, Bredehorn T (Hrsg) Augenbanken. Walter de Gruyter, Berlin, New York, S 43–46
6. Mourits DL, Hartong DT, Lissenberg-Witte BI, Bosscha MI, Tan HS, Moll AC (2018) Cosmetic results of enucleation and/or external beam radiation therapy in 195 retinoblastoma survivors. Acta Ophthalmol 96:631–640
7. Rokohl AC, Koch KR, Trester M, Heindl LM (2018) Augenprothesen aus Kryolithglas bei korallinen Hydroxylapatitimplantaten als Bulbusersatz nach Enukleation. Ophthalmologe 115:793–794

Iridectomy

17

Erik Chankiewitz and Frank Wilhelm

Contents

17.1 Introduction

Iridectomy refers to the excision of a piece of the iris. Depending on the technical approach, a corresponding coloboma results (Fig. 17.1).

Performing an iridectomy is one of the fundamental skills of any surgically active ophthalmologist and is therefore typically part of the training to become a specialist in ophthalmology as the "smallest intraocular procedure." The oldest surgical procedure in glaucoma treatment was introduced as early as the 19th century by Albrecht von Graefe and is now predominantly performed with the Neodymium: YAG laser as laser iridotomy [1]. It is the method of choice for angle-closure glaucoma as a prophylaxis for pupillary block. However, for this, the cornea must be sufficiently transparent to allow the transmission of laser energy to the iris. Additionally, any pre-existing anterior synechiae can be resolved during a surgical iridectomy [3]. It has been shown that, at least after three years, there is no significant difference between the two procedures [2].

Today, this procedure is an important step in many complex operations to achieve the desired functionality, such as in trabeculectomy, or essential to prevent postoperative complications, among others in Descemet endothelial membrane keratoplasty (DMEK) and penetrating keratoplasty, as Ando-iridectomy in silicone oil fillings after PpV, as well as in the implantation of iris-clip lenses or add-on lenses, and many more.

In this article for beginners in eye surgery, only the surgical iridectomy to prevent a pupillary block is discussed. The goal is to create a sufficiently large opening in the peripheral iris between the posterior and anterior chambers so that the aqueous humor can flow from the posterior chamber to the anterior chamber bypassing the pupil. This is usually done in the upper half of the iris. This can prevent later glare, as the upper eyelid covers the iris defect.

E. Chankiewitz (✉)
Augenklinik, Städtisches Klinikum Braunschweig gGmbH, Braunschweig, Germany
e-mail: erik@chankiewitz.de

F. Wilhelm
Universitätsklinikum Halle Saale, Greifswald, Germany

F. Wilhelm (ed.), *Ophthalmic Surgery for Beginners*, https://doi.org/10.1007/978-3-662-70287-1_17

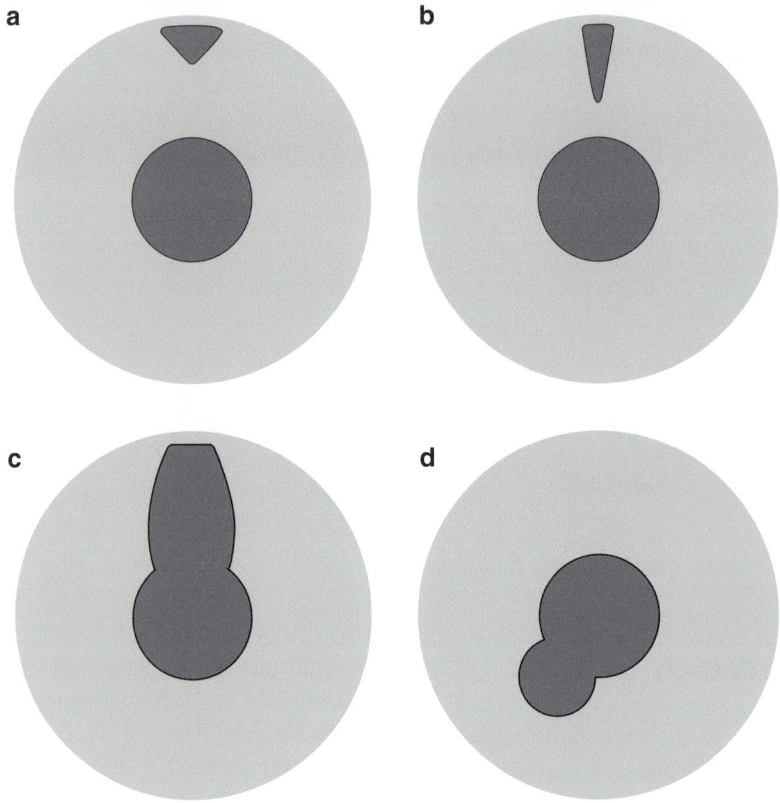

Fig. 17.1 **a–d** Representation of the basic types of surgically achieved colobomas after basal (**a**), more peripheral (**b**), sector-shaped (**c**), central (**d**) iridectomy. [According to 4]

Before starting the iridectomy, the eye must be carefully examined to determine the ideal position.

▶ Areas with strong peripheral corneal vascularization, prominent iris vessels, iris stroma with little structure (unlike laser iridectomy), or in the area of iris nevi are particularly unsuitable.

▶ Before the procedure, the pupil should be constricted with a series of pilocarpine eye drops.

A limbus-parallel corneal incision approximately 1.5 to 2 mm long is made as vertically as possible through the cornea and close to the limbus (Fig. 17.2). This incision should not be conical (outer and inner openings are the same size) and not tunneled (Chap. 13). After perforating the cornea, some aqueous humor spontaneously egresses, and the anterior chamber slightly flattens. Now, using an iris forceps or a fine tying forceps, the iris tissue near the iris root is securely grasped. It is gently pulled outward above the corneal level and the prolapsed iris tissue is cut off flat with a single snip of scissors. A slight distortion of the pupil towards the paracentesis is usually observed.

▶ It is important to grasp enough tissue so that the anterior and posterior layers of the iris are securely cut through, but not so much that a large opening results, which could later cause glare. Moderate bleeding and pigment dispersion into the anterior chamber can occur and are immediately rinsed out with BSS. Usually, parts of the iris tissue trapped in the incision fall back into the anterior chamber. Finally, the incision is sealed by slight

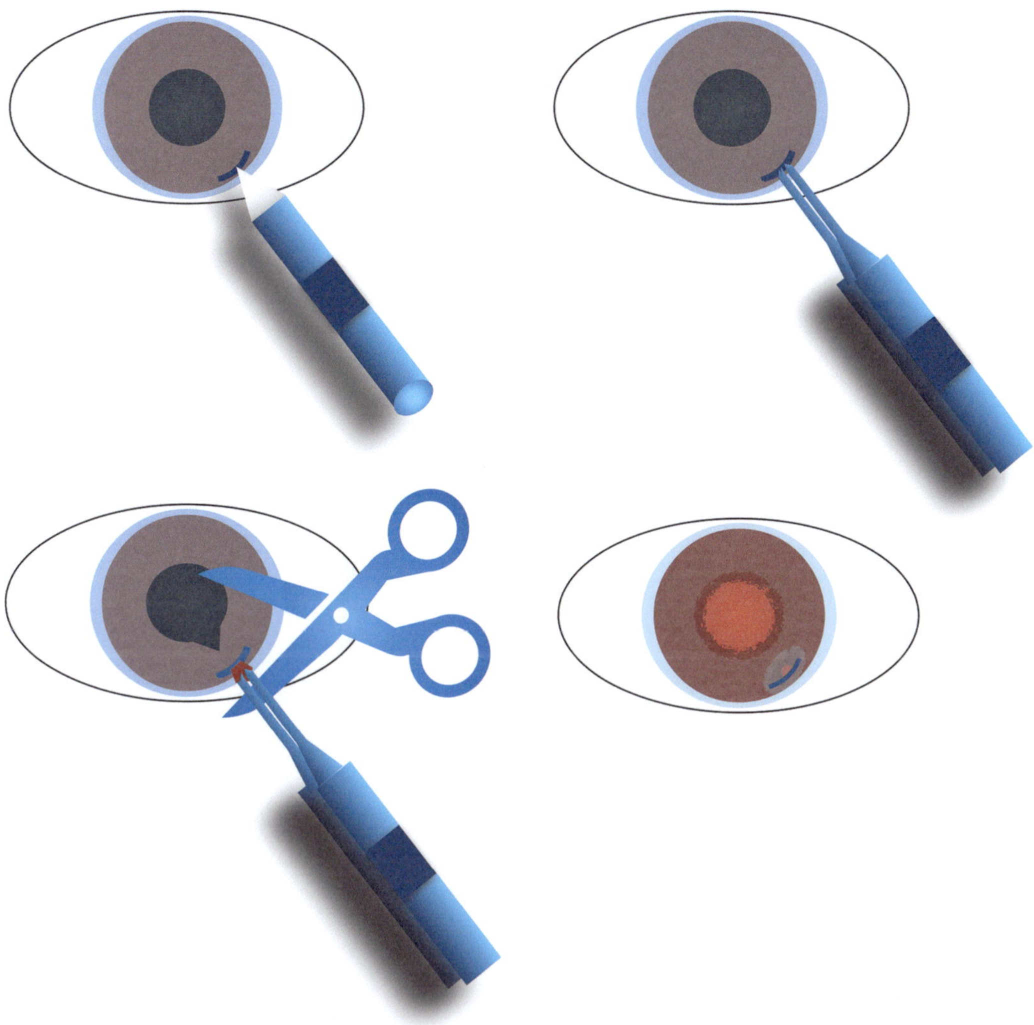

Fig. 17.2 Schematic representation of the procedure of a basal iridectomy

hydrating of the stroma using an intrastromal injection of BSS, and any potential bleeding is stopped by slightly increasing the intraocular pressure.

▶ In retro-illumination, the iridectomy appears red, indicating a full-thickness opening of the iris.

If the iridectomy is too large, it can lead to increased sensitivity to glare postoperatively. Reaching the dilator muscle of the pupil through the excision results in pupil motility disorders. Due to the irritation of the iris tissue during the procedure, it can sometimes lead to a severe inflammatory reaction, especially in younger people, which is why postoperative steroid eye drops are essential. These also prevent the partially pronounced synechiae with the anterior lens surface after laser or surgical iridectomies. To prevent a consecutive increase in intraocular pressure due to increased pigment dispersion and the resulting accumulation in the chamber angle, postoperative controls for biomicroscopy of the anterior eye segments with tension controls are necessary.

References and Further Reading

1. Congdon NG, Friedman DS (2003) Angle-closure glaucoma: impact, etiology, diagnosis, and treatment. Curr Opin Ophthalmol 14:70–73
2. Fleck BW, Wright E, Fairley EA (1997) A randomised prospective comparison of operative peripheral iridectomy and Nd: YAG laser iridotomy treatment of acute angle closure glaucoma: 3 year visual acuity and intraocular pressure control outcome. Br J Ophthalmol 81:884–888
3. Funk J (2009) Antiglaukomatöse Laserchirurgie Was war? Was ist? Was wird? Ophthalmo Chir 21:25–32
4. Mackensen G (1989) Chirurgie der Iris und des Ziliarkörpers. In: Mackensen G, Neubauer H (Hrsg) Augenärztliche Operationen, Teil 1. Springer, Berlin, pp 603–649

Intravitreal Injections 18

Klaus Mayer, Christoph Schmidt and Uwe Wilhelm

Contents

An intravitreal injection at the slit lamp is not permissible and should be performed in a certified operating room!

18.1 Material and Instrument List

The following instruments and materials should be prepared before the procedure. The list is a recommendation intended to standardize the procedure and minimze the risk of infection (Chap. 5):

- PVP-iodine solution 5% and 10%
- Eye drops for topical anesthesia, e.g., Conjuncain® (Oxybuprocaine 0.4%, Mann, Berlin, Germany)
- Eyelid speculum
- Surgical eye forceps or colibri forceps
- Sterile microscope buttons/microscope handles
- Sterile eye dressing, (if necessary, hourglas dressing)/capsule dressing
- Adhesive strips
- Table cover
- Surgical gloves for assistant
- Surgical gloves for surgeon
- Surgical gown for assistant
- Surgical gown for surgeon
- Two cigarette swabs
- An eye marker (compass 3.5/4.0 mm) or equivalent
- An eye drape (with incision film)
- Paracentesis knife (in reserve)

K. Mayer (✉)
Augenpraxisklinik im Alleecenter, Remscheid, Germany
e-mail: kla.mayer@t-online.de

C. Schmidt
Augenärztliche Gemeinschaftspraxis „Augen im Zentrum“, Greifswald, Germany

U. Wilhelm
MVZ Roswitha und Daniel Krause, Dortmund, Germany

F. Wilhelm (ed.), *Ophthalmic Surgery for Beginners*, https://doi.org/10.1007/978-3-662-70287-1_18

Eyelid speculum, compass, and forceps can be used as reusable or disposable instruments. Disposable instruments can also be obtained as a complete package along with the additionally required disposable materials from various suppliers of surgical materials.

18.2 Patient Selection for Beginners

For beginners, it is advisable to start with pseudophakic eyes. Steroid implants (Ozurdex®, Allergan, Dublin, Ireland, and Iluvien®, Alimera Sciences, Alpharetta, USA) should be avoided at the beginning due to the larger cannula diameter and the slightly higher risk of complications.

The first injections should be performed under the supervision of an experienced surgeon.

18.3 Verification of Indication and Identity

Before each procedure, the surgeon must verify the patient's identity and ensure the correct side of the operation. Furthermore, they must confirm the correct indication.

▶ For the first indication, a fluorescein angiography is required. Indications during the course can also be determined via OCT.

Since many procedures are performed consecutively in many surgical centers, a routine must also ensure that there are no mix-ups with the medications. Direct personal communication with the patient provides the final assurance.

The surgeon must ensure that the cold chain has been maintained when providing the medications. This is relevant for anti-VEGF medications. Iluvien and Ozurdex do not need to be stored refrigerated.

18.4 Preparation of the Eye

Before the procedure, a medicinal mydriasis is performed with, for example, Mydriaticum Stulln® UD AT (Tropicamide, Pharma Stulln,

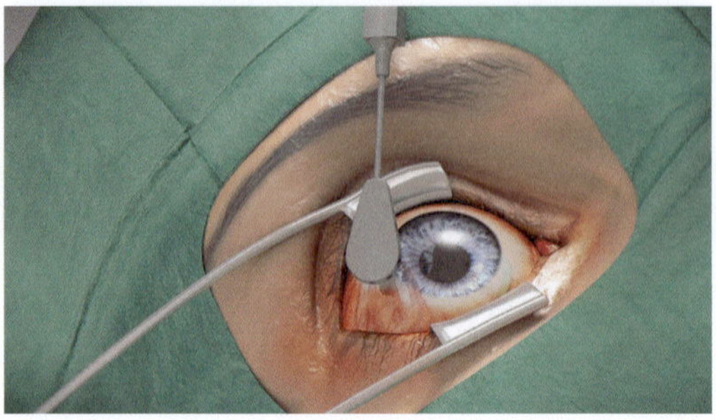

Fig. 18.1 Irrigation of the conjunctiva with PVP-iodine. (© Bayer AG)

Stulln, Germany). Furthermore, the eye receives a topical anesthesia with, for example, Conjuncain®. To achieve good anesthesia, at least three series should be administered at intervals of five minutes.

Once good topical anesthesia is achieved, local PVP-iodine 5% irrigation can be performed (Fig. 18.1). This is mandatory before every intravitreal injections. A contact time of at least three minutes is common. The irrigation is often perceived as unpleasant by the patient, which is why the topical anesthesia must be performed beforehand. Conjunctival disinfection with PVP-iodine is considered the gold standard. However, if there is a PVP-iodine intolerance, polihexanide 0.04% can also be used after informing the patient [6]. The extended contact time of 20 minutes and multiple applications must be considered during preparation! The disinfection of the periocular skin and eyelashes is performed with PVP-iodine 10%. The wiping of the eyelashes, eyelid margins, and periorbital skin is done twice with a sterile forceps and a sterile swab. It is important to ensure that no massage of the Meibomian glands occurs! If there is an intolerance to PVP-iodine, Octenisept can alternatively be used for the skin. However, when using colorless Octenisept, it is not apparent to the surgeon how well the surface disinfection was performed.

18.4.1 Preparation of the Syringe

It is best to use a pre-filled syringe. Pre-filled syringes reduce the risk of contamination and also facilitate the surgical process with a higher number of patients. If the medication still needs to be drawn up, a filter needle is used for this purpose. Ideally, a 30G-x-½-inch needle is used as the injection needle. This is sufficiently thin to allow for a leakage-free wound closure and with a low risk of scleral perforation. A Luer-Lock connection is important for a secure connection between the needle and the syringe. An injection volume of 0,05 or 0,1 . ml is common. To remove excess medication and bubbles, you can tap the upright syringe slightly and then push the plunger up to the 0,05 or 0,1 ml mark.

18.4.2 Draping the Eye

In the operating room, a renewed check of the patient's name and side must be performed before the injection.

The procedure is performed after surgical hand disinfection and with sterile gloves.

The eye is now draped with a sterile drape. If fenestrated drapes are used, an additional incision film is necessary. Generally, specially prepared fenestrated drapes with adhesive film and perforation line are used so that the eyelids and eyelashes can be well covered. Before applying the film, excess disinfectant is removed with a sterile swab to ensure better adhesion. For better positioning of the film, the lower eyelid is slightly moved downward with a cigar swab until a slight ectropion position is achieved. The patient looks up while the film is applied. The film is lightly pressed, and the drape is unfolded. The drape should be positioned towards the anesthesia bar so that there is sufficient distance between the mouth and the drape.

An eyelid speculum is used to keep the eye securely open. Good spreading is important for free access to the injection without the risk of touching the eyelid margin and cilia with the sterile needle tip during the procedure. Eyelid speculums with closed metal wings can be used to hold back the cilia.

18.5 Use of an Operating Microscope

▶ The intravitreal injection is a microsurgical procedure, so it is recommended that this surgery be performed under a surgical microscope.

If a supine position of the patient is not possible, an intravitreal injection can also be performed without a microscope in individual cases.

The microscope lighting should be set low so that the patient is not too dazzled and the eye can be kept still better. Ideally, the patient is asked to fixate on the microscope light to keep the eye straight and still.

Depending on where the injection is to be made, the patient can also be given a different direction to look.

18.6 Choice of the Appropriate Injection site

The injection is performed in the area of the pars plana and is located between 3.5 to 4 mm behind the limbus [4]. When choosing the location, various factors must be considered. Ideally, a site that is freely accessible in the straight-ahead view and thus provides enough distance from the lid margin and eyelashes is chosen. A temporal injection site has the advantage that the pars plana is widest there and thus offers a bit more safety access. The injection site can also be changed with repeated injections to avoid structural changes in the sclera. Thin areas of the sclera can be recognized by a bluish discoloration. Such areas should be avoided. Possible peculiarities such as a retinoschisis or a filtering bleb must also be considered when choosing the site. An inferior injection site has the advantage that, in the event of a defensive reaction with Bell's phenomenon, the eye does not move towards the needle, thus reducing the risk of lens injury.

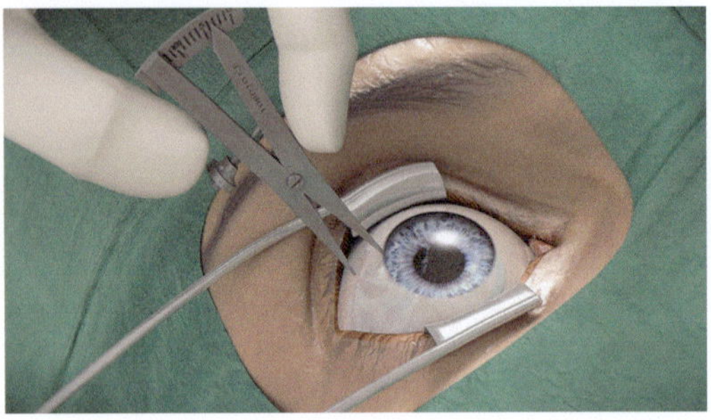

Fig. 18.2 Marking of the injection site. (© Bayer AG)

The injection site is marked with a caliper set to 3.5 or 4 mm (Fig. 18.2). The marking is done with light pressure from the caliper on the sclera. The marking by the caliper then appears as a small, dark gray, dot-like discoloration of the sclera. Similar plastic markers are included with disposable materials. If the injection is too anterior, there is a risk of lens injury; if it is too posterior, there is a risk of causing retinal injury[1].

18.7 Administration of the Injection

The globe is held with tweezers. Tenon's capsule, episcleral tissue, and the conjunctiva are firmly anchored to the sclera at the limbus. There, the bulb can be safely guided with the tweezers (Fig. 18.3). The grip with the tweezers also simultaneously checks whether the anesthesia is sufficient. There is always the risk that the patient may startle and turn their head or eye away. As an alternative to fixing the eye with tweezers, one can also use the compass. Here, the compass is used for distance measurement and simultaneous fixation of the eye, with one tip pressed on the limbus and the second tip pressed parallel to the limbus on the sclera. The injection is then performed directly at the end of the compass tip fixed on the sclera. To facilitate keeping the eye still, the patient can also be given a fixation target if necessary.

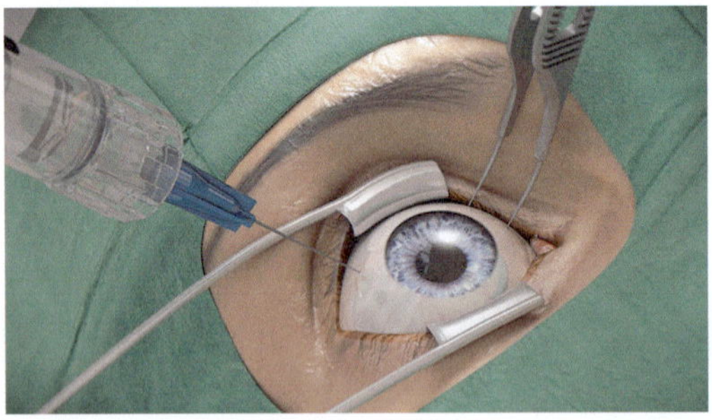

Fig. 18.3 Guiding the eye with tweezers during the injection. (© Bayer AG)

The perforation is performed with the beveled side and slightly obliquely to the sclera lamellarly under even pressure. A stepwise injection with displacement of the conjunctiva was initially recommended. However, this has not generally been adopted. After perforating the sclera, the syringe is finally aimed at the center of the eyeball (Fig. 18.4). This avoids damage to the lens.

When administering a steroid implant, a shallower injection angle can ensure a more secure wound closure. With the larger diameter of the Ozurdex cannula, a more reliable pain reduction can be achieved with an additional subconjunctival anesthesia before the injection.

The patient should be informed that they may see vitreous floaters in the form of "clouds." In the case of a small air bubble in the vitreous cavity, the patient can be reassured about the harmlessness of the "small black ball," and that the effect will disappear after one to two days.

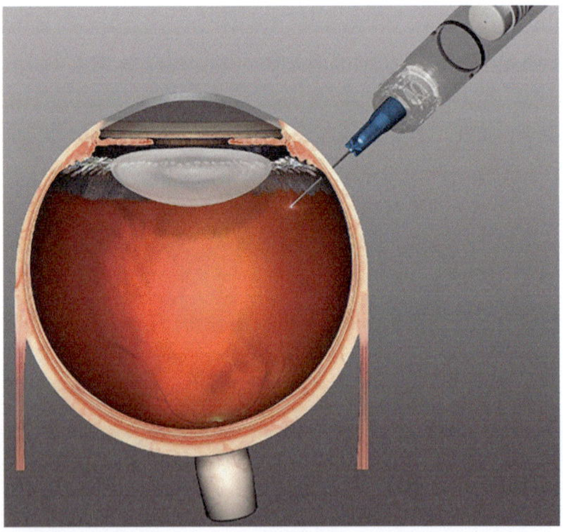

Fig. 18.4 Injection via the pars plana. (© Bayer AG)

18.7.1 Post-Injection Checks

Following the injection, vision is checked with hand movements to rule out a pressure-induced central artery occlusion. A critical increase in intraocular pressure is generally not to be feared with an injection volume of 0,05 up to 0,1ml. Nevertheless, a paracentesis lance should be kept on standby to surgically reduce the pressure via paracentesis if necessary. It should be noted that in poorly controlled glaucoma, the small amount of 0.05 up to 0,1 ml can still increase postoperative intraocular pressure. Preoperative administration of 250 mg acetazolamide intravenously or orally can prevent this. In some surgical centers and eye clinics, intraocular pressure is checked after the injection using non-contact tonometry. Additionally, retinal blood flow (pulsation over the disc) and the position of the medication implant in the vitreous cavity can be checked with an ophthalmoscope if necessary. Often, an eye bandage with or without antibiotic ointment is applied afterward. However, many surgical centers now forgo this. Postoperative topical antibiotic treatment is generally no longer recommended according to the guidelines of the DOG and the German Retinological Society [2, 5].

18.7.2 Possible Complications

Rarely, a residual effect of the local anesthesia and a possibly compressing bandage on the cornea can lead to an erosion. For a small erosion, viscous artificial tears and eye ointment are sufficient. In the case of a larger erosion, a bandage lens or a simple soft daily contact lens provides rapid relief. The patient is then scheduled for a follow-up the next day.

A postoperative hyposphagma is commonly observed and is generally harmless.

An iatrogenic cataract due to lens injury is rare. However, if it occurs, the required cataract surgery is not simple, as the lens capsule has a pre-existing damage. The administration of steroid medications often accelerates cataract progression.

Mild vitreous opacities can be observed by patients during an intravitreal injection. However, severe vitreous hemorrhages are rare.

▶ Endophthalmitis is the most feared complication after an intravitreal injection.

Depending on the study, the rate of endophthalmitis after intravitreal injections ranges between 0.019 and 1.4% [5, 7].

18.8 Aftercare

The surgeon's last question to the patient is always whether the postoperative follow-up is ensured.

The first follow-up is usually conducted between the second and fourth postoperative day. Endophthalmitis is generally only visible on the second or third postoperative day. With steroid implants (Ozurdex® and Iluvien®), further checks to monitor intraocular pressure are required during the postoperative course.

References and Further Reading

1. Bartz-Schmidt KU, Ziemssen F (2008) Intravitreale Pharmakotherapie. Schattauer, Stuttgart
2. Bhatt SS, Stepien KE, Joshi K (2011) Prophylactic antibiotic use after intravitreal injection: effect on endophthalmitis rate. Retina 31:2032–2036
3. Bundesärztekammer (2018) Weiterbildungsordnung. Berlin
4. DOG (2007) Empfehlung der Deutschen Ophthalmologischen Gesellschaft, der Retinologischen Gesellschaft und des Berufsverbandes der Augenärzte Deutschlands für die Durchführung von intravitrealen Injektionen (IVI)
5. DOG (2013) Stellungnahme der DOG, Endophthalmitis Prophylaxe bei intravitrealer operativer Medikamenteneingabe (IVOM)
6. Hansmann F, Kramer A, Ohgke H, Strobel H, Müller M, Geerling G (2005) Lavasept als Alternative

für PVP-Iod zur präoperativen Antiseptik in der Ophthalmochirurgie. Ophthalmologe 102:1043–1050
7. McCannel C (2011) Meta-analysis of endophthalmitis after intravitreal injection of anti-vascular endothelial growth factor agents: causative organisms and possible prevention strategies. Retina 31:654–661
8. Wenzel M, Dick HB, Scharrer A, Schayan K, Agostini H, Reinhard T (2020) Intraokulare Operationen: Ergebnisse der Jahresumfrage 2019/2020 von DGII, DOG, BVA und BDOC. In: 34. Kongress der Deutschprachigen Gesellschaft für Intraokularlinsen-Implantation, Interventionelle und Refraktive Chirurgie. DGII, Mainz, S 55–58

19 Emergency Vitrectomy for Beginners in Endophthalmitis—The Core Vitrectomy

Arne Viestenz, Wolfgang Schrader, Anja Viestenz and Frank Wilhelm

Contents

Endophthalmitis is one of the most vision-threatening emergencies and is considered a clear emergency surgery indication in ophthalmology. Young ophthalmic surgeons are faced with the challenge of quickly and efficiently conducting the medical history, diagnostics, team coordination, and surgical decision-making. The operation should be performed as soon as possible to preserve any remaining vision.

A. Viestenz (✉) · A. Viestenz
Klinik und Poliklinik für Augenheilkunde, Universitätsklinikum Halle/Saale, Halle/Saale, Germany
e-mail: sekretariat.augenklinik@uk-halle.de

A. Viestenz
e-mail: sekretariat.augenklinik@uk-halle.de

W. Schrader
Augenzentrum Würzburg, Würzburg, Germany
e-mail: mail@profschrader.de

F. Wilhelm
Universitätsklinikum Halle Saale, Greifswald, Germany

19.1 Signs of Endophthalmitis

Typical signs of endophthalmitis are: pain, photophobia, epiphora, conjunctival and ciliary injection—also with conjunctival chemosis, periorbital soft tissue swelling, hypopyon, iris hyperemia, vitreous infiltrates and retinal infiltrates, vision loss. Not all of these signs need to be present; for example, only 75% of patients with endophthalmitis experience pain—especially in patients with neuropathy (e.g., in diabetes mellitus or after cerebral/orbital radiation, taking analgesics), pain is not a reliable leading symptom for endophthalmitis (Fig. 19.1).

▶ The absence of pain does not rule out endophthalmitis!

It is especially important for young surgeons to diagnose endophthalmitis. Sometimes no fundus details are visible. Standardized ultrasound of the eye is helpful here. All four quadrants of the globe must be examined in a standardized manner using sonography. In the B-scan, the position with the greatest accumulation of infiltrates is identified. At this position with the most

F. Wilhelm (ed.), *Ophthalmic Surgery for Beginners*, https://doi.org/10.1007/978-3-662-70287-1_19

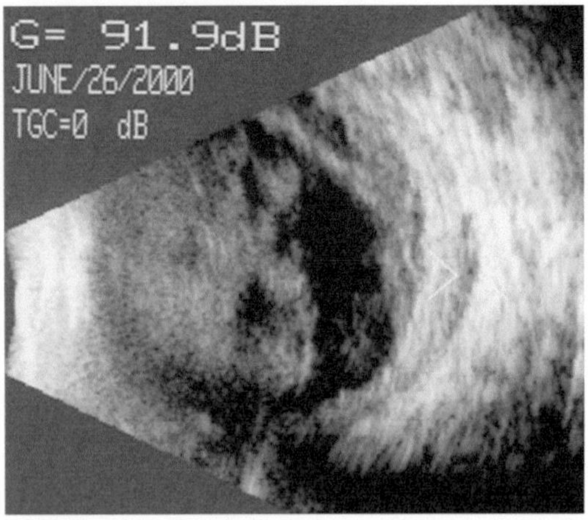

Fig. 19.1 Ultrasound (B-scan) demonstrating massive intravitreal infiltration

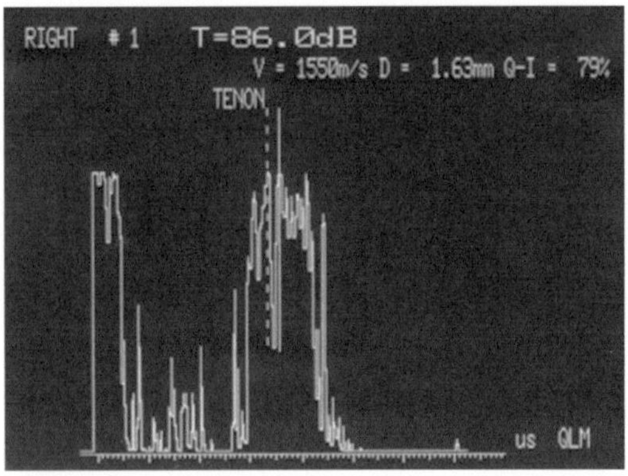

Fig. 19.2 A-scan with vitreous buzz (78 dB = tissue sensitivity T, T+9 dB would be 87 dB). The ultrasound buzz starts below the endophthalmitis lower limit for endophthalmitis

densities (highly reflective structures in the vitreous), the vitreous infiltration is then measured using the standardized A-scan probe (tissue sensitivity T+9 dB = endophthalmitis threshold). If swirling spikes are found in the vitreous space below this threshold, this, combined with clinical findings and medical history, indicates the presence of endophthalmitis (Fig. 19.2).

19.1.1 Medical History

A thorough medical history also helps:

- Do you have pain? Since when?
- Have you had eye surgery or any surgery in the past few weeks? Did you possibly not wear your eye shield or did it slip while sleeping?
- Do you have an artificial heart valve?
- Do you have open sores on your body or in your mouth?
- Have you had an eye injury in the past few days or worked in the garden or workshop and got something in your eye?
- Do you suffer from diabetes mellitus?
- Do you take immunosuppressants?
- Are you infected with HIV/AIDS?
- Do you work in agriculture or a riding stable/do you have pets?
- Do you suffer from a tumor or have you been treated with radiation or chemotherapy?
- For patients in the intensive care unit, it is important to inspect venous or intra-arterial accesses/indwelling catheters—these could be entry points for, e.g., Candida. In the case of confirmed endophthalmitis, the intravascular accesses must be re-established and the catheter tip must be microbiologically analyzed.

19.1.2 Timing of Surgery

The surgery should be performed promptly, i.e., preferably within the next two hours. This means that under central OR conditions, the surgeon must emphasize the urgency of the procedure, and the next available OR slot must be provided. If endophthalmitis is present, an infusion with antibiotics should already be administered systemically (see Magdeburg three-stage scheme by Prof. Wolfgang Behrens-Baumann). If the patient has consumed food within the last six hours, the risks and benefits must be weighed. An ileus induction by the anesthesia team allows the operation to be performed within two hours.

19.1.3 Proper Posture and Monitoring Before Surgery

A supine position is obsolete for the patient before the surgical procedure. This causes cytokines, leukocytes, and germs to sink to the posterior pole and can thus induce a hypopyon on the macula. This toxic accumulation leads to massive inflammation in the macula and not infrequently to vascular occlusion with drastically reduced visual prognosis.

Temperature measurements should be performed regularly (at least 3 times/day) and if there is an elevated temperature or fever, blood should be analyzed for germs (blood culture) to detect and quickly treat sepsis. A conjunctival or corneal swab is performed with the requirement for germ detection and resistance testing. It is also worthwhile to name the planned or used antibiotics. A Hertel-exophthalmometry is also useful. In the case of orbital cellulitis or the progression of endophthalmitis to panophthalmitis with orbital phlegmon, the early comparison of exophthalmometer values can be diagnostically valuable.

A local therapy (every fifteen minutes) with antibiotic eye drops (also "fortified") combined with polyhexanide eye drops should be performed before the surgery. Depending on the preoperativ findings in addition to the widening of the pupil it can be necesssary to perform the scraping of the corneal epithelium.

19.1.4 Local Anesthesia or General Anesthesia?

The inflammation changes the pH value towards the acidic range, so the effectiveness of local anesthetics decreases. To spare the patient with endophthalmitis additional and unnecessary pain, general anesthesia is preferred.

19.1.5 Procedure in the Operating Room

To specifically treat the infection, the germ must be identified.

After disinfecting the surgical area and sterile draping, there are two options for tissue sampling:

1. from the anterior and posterior chambers, respectively.
2. from the vitreous cavity.

While anterior chamber puncture usually yields only 200 µl of aspirate, a volume of 4 to 5 ml can often be obtained from the vitreous, increasing the chances of detecting the germs.

It is crucial that no antibiotics or antifungals are added to the infusion.

The authors recommend the following procedure:

1. Before the start of the operation: Team time-out.
2. In general anesthesia, the periocular region (10% PVP-iodine) and the conjunctiva (5% PVP-iodine) are disinfected. In the case of an open wound of the eyeball, the conjunctiva and cornea are disinfected only with 1% PVP-iodine.
3. Three trocars are inserted at a distance of 3 to 4 mm behind the limbus (Figs. 19.3 and 19.4).
4. The infusion tube with the adapted three-way stopcock is filled only with BSS. Now, if necessary, the IOP can be managed with a syringe filled with BSS.
5. Anterior vitrectomy via pars plana is performed through a trocar.
6. A syringe (e.g., 3 ml) is adapted to the suction tube of the vitrectome and carefully aspirated under rapid cuts of the vitrectome (at least 4000 cuts/minute). Ideally, two syringes are obtained: one for the search for bacteria with a resistance profile and one for the analysis of fungi (fungal PCR and culture).

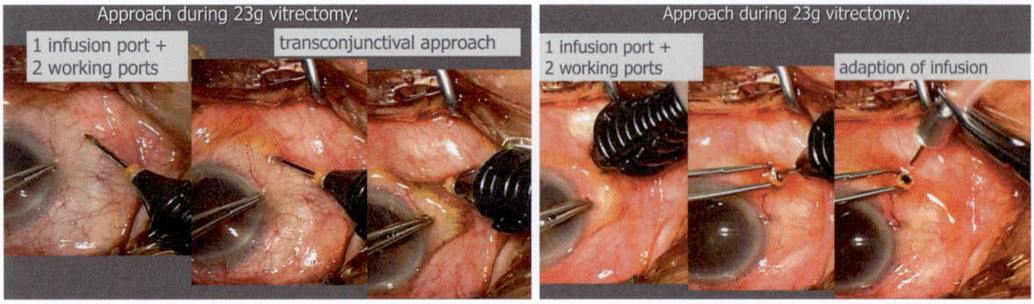

Fig. 19.3 Transconjunctival positioning of trocars. The conjunctiva will be displaced with the tip of the trocars with a distance of 3–4 mm from the limbus and with an angle of approximately 45 to 80 degrees as stepwise line through the sclera into the vitreus cavity.

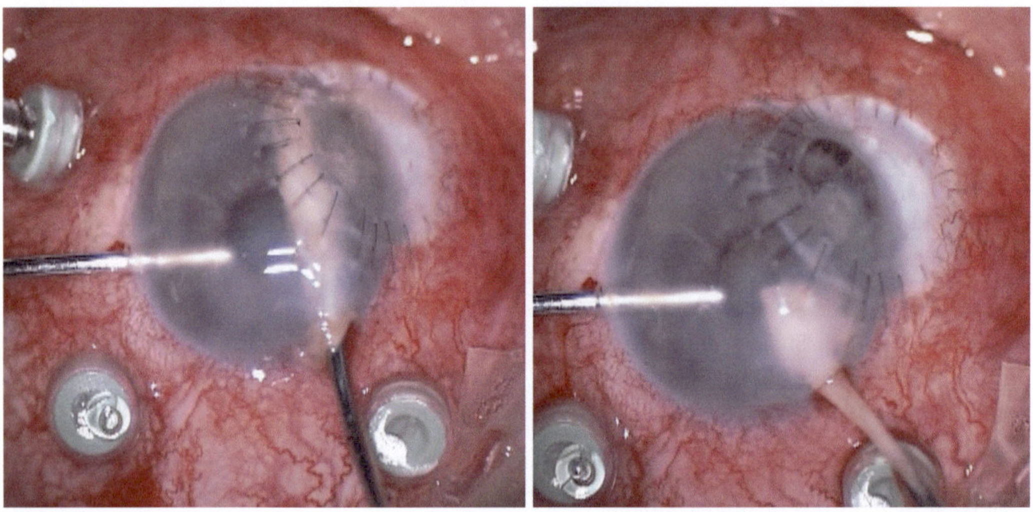

Fig. 19.4 Removal of a hypopyon from the anterior chamber with a 23 g forceps. The hypopyon will be sent for microbiological analysis.

7. The syringe is sealed and sent for microbiological analysis.
8. Pus in the anterior chamber: Chamber water is obtained via a paracentesis with the Sautter cannula. If there is a tough hypopyon in the anterior chamber, it is removed with forceps or tube-guided forceps (Fig. 19.5).
9. Gentamycin is one option that can be used during vitrectomy additionally in BSS-solution (Fig. 19.6).
10. Under continuous infusion, the anterior vitrectomy can now be continued from both upper trocars.
11. The vitreous body should be handled gently. However, in areas without visible retinal infiltrates, it is important to achieve posterior vitreous detachment. Great care should be taken in areas where visibility is limited (Fig. 19.7).
12. Careful water-air exchange (only about 20% of the vitreous volume). This fills the vitreous cavity from the lens to under the trocars with air.

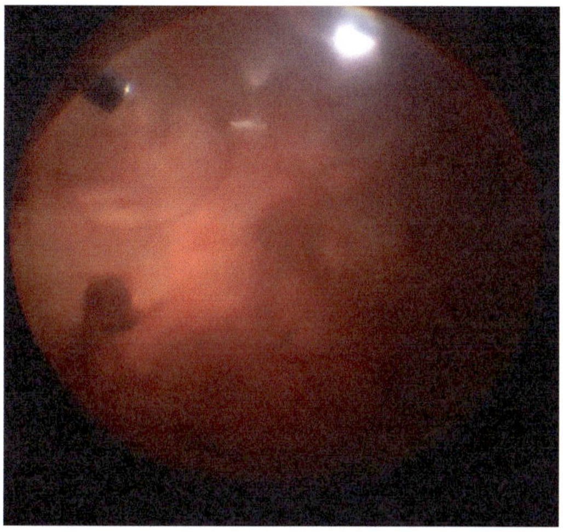

Fig. 19.5 Endophthalmitis after an injury due to a wooden stick. Ophthalmoscopy shows only blurry retinal vessels. The vitreous cavity is filled with blood and strains of bacterial colonies.

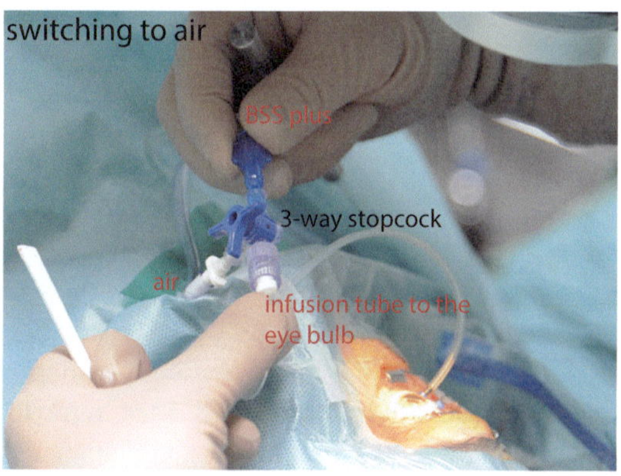

Fig. 19.6 Work with the 3 way port: one tube is connected with the globe, the surgeon may choose between BSS or air supply.

13. Now, 0.1 ml of vancomycin and 0.1 ml of ceftazidime are administered into the vitreous cavity. In case of a strong suspicion of fungal endophthalmitis, voriconazole and amphotericin B are administered intravitreally. The superficial air administration prevents the antibiotics or antifungals from escaping outward (Fig. 19.5).
14. Removal of the trocars and, if necessary, suturing with Vicryl 7-0 EKN in case of air leakage.
15. Subconjunctival administration of steroids and antibiotics/antifungals.
16. Bandage with antibiotic and steroid eye ointment, postoperative local therapy should definitely be continued in the ward!

With a bit more surgical experience, the posterior vitreous cavity can be vitrectomized using the BIOM or a contact lens. The inexperienced are well advised not to aspirate or peel off the deposits on the retina.

After the surgery, the Magdeburg step scheme 3 (endophthalmitis) should be continued. After receiving the antibiogram/resistogram, targeted antibiotic therapy must be administered.

In the following days, the degree of infiltration in the vitreous cavity should be measured daily (preferably 2 to 3 times) using ultrasound. If the decibel threshold decreases, this is an indication of a worsening condition. Consequently, vancomycin and ceftazidime can be re-administered into the vitreous cavity as intravitreal injections after one to three days (Fig. 19.8).

19.1.6 Special case: Endophthalmitis after Intravitreal Injections or pars plana vitrectomy

In contrast to endophthalmitis in cataract surgery, postoperative endophthalmitis in the posterior segment usually initially presents with the accumulation of pus, while the anterior segment may appear uninflamed in the initial phase of endophthalmitis after intravitreal injections or ppV. Examination of the eye in mydriasis is absolutely indicated if post- intravitreal injection endophthalmitis is suspected! Patients often only become sensitive to pain after a longer interval.

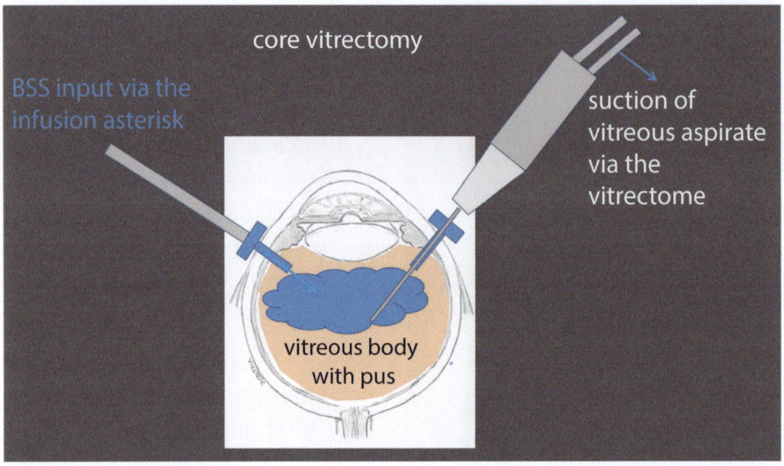

Fig. 19.7 Vitreous probe during core vitrectomy. The vitrectom should be used with a high cutting rate (min. 4000 cuts/min) to avoid tractional forces onto the retina with retinal breaks. The vitrectomy probe should be moved very slowly during the shaving procedure of the vitreus base.

A risk factor for post-intravitreal injections endophthalmitis is the so-called "iodine allergy", which is usually just a contact intolerance of the skin. Sometimes the exposure time of Serasept or polyhexanide (Lavasept 0.04%, applied 3 times every 10 minutes) was not long enough, so the germs were not sufficiently reduced.

19.1.7 What to do if I have never performed a vitrectomy?

In this case, it must be weighed whether the rapid transfer of the patient to a clinic with a vitrectomy service would be better, or whether at least the administration of vancomycin and ceftazidime as intravitreal injection in the procedure room under gel anesthesia should be performed to reduce the proliferation of germs before transferring the patient to a vitrectomy center. In any case, the vitrectomy center should be pre-informed to avoid so-called transfer liability.

Ultimately, the aspiring ophthalmic surgeon should practise the handling of the surgical instruments and control of the machines in the wet lab including vitrectomy.

19.1.8 Special Features: COVID and Endophthalmitis

In the initial phase of the COVID pandemic, the authors observed an increase in endophthalmitis cases (by a factor of 8 after intravitreal injection), often caused by a contaminated mouth-nose protection (MNP), but also by an unsanitized dental status, allowing an airflow over the operated eye through the mask. The bandage is, in our opinion, essential for one day after intravitreal injection when wearing an MNP.

If the patient has endophthalmitis and tested positive for COVID, the risk of general anesthesia must be weighed with the anesthesia team. The surgical team can operate under maximum protection (protective clothing, FFP3 mask) (Fig. 19.9, Tables 19.1 and 19.2).

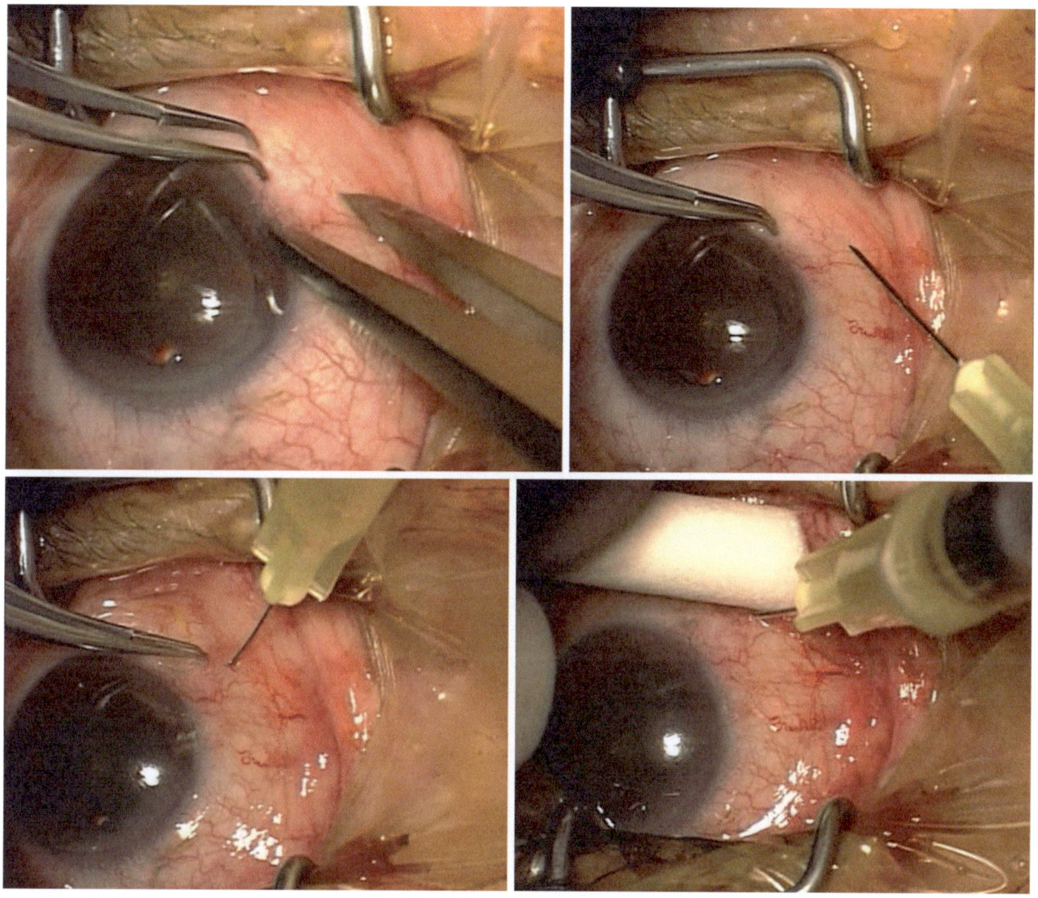

Fig. 19.8 Application of intravitreal injections with vancomycin and ceftazidime (0.1 ml each). The distance will be marked 3 up to 4 mm from the limbus at the sclera (3 mm in aphakic eyes/3.5 mm in pseudophakic eyes/4 mm in phakic eyes). The injection canula will displace the conjunctiva to the middle of the marked scleral point. The cannula will be inserted in a 45° angle into the sclera and moved more perpendicular into the vitreous cavity. Antibiotics will be injected into the vitreous cavity after this maneuver. The cannula will be removed and the conjunctiva will be closed with a e.g. sterile cotton tip. Alternatively, the antibiotics may be injected during a vitrectomy through the trocars.

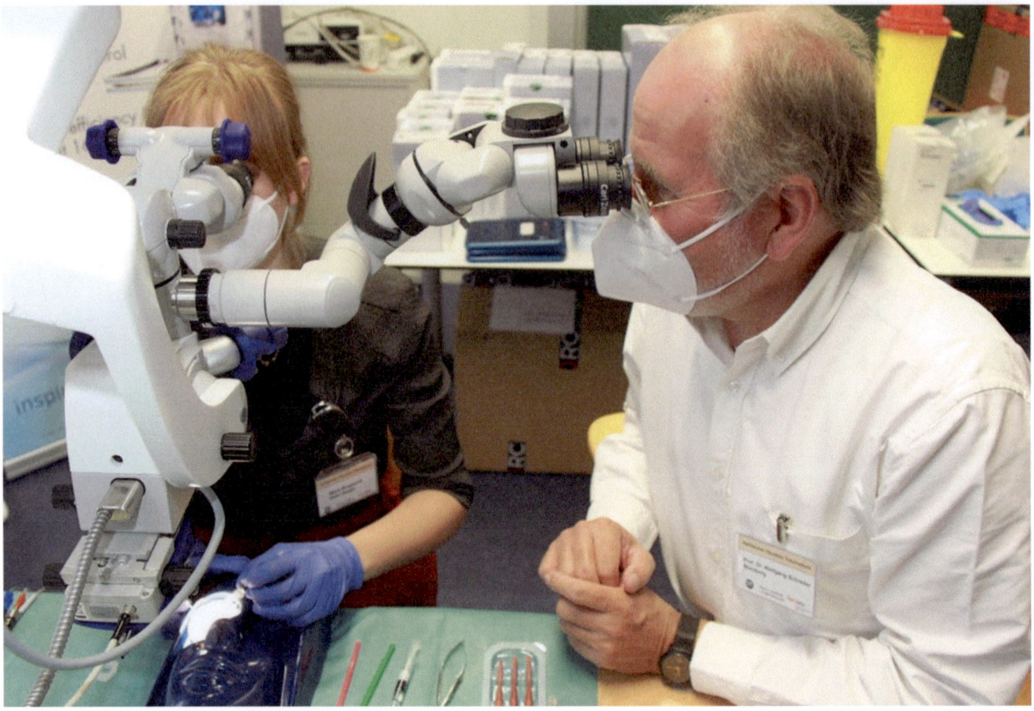

Fig. 19.9 WetLabs using OR microscopes and OR machines are the best preparing stress test for exhausting situations during surgery (crossref. Chap. 7.2). For example: The Halle Ophthalmo-Trauma Course (HOT) of the DOG and the International Society of Ocular Trauma, Prof. Schrader trains a resident.

Table 19.1 Injection of antibiotics into the anterior chamber or vitreous cavity in endophthalmitis. The dosage of the IVI-medication must be reduced to a level 1/4 to 1/5 if gas or silicone oil into the vitreus cavity.

Active ingredient	Administration in AC or VC with approx. 4/5 BSS filling
Vancomycin	1 mg in 0.1 ml
Ceftazidime	2.25 mg in 0.1 ml
Dexamethasone	400 μg in 0.1 ml
Voriconazole	100 μg in 0.1 ml
Amphotericin B	5–7.5 μg in 0.1 ml

Table 19.2 Systemical antibiotics (maximum therapy according to Magdeburg Three-Stage Plan according to Behrens-Baumann)

	Against gram-positive bacteria	Against gram-negative bacteria
Preparation	Vancomycin (e.g., Vancomycin Lederle)	Ceftazidime (e.g., Fortum)
Daily dose	2 × 1 g iv	3 × 2 g
In case of resistance	Daptomycin (Cubicin) 1 × 1500 mg iv	Imipenem

www.kaug.ovgu.de/Zuweiser/Leitlinien

References and Further Reading

1. Barry P, Behrens-Baumann W, Pleyer U, Seal D (2007) ESCRS Guidelines on prevention, investigation and management of post-operative endophthalmitis. Version 2. Published by The European Society for Cataract & Refractive Surgeons. ISBN 0-9550988-0-7
2. Behrens-Baumann W (2004) Antiinfektiva bei Augenverletzungen. Klin Monatsbl Augenheilkd 221:674–676
3. Behrens-Baumann W, Augustin A, Dick B, Fabian E, Huber-Spitzy V, Klauß V, Kramer A, Pitten FA, Pleyer U, Zeitz J (2003) Leitlinie zur Prophylaxe und Therapie von Endophthalmitiden. Hyg Med 28:447–460. (Erratum 511), (Leitlinie der Deutschsprachigen Gesellschaft für Intraokularlinsen-Implantation und refraktive Chirurgie, DGII 2005)
4. Behrens-Baumann W (2011) Zur Prophylaxe und Therapie der postoperativen Endophthalmitis.

ESCRS-Studie und „Early Vitrectomy Study“ in der Kritik. Ophthalmologe 108:1062–1066
5. Behrens-Baumann W, Finis D, MacKenzie C, Roth M, Geerling G (2015) Keratomykose – Therapiestandards und aktuelle Entwicklungen. Klin Monatsbl Augenheilkd 232:754–764
6. Endophthalmitis Vitrectomy Study Group (1995) Results of the Endophthalmitis Vitrectomy Study. A randomized trial of immediate vitrectomy and of intravenous antibiotics for the treatment of postoperative bacterial endophthalmitis. Arch Ophthalmol 113:1479–1496
7. Kuhn F, Mester V, Morris R (2004) A proactive treatment for eyes with perforating injury. Klin Monatsbl Augenheilkd 221:622–628
8. Narang S, Gupta V, Dogra MR, Pandav SS, Das S (2003) Role of prophylactic intravitreal antibiotics in open globe injuries. Indian J Ophthalmol 51:39–44
9. Pleyer U, Mondino BJ, Adamu SA et al (1992) Immune response to staphylococcus epidermidis-induced endophthalmitis in a rabbit model. Invest Ophthalmol Vis Sci 33:2650–2663
10. Roth M et al (2019) Das Deutsche Pilz-Keratitis-Register. Erste Ergebnisse einer multizentrischen Erhebung. Ophthalmologe. https://doi.org/10.1007/s00347-019-0871-9
11. Schrader W (1990) Endogene Candidaendophthalmitis. Frühzeitige Diagnose und frühzeitige Vitrektomie. Fortschr Ophthalmol 87:331–335
12. Schrader WF (2004) Epidemiologie bulbuseröffnender Augenverletzungen: Analyse von 1026 Fällen über 18 Jahre. Klin Monatsbl Augenheilkd 221:629–635
13. Viestenz A, Schrader W, Behrens-Baumann W (2008) Traumatic Endophthalmitis Prevention Trial (TEPT). Klin Monatsbl Augenheilkd 225:941–946
14. Viestenz A, Wilhelm F, Schrader W (2018) Einführung in die OphthalmoChirurgie – Teil 9: Verletzungen des Auges – was ist zu tun bei der Erstversorgung? Ophthalmo Chir:317–324
15. Viestenz A, Schrader W, Wilhelm F, Behrens-Baumann W (2022) Vitrektomie. In: Schargus M (Eds) Einführung in die Ophthalmochirurgie. Dr. Reinhard Kaden, Mannheim, pp 189–200
16. Viestenz A, Heichel J, Viestenz A (2022) Hygiene und Sterilität im OP. In: Schargus M (Eds) Einführung in die Ophthalmochirurgie. Dr. Reinhard Kaden, Mannheim, pp 217–224
17. www.kaug.ovgu.de/Zuweiser/Leitlinien

My First Phaco—How Do I Prepare?

20

Christian Schäferhoff and Thomas Neuhann

Contents

C. Schäferhoff (✉)
Esslingen, Germany
e-mail: schaeferhoff@me.com

T. Neuhann
München, Germany
e-mail: prof@neuhann.de

20.1 Preparation before Surgery

A precise knowledge of the anatomy as well as the individual surgical steps is essential for the success of the operation (Chap. 2). Complications, which always occur (no matter

F. Wilhelm (ed.), *Ophthalmic Surgery for Beginners*, https://doi.org/10.1007/978-3-662-70287-1_20

how much one has operated), can also be managed in this way. Ideally, one has attended wet labs before the first phacoemulsification and observed and assisted as much as possible with their mentor. The preparation as a surgeon is addressed in Chap. 7.

One must also be thoroughly familiar with devices such as the phaco machine, the instruments, and the microscope.

It is advisable to approach cautiously. It is worth investing the time to assist as an "OR nurse." This provides security regarding the surgical procedure and the instruments. It is helpful to watch as many operations as possible by experienced surgeons through the observer. Experience shows that it is easier to learn cataract surgery step by step. After learning to drape a patient sterilely and insert the lid speculum, one can begin to perform the paracenteses. Once the beginner masters this safely, the first injections of suprarenin and viscoelastic can be practiced. This is followed by the performance of the capsulorhexis until all surgical steps have been learned. Detailed descriptions can be found, for example, in "Cataract and Lens Surgery in Ophthalmology" by M. Shajari, B. Zuberbühler's "Cataract Surgery," or "Phacoemulsification and Intraocular Lens Implantation" by M. C. Knorz.

20.2 Microscope

Before starting the operation, one should sit down calmly and comfortably and adjust the microscope to their needs. Since operations take longer at the beginning, this avoids tension. Most microscopes can be operated with a footswitch, allowing refocusing even while working in the eye.

▶ Dry runs (non-sterile) with the surgical microscope before the first operation are strongly recommended.

The structure and function of the surgical microscope are described in detail in Sect. 4.1.

20.3 Phaco Machine

Every surgeon should perfectly know the technique of the phaco machine, the setting parameters, and their significance. The phaco machine should initially be set conservatively for a beginner. With increasing experience, the settings can become more advanced and aggressive. In our experience, the representatives of the machine manufacturers are very cooperative and are happy to assist with the first operations. The phaco device controls the irrigation (i.e., the flow of fluid into the anterior chamber), the strength of aspiration (i.e., the suction of lens fragments and fluid), and the strength and frequency of the ultrasound necessary for the emulsification of lens particles. The phaco machine is controlled via a footpedal which either activates the irrigation first, then the aspiration, and the phacoemulsification with increasing strength from top to bottom, or activates the irrigation first, then increasingly the aspiration in two stages from top to bottom, and activates the phacoemulsification by tilting the footswitch to the side. The interaction between irrigation and aspiration is called fluidics. This ensures a stable anterior chamber. The fluidics influence the "followability," i.e., the bringing of lens parts to the phaco tip, and the "holdability," i.e., the ability to fix a lens fragment sucked onto the phaco tip to emulsify it afterwards. To support this, the fluid flow is directed so that the fluid flows out of the side openings of the sleeve and flushes lens fragments towards the phaco tip through a circular fluid movement. Further details can be found in Sect. 4.2 on the phaco machine.

20.4 Selection of Patients

When selecting the first patients, a few points should be considered:

- The cataract should be moderately advanced. If the cataract should be moderately advanced. If the cataract is too dense, complications are more likely: During capsulorhexis, the red reflex may be missing, making it difficult to see the rhexis edges. The higher phaco energy required for lens emulsification can lead to endothelial damage of the cornea. Additionally, the pressure on the zonular fibers during phacoemulsification can be too high, making normal posterior chamber lens implantation impossible, as the capsular bag can no longer hold the artificial lens

- If the cataract is too "soft," dividing the nucleus can be difficult because there is no good counterforce for the instruments.
- Especially as a beginner, one should avoid indications with an above-average success expectation, such as a clear lens exchange and the implantation of premium lenses, as the patients' expectations are very high for such procedures.
- The pupil should dilate sufficiently, as cataract surgery becomes more complicated with a narrow pupil due to the poorer view.
- Comorbidities, such as cornea guttata or pseudoexfoliation syndrome, which can be associated with loose zonules, make pressure increases more likely and the rhexis more prone to tearing outward, should be reserved for more advanced colleagues. Previous surgeries, such as vitrectomized eyes where the vitreous body is missing as a counterforce, also make zonular fiber injuries more likely. Previous trauma can also loosen the zonular fibers, and even with careful surgery, vitreous prolapse can occur.

▶ For the first cataract surgeries, the selection of patients should be done carefully and in consultation with the mentor!

20.5 Checking the Indication

Before starting the surgery, it must be ensured that the correct patient with the correct IOL lens is operated on the correct eye. The best way to check this is to have the patient state their name, date of birth, and the eye to be operated on, and compare this with the documents.

20.6 Draping the Patient

There are different drapes. Most have an adhesive film that is stuck to the disinfected area. Then the film must either be cut open or, if already preperforated, torn open. As with all further steps, strict adherence to hygiene is essential. Chap. 3 describes asepsis and antisepsis in the OR.

20.7 Inserting the Eyelid Speculum

When inserting the eyelid speculum, have the patient look down and slide the upper arm of the speculum under the upper eyelid. In the next step, the patient looks up, and the lower arm is slid under the lower eyelid. This eye movement avoids corneal injuries.

▶ As little manipulation as possible should be done on the eyelids, as this can express bacteria into the conjunctival sac and thus into the surgical area.

An overview of different eyelid speculums can be found in Sect. 5.5.2.

20.8 Paracentesis

Paracenteses are needed to inject viscoelastic, saline solution, or VisionBlue into the eye, as well as to introduce smaller instruments into the eye, such as the Push-Pull during phacoemulsification and, if necessary, a bimanual irrigation and aspiration. The size of the paracenteses depends on the instruments to be used or the diameter of the bimanual suction-irrigation (Chap. 13).

The number and location of the paracenteses depend on the subsequent planned surgical steps.

Typically, the paracentesis is performed 60°–90° offset from the planned main incision. The eye is fixed with a forceps (e.g., colibri forceps) with the second hand. The incision should be horizontal, parallel to the iris, and peripheral through the cornea. If the incision is too peripheral, the iris can be injured by the paracentesis knife, or the iris may push towards or through the incision over time. This risk is especially present with a floppy iris. Additionally, an incision leak can cause the conjunctiva to be undermined and inflated.

If the incision is too central, the patient can be disturbed by corneal scars. A nonoblique incision is more difficult to seal.

20.9 Main Incision

Nowadays, a clear cornea or limbal corneal incision is usually performed. The phaco tunnel should be self-sealing and is usually stepped. An angled keratome is typically used (Chap. 13). The blade has a width of approximately 2.5 mm. The incision width must be matched to the size of the phaco tip. First, one punctures the cornea or the cornea-near sclera at the peripheral edge at a 70° angle to the corneal surface, then guides the blade 2 mm parallel to the corneal surface, and then punctures vertically into the anterior chamber. Due to this stepping, the incision can self-seal through the intraocular pressure on the inner lip of the wound. During the incision, the eye should be fixed, for example, with a colibri forceps. The location must be chosen so that the phacoemulsification can be performed comfortably. Sclerocorneal or scleral incisions are nowadays mostly performed only for selected indications, such as the implantation of a non-foldable lens. If the clear cornea incision is performed too short, it is difficult to seal. The more peripheral the tunnel incision, the lower the astigmatic effect. An overview of the incision instruments can be found in Chap. 5.

20.10 Viscoelastics

Viscoelastics are substances that are, on the one hand, viscous, i.e. thick, and on the other hand, elastic (Chap. 11). They serve to maintain the stability of the eye. Due to their viscosity, the eye does not collapse when paracenteses or main incisions are opened with instruments. They are divided into cohesive and dispersive viscoelastics. Sodium hyaluronate, chondroitin sulfate, and hydroxypropyl methylcellulose are used. Cohesive viscoelastics are more stable in their form, while dispersive ones are somewhat more fluid.

20.11 Preparation of the Capsulorhexis

To optimally perform the capsulorhexis, the pupil must be sufficiently dilated. Preoperatively, this can be done locally with tropicamide (Mydrum) and phenylephrine (Neosynephrine) eye drops. Intraoperatively, epinephrine (Suprarenin, diluted 1:10) or Mydrane (a combination of tropicamide, phenylephrine, and lidocaine) is injected. This is injected into the anterior chamber through a paracentesis. If the pupil is not sufficiently dilated, the Malyugin ring or iris retractors are available. To prevent the anterior chamber from collapsing, a viscoelastic is injected afterward. Hyaluronic acid derivatives or methylcellulose are commonly used. In Chap. 11, intraocularly used medications are discussed in detail.

20.12 Capsulorhexis

The capsulorhexis suggested by Neuhann is still the standard for opening the anterior capsule. This can be performed either with a curved cannula or forceps needle. The ideal size of the capsulorhexis is approximately 5 mm in diameter. This ensures that the posterior chamber lens, which usually has an optic diameter of 6 mm, is circularly covered by the anterior capsule. If the opening is smaller, capsular phimosis with tearing of the zonular fibers can occur due to scarring of the capsular bag. If the opening is too large, the posterior chamber lens can more easily dislocate into the anterior chamber or tilt, causing higher-order aberration errors. If one punctures too deeply into the lens, the lens can swell, and the edge of the rhexis is no longer visible. If the rhexis runs too far outward, the folded edge of the rhexis is pulled centrally. If there is a tear in the anterior capsule, the tear can extend to the posterior capsule, resulting in vitreous prolapse and the sinking of lens remnants into the vitreous cavity.

▶ In principle, the rhexis can be best controlled if one pulls the capsule close to the edge of the rhexis towards the center with a needle or forceps.

20.13 Hydrodissection and Hydrodelineation

Hydrodissection is the separation of the lens cortex from the lens capsule. This is necessary so that the nucleus can be properly processed. A blunt irrigation cannula is guided under the edge of the rhexis. The dissection is performed by careful irrigation with a saline solution. Ideally, one can see the fluid wave flowing over the anterior capsule and the lens equator between the posterior capsule and the lens towards the irrigation cannula. If this is not the case, one should start again at another point and irrigate again. The nucleus should be able to be rotated within the capsular bag. If irrigated too forcefully, the pressure that builds up in the capsular bag can cause the posterior capsule to rupture. If too much volume is injected, the lens nucleus can luxate forward, which can result in a tear of the anterior capsule. In this case, the lens should be pushed back either with the irrigation cannula or with viscoelastic. After the dissection, hydrodelineation follows. The lens cortex is penetrated while irrigating and the lens nucleus is separated from the lens capsule. One should see the fluid waves flowing in the interface here, too. This also makes it easier to process the nucleus. Figure 20.1 shows the hydrodissection.

▶ Extensive hydrodissection and hydrodelineation are crucial prerequisites for gentle work within the capsular bag!

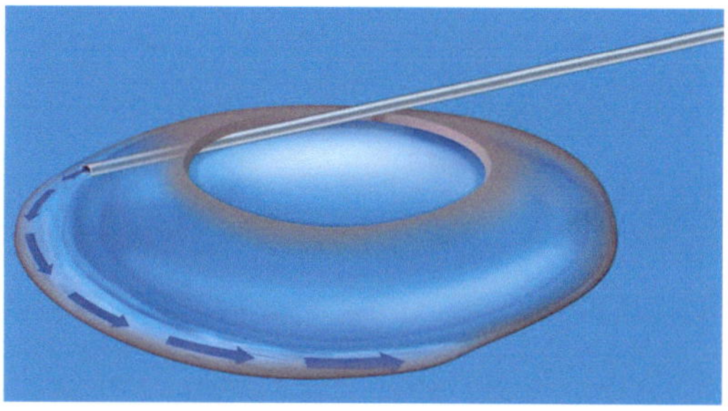

Fig. 20.1 Separation of the lens capsule from the lens during hydrodissection

20.14 Phacoemulsification, Divide and Conquer

In phacoemulsification, there are various techniques by which the lens is fragmented and aspirated. The phaco tip works through the lateral outflow of saline solution, which flows back circularly to the tip of the phaco tip and is supposed to carry lens fragments with it. This is shown in Fig. 20.2. Firmer fragments are supposed to dock onto the phaco tip and are then

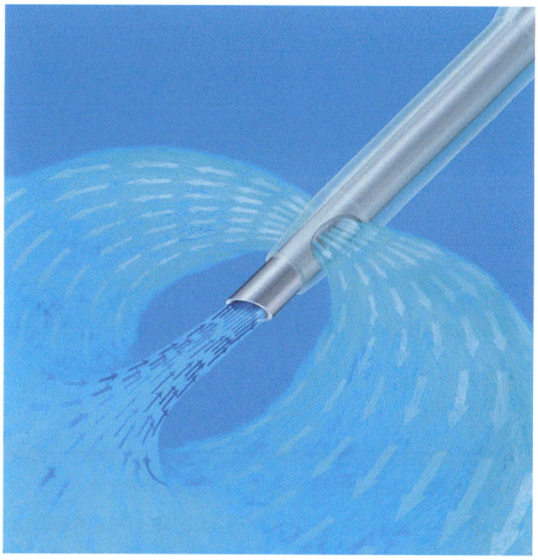

Fig. 20.2 Circular fluid flow from the lateral openings of the sleeve to the phaco tip

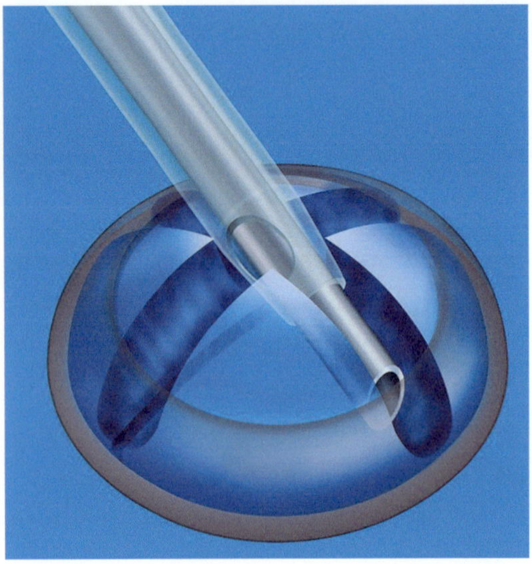

Fig. 20.3 The correct division of the lens into four fragments. Based on the thickness of the phaco tip, the depth of the trench in relation to the lens can also be estimated

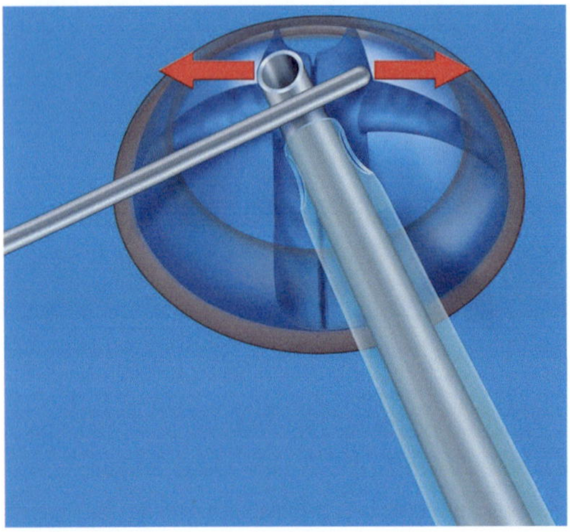

Fig. 20.4 The fragmentation of the lens with crossed instruments

emulsified with ultrasound. It has proven beneficial for beginners to work bevel-up (the opening of the phaco tip points upwards), as the posterior capsule is less likely to be aspirated.

For beginners, the "Divide-and-Conquer" technique is the most suitable. First, the lens is divided in the middle by a trench using the phaco tip. This should be at least ¾ of the lens thickness deep. Figure 20.3 shows the correct division. Since the lens is approximately 6 mm deep in the center and decreases in thickness towards the edge, and the width of the phaco tip is about 1 mm, one can estimate intraoperatively how deep the trench has been "dug" in the center of the lens. However, the lens thickness can vary depending on age and cataract. If the trench is deep enough, one attempts to divide the lens by manipulation with a second instrument, e.g., a Push-Pull. An overview of the instruments can be found in Chap. 5. Figures 20.4, 20.5, and 20.6 show the "cracking" of the lens. If the instruments are placed too high, the lens will not be cracked but only flipped downwards, which can tear the posterior capsule. This is shown in Fig. 20.7.

If this is successful, the lens is rotated and one half is divided again. The technique of rotating the lens is shown in Fig. 20.8. This quarter can then be aspirated and phacoemulsified. It is best to dock the fragment in the middle or in the lower third. This is shown in Figs. 20.9 and 20.10. Only with complete occlusion can the lens be emulsified. It has proven effective to protect the capsule and iris with a second instrument by positioning it under and behind the lens fragment when a lens fragment is aspirated by the phaco tip. This way, even if there is a sudden increase in vacuum because either the occlusion is suddenly interrupted or the fragment is completely removed, the posterior capsule is not sucked into the phaco tip. During phacoemulsification, the fragment to be emulsified must first be firmly aspirated to the phaco tip, otherwise it will be pushed away by the water flow. Only then can it be emulsified. With a second instrument, the lens fragments may need to be rotated into the correct position. If the phaco tip is applied too high on the core fragment, the posterior capsule can be torn by a sharp edge of the lens core. This is shown in Fig. 20.11.

The goal is to create an occlusion of the aspiration opening by a lens fragment so that the vacuum can build up. The irrigation should at this moment only replace the fluid that escapes through the incision. Once the lens fragment is fixed by the vacuum, one begins to break it

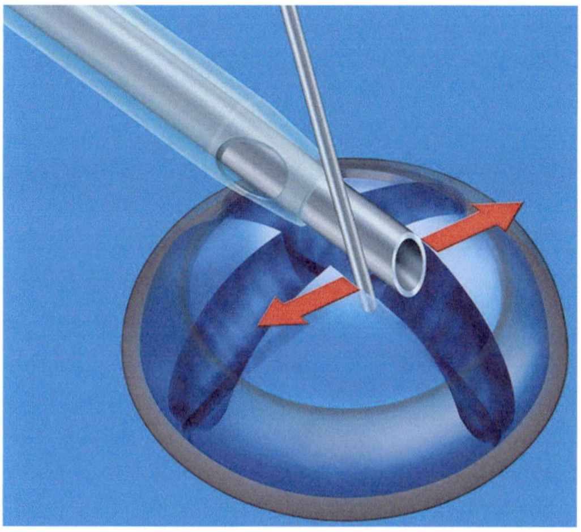

Fig. 20.5 The fragmentation of the lens with parallel-guided instruments

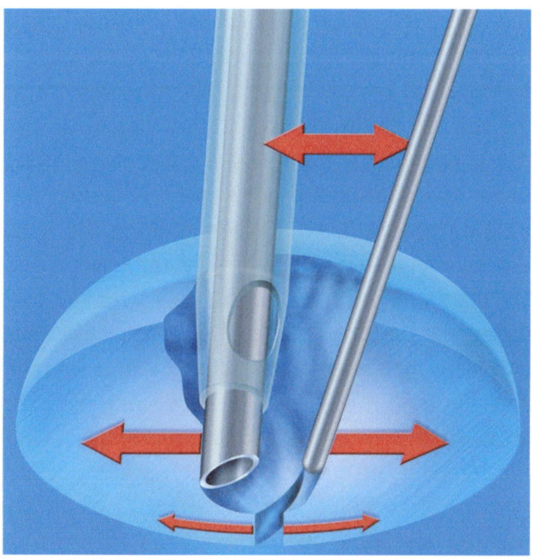

Fig. 20.6 The "cracking" of the lens using the phaco tip and a second instrument

down and aspirate it through emulsification. If contact with the lens fragment is lost or the fragment is emulsified, the vacuum drops abruptly and the aspiration increases rapidly. The latter is referred to as a "surge" and can lead to a collapse of the anterior chamber.

An alternative technique is "stop & chop." As with "divide and conquer," a trench divides the lens into two halves, which are "cracked." The halves are rotated about 50° and each half is divided into several small fragments and emulsified. In the "direct chop" technique, the phaco tip is deeply embedded in the center, the auxiliary instrument is guided to the opposite side under the lens, and both instruments are worked against each other.

▶ When learning phacoemulsification, the "divide-and-conquer" technique is preferred for beginners. The first trench (depending on the core's consistency) should be sufficiently deep and as centered as possible so that it halves the core.

20.15 Irrigation/Aspiration

Once the lens core is removed, irrigation and aspiration are easiest for the beginner with a bimanual irrigation-aspiration system. The instruments are inserted through the paracenteses. The aspiration is placed under the edge of the anterior capsule and the lens cortex is aspirated. Then the cortex is "peeled" towards the center. This also loosens the cortical remnants on the posterior capsule. Cell residues and deposits on the capsule can be carefully mobilized with the roughened underside of the instruments and then aspirated. Remaining lens residues can lead to inflammatory reactions and cause a pressure increase due to swelling.

▶ If the posterior capsule is accidentally aspirated, the aspiration is immediately stopped (switch to "reflux" if necessary). If the aspiration handpiece is pulled back in this situation, a capsule defect occurs.

20.16 Polishing the Capsule

Using a blunt irrigation cannula, the posterior capsule is polished with a hard water jet of NaCl solution. This serves as a prophylaxis against posterior capsule opacification. Care must be taken to ensure that the pressure

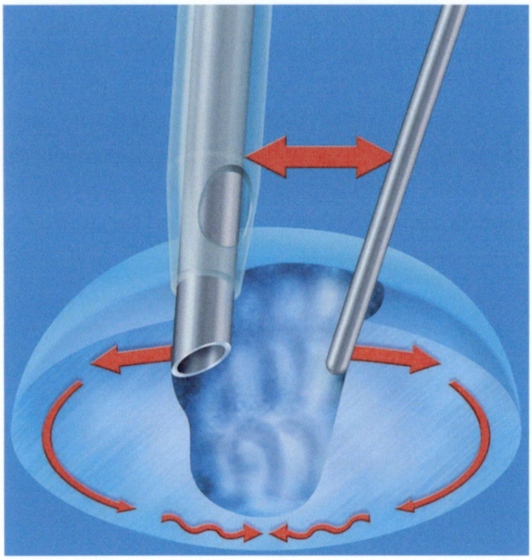

Fig. 20.7 The incorrect attempt to divide the lens with instruments placed too high. As a result, pressure is only applied to the lower part of the lens, compressing it in this area instead of dividing it, similar to a hinge

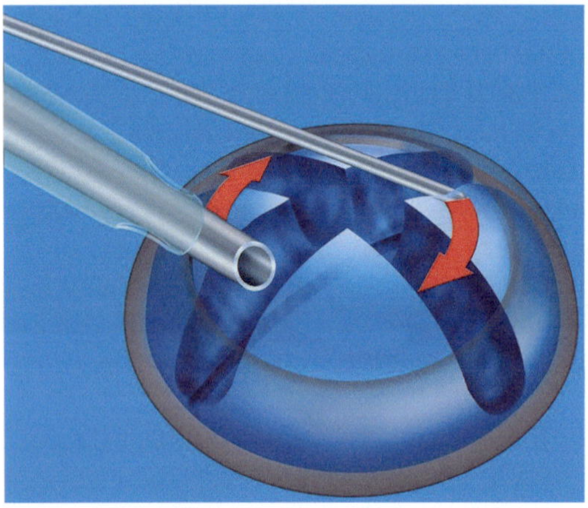

Fig. 20.8 The figure demonstrates rotating the lens core into the correct position using the phaco tip and an auxiliary instrument

exerted by the irrigation is not too high, so that the posterior capsule is not damaged. It should also be ensured that the irrigation cannula is not tilted and is securely attached to the syringe. Otherwise, the built-up pressure can injure all structures in the eye if the cannula is dislodged. Polishing the posterior capsule with a roughened aspiration handpiece has also proven effective.

20.17 Implantation of the Posterior Chamber Intraocular Lens

Many lenses are now delivered "preloaded," so the shooter used to implant the lens can be prepared with just a few steps. Depending on the lens type, there are different techniques. Here, too, reference should be made to the representatives of the lens manufacturers. There are shooters for rotating or pressing. The rotating shooters are easier to control. Once all cortical remnants are removed and the posterior capsule is polished, viscoelastic is introduced into the anterior chamber and the capsular bag, the tip of the shooter's cartridge is inserted into the phaco tunnel up to the middle of the capsular bag, and rotation begins. The slow release of the lens from the cartridge allows precise control to ensure that the anterior haptic lies directly under the anterior capsule and the lens does not unfold "upside down." When rotating the lens, the shooter can also be slowly retracted a bit. By manipulating the opening lens with the cartridge, the posterior haptic of the intraocular lens can be pushed under the anterior capsule into the capsular bag. If this does not succeed, it can also be done before aspirating the viscoelastic with the bimanual irrigation-aspiration system or the viscoelastic needle. This is achieved by slightly rotating the lens and simultaneously pressing the posterior haptic down a bit. When using a press injector, care must be taken to implant the lens slowly and evenly. If resistance suddenly decreases during implantation, the sudden pressure can injure the iris or capsule. The intraocular lens can also be implanted using a folding forceps. In this case, the lens is folded to about half its diameter and must be implanted through a correspondingly larger incision of about 3 mm. For the implantation of non-foldable lenses, the incision must be enlarged to the size of the optic, usually about 5–6 mm. The last two methods

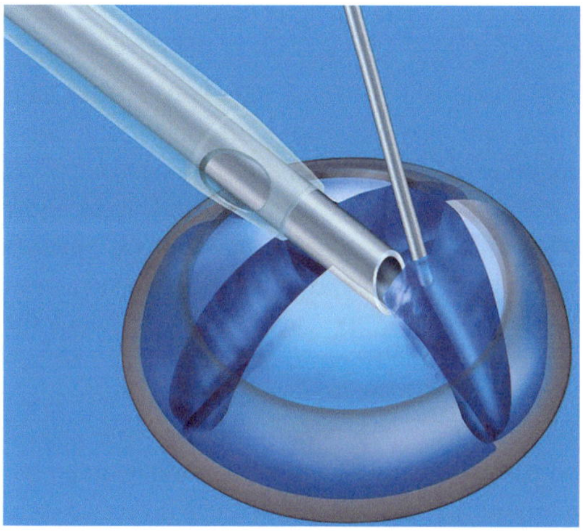

Fig. 20.9 The correct aspiration of a lens fragment in the lower third while protecting the posterior capsule with a second instrument

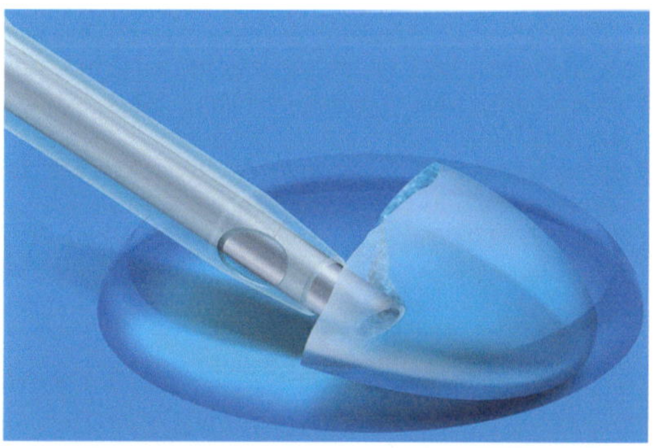

Fig. 20.10 The correct docking of the phaco tip to the lens in the lower third. This fixes the lens core without stressing the capsular bag

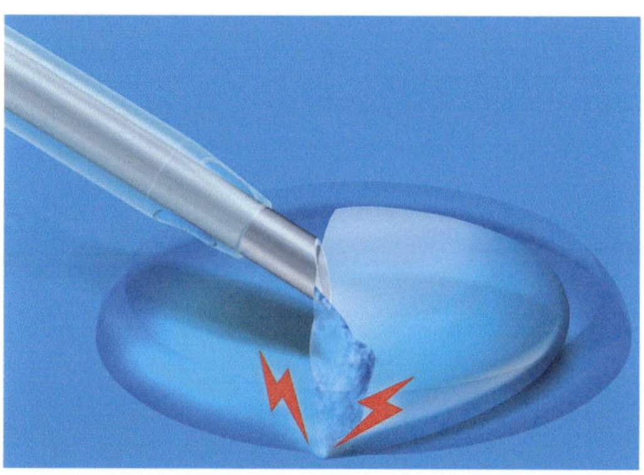

Fig. 20.11 If a lens half is aspirated incorrectly in the upper third, a potentially sharp lower edge can tear the posterior capsule due to tilting of the lens

have become very uncommon due to the significantly easier implantation with the injector. An overview of intraocular lenses is provided in Chap. 10.

20.18 Removing the Viscoelastic

Removing the viscoelastic is particularly important because any remaining residues in the eye can lead to a massive increase in pressure, usually within the first two days. Through the paracenteses, the viscoelastic can be conveniently flushed out with the bimanual irrigation-aspiration system. Behind the lens, it is best to flush from both sides with irrigation, as the posterior capsule can be aspirated and torn with the aspiration handpiece.

20.19 Sealing the Incision and the Paracenteses

The paracenteses are sealed by entering the incision with a syringe filled with NaCl solution and hydrating the stroma (by injecting fluid into it) to swell until it turns slightly whitish. The main incision usually does not need to be sealed. If necessary, the sealing of the phaco tunnel can be checked by applying pressure to the wound. If a fistula results from the main incision, a small air bubble can be inserted into the anterior chamber. In the upright position of the patient, with an incision in the upper area, the lower lip is pressed against the upper lip, thereby sealing the incision.

20.20 Postoperative Antibiosis

According to the guidelines of the German Ophthalmological Society (GOS), it is recommended to administer cefuroxime into the anterior chamber at the end of the operation and to treat locally with a combination of antibiotic and steroid eye drops. Examples include Dexa-Gentamicin eye drops, Isoptomax eye drops, or Inflanefran forte eye drops with, for example,

Ofloxacin eye drops or Oftaquix eye drops. Mydriatics such as Cyclopentolate eye drops, BoroScopol eye drops, or Atropine eye drops are usually not necessary but can be given prophylactically to patients with known iritis. For steroid responders, non-steroidal anti-inflammatory drugs such as Nevanac eye drops, Yellox eye drops, or Voltaren eye drops can also be used.

20.21 Femtosecond Laser Cataract Surgery (see also Sect. 21.2)

In 2008, Nagy clinically applied a femtosecond laser in the context of cataract surgery. The use of the femtosecond laser can reduce the operative risk through more precise procedure. With the laser, self-sealing corneal incision profiles can be created, a more precise circular opening of the lens capsule for central lens positioning, targeted fragmentation of the lens, which reduces the ultrasound energy during phacoemulsification, and arcuate keratotomy to influence corneal astigmatism can be performed. Not all steps need to be performed with the laser. The execution of corneal incisions is controversially assessed by some surgeons, as the incisions can only be made corneally, not limbal. In principle, the use of the femtosecond laser facilitates cataract surgery. During capsulotomy with the femtolaser, one must check whether the "rhexis" is complete. Hydrodissection must be carried out very carefully. "Cracking" the nucleus is usually no longer possible or necessary, as the fragments can be individually aspirated. During phacoemulsification, one should be particularly cautious due to the pre-fragmentation of the lens nucleus and use little energy to protect the posterior capsule.

Further Reading

1. „Katarakt- und Linsenchirurgie in der Augenheilkunde" by M Shajari, 2023, ISBN - 13: 978-3662624579
2. „Kataraktchirurgie" by B Zuberbühler, 2008, ISBN - 13: 978-3540799436
3. „Phakoemulsifikation und Intraokularlinsen-Implantation" by M C Knorz, 2004, ISBN-13 : 978-3922777670

The First Surgeries Are Completed, What Comes Next?

21

Thomas Hammer, Frank Wilhelm, Armin Scharrer, Alexander Petzold, Erik Chankiewitz, Arne Viestenz, Heiko Philippin, Karin Knoll and Martin Nentwich

Contents

The first operations under the supervision of a mentor have been successfully completed. Now it is time to gain experience, get routine into the processes, and continue to develop. The following chapter will explain that careful planning of interventions – especially in complicated initial situations – can be as helpful as in the management of complications.

To expand their surgical spectrum, every surgeon should continuously inform themselves about innovations and try to observe experienced colleagues in the operating room. In this

T. Hammer
Klinik und Poliklinik für Augenheilkunde, Universitätsklinikum Halle/Saale, Martin-Luther-Universität Halle-Wittenberg, Halle/Saale, Germany
e-mail: thomas.hammer@uk-halle.de

Augenarztpraxis, Augenzentrum "Frohe Zukunft", Halle/Saale, Germany

F. Wilhelm (✉)
Greifswald, Germany

A. Scharrer
DOC—Deutsche Gesellschaft für Ophthalmochirurgie e.V. Neuwieder Straße 9, Nürnberg, Germany
e-mail: armin.scharrer@augen-scharrer.de

A. Petzold
Augenzentrum am Johannisplatz, Leipzig, Germany

E. Chankiewitz
Augenklinik, Städtisches Klinikum Braunschweig gGmbH, Braunschweig, Germany
e-mail: erik@chankiewitz.de

A. Viestenz
Klinik und Poliklinik für Augenheilkunde, Universitätsklinikum Halle/Saale, Halle/Saale, Germany

H. Philippin
Klinik für Augenheilkunde, Universitätsklinikum Freiburg, Freiburg, Germany
e-mail: heiko.philippin@uniklinik-freiburg.de

International Centre for Eye Health, London School of Hygiene & Tropical Medicine, London, Großbritannien

CBM e. V., Bensheim, Germany

K. Knoll
Christoffel-Blindenmission Deutschland e. V., Bensheim, Germany
e-mail: karin.knoll@cbm.org

M. Nentwich
Augenklinik, Universitätsklinikum Würzburg, Würzburg, Germany
e-mail: nentwich_m@ukw.de

F. Wilhelm (ed.), *Ophthalmic Surgery for Beginners*, https://doi.org/10.1007/978-3-662-70287-1_21

context, ophthalmic surgical activities in developing countries pose a particular challenge and offer a wealth of experience.

21.1 Complication Management

Thomas Hammer, Frank Wilhelm and Armin Scharrer

Mastering a complication begins with the surgical planning. It is important from the first contact to assess the patient's compliance and then decide which form of anesthesia is best for them for the planned procedure, and if in doubt, opt for general anesthesia. It is also important in advance to assess the patient's general condition and resilience in consultation with the general practitioner as part of the operation (Chap. 8). This can prevent unforeseen reactions from the patient and incidents in the operating room. It is also necessary to record the medications the patient is taking or has taken in the past. From this, it can be concluded, for example, whether the iris is affected and whether a narrow pupil or a "Floppy Iris" is to be expected intraoperatively. It may also be necessary, as part of the planning of a procedure involving the cutting of blood vessels, to suspend anticoagulant therapy in advance and in consultation with the general practitioner. The complication management does not end with the completion of the surgical procedure in the operating room. It also includes consistent early postoperative care to promptly identify problems up to and including endophthalmitis and adjust the therapy accordingly [1]. Collegial contact with the follow-up physician is necessary to recognize and manage late complications, for example, after intraocular lens implantations, as early as possible [7].

The basis for successful surgery in the eye operating room is the precise coordination between the surgeon and the assistant. Coordination with each other and mutual knowledge of the procedures is the basis for avoiding surprises. For example, every cannula handed to the surgeon should be checked for patency beforehand. If this is done immediately before use, any air remaining in the cannula is also removed. Without this coordination, the surgeon cannot inject gently, or an air bubble can enter the anterior chamber and obstruct the view during intraocular surgery.

If it becomes necessary to deviate from the planned course, every eye surgeon must be able to draw on a broader repertoire. It makes sense to familiarize oneself with the "old techniques" in advance to adapt the approach as needed. For beginners, it is particularly valuable to have an experienced teacher by their side in this situation, who can provide guidance and, if necessary, take over the continuation of the procedure.

In principle, every surgeon is well advised to restore a "known" situation in the event of a deviation from the norm, so that the procedure can continue in the usual manner.

For this, it is absolutely necessary for the surgeon to know exactly what material resources are available in the operating department. This includes devices and instruments as well as various consumables (Chaps. 4 , 5 , 6 , 10, and 11).

21.1.1 What to do in case of (nonexpulsive) bleeding?

It was already mentioned at the beginning that it must be known whether the patient is taking "blood-thinning medications". If this is the case, the further procedure depends on the execution of the planned intervention.

In a regular phacoemulsification with clear-cornea access, access under topical anesthesia, the treatment with anticoagulants does not generally need to be interrupted, as no blood vessels are severed.

In cases where additional intraocular manipulations - for example, on the iris - are planned or in the bulbus opening laceration involving the conjunctiva and sclera, a peribulbar anesthesia is performed, as well as in all other procedures on vascularized tissues—especially on the eyelids—it is recommended to interrupt the anticoagulant therapy in collegial consultation with the general practitioner (Chap. 9).

If bleeding occurs intraoperatively, the following principles should be observed and applied simultaneously:

1. Stay calm,
2. Control the patient's blood pressure—lower it if necessary with medication,
3. Locate the source of the bleeding,
4. Stop the bleeding.

If this bleeding occurs intraocularly, the first measure can be to increase the irrigation pressure, i.e., raise the bottle height. Care must be taken not to provoke a prolapse—for example, of the iris—through the accesses. Alternatively, an initial attempt can be made to tamponade the bleeding source by instilling a (high-molecular) viscoelastic in the area of the bleeding source. After that, the "problem area" can usually be better visualized and the cause found.

Extraocularly, this tamponade is performed with a suitable instrument, with swabs proving effective here. Depending on the source, the bleeding may cease after sufficient compression or—by rinsing with BSS (Chap. 11) be so well visualized that it can be stopped by targeted and dosed thermocoagulation. Here, the principle of ophthalmic surgery "As much as necessary and as little as possible!" must be particularly observed!

A similar approach is taken in eyelid surgery. Here, it may be necessary to locate the severed vessel by clamping it with a suitable instrument and finally stopping the bleeding source with a suture.

21.1.2 Complication management in cataract surgery

During a cataract operation, various moments can challenge both an inexperienced and an experienced surgeon. It is important to know the steps necessary to resolve the issue and then implement them quickly without allowing hectic movements or startled reactions. Since it is not possible to cover all potential problems, this section will exemplarily address common complications in cataract surgery and provide tips for managing them.

To avoid making operations unnecessarily complicated, it is important to check the patient's positioning before the start of the surgery, i.e., the horizontal head position and the proper seating of the eyelid speculum with the eyelashes held back. If there is a situation where the eyebrows are very prominent or the bulbus is very deep, the head can be slightly hyperextended or rotated slightly to the opposite side (Chap. 8).

21.1.3 What approach is advisable for a narrow pupil?

Cataract surgery in patients with a small pupil should not be performed by a beginner and can also be a particular challenge for the experienced surgeon. Therefore, it must be determined in advance whether the diagnostic pupil dilation is already limited during the preliminary examination. It is also necessary to clarify whether there has been a glaucoma therapy with miotics (usually Pilocarpine°) in the past, synechiae of the iris, or a pseudoexfoliation syndrome. Information on systemic therapy that affects the iris, preferably with Tamsulosin° and similar medications (Chap. 8), must also be collected. If the pupil is so narrow at the beginning of the procedure that further action is too risky, there are various options to reduce the risk, considering the primary pupil width and the surgeon's experience. In these cases, it is advisable to use pupil-dilating drugs such as adrenaline or Mydrane° (Chap. 11) intracamerally. If posterior synechiae are present, an attempt should be made to bluntly separate them. This can be done particularly gently by introducing a viscoelastic into the anterior chamber.

This process can then be repeated by placing the opening of the injection cannula in the center of the pupil, thereby pushing the iris further peripherally.

If sufficient mydriasis does not result, a temporary mechanical expansion using iris retractors [2] or pupil expanders [4] may be necessary.

Most precautions and manipulations for pupil dilation should, if possible, be performed topically with medication or through paracenteses and the creation of the phaco tunnel. If the introduction of an iris expander through the incision is planned, special attention should be given to this!

21.1.4 How do I proceed with problems with the incisions?

If the introduction of instruments through the paracenteses or the tunnel is not exactly in the direction of the cut, they can easily get caught in the stromal lamellae, as well as at limbal and post-limbal incisions involving the conjunctiva. In these cases, widening the incision with the help of a viscoelastic can be helpful, while simultaneously probing the access with the injection cannula. An expansion of the tunnel might result in a tunnel insufficiency, as the extent of the incision is matched to the dimensions of the phaco tip by the width of the phaco lance. It should also be considered that the sleeve may be worn out and therefore sits loosely on the tip, which is why it needs to be replaced.

Tunnel insufficiency can occur especially in the early stages [3], when there is not much experience with performing corneal incisions (Chap. 13), or later after an intraoperatively necessary expansion of the anterior chamber opening. In these cases, placing a temporary suture (possibly several) has proven effective. Monofilament suture material (Nylon 10/0, Chap. 12) is used for this purpose. These "situational sutures" serve to stabilize the anterior chamber during the further course of the operation and to ensure safe intraocular manipulation. These are usually removed at the end of the procedure but can also be left in place if necessary, to be removed later during postoperative checks (considering astigmatism). If the tightness of the tunnel is not certain, the instillation of an air bubble into the anterior chamber can be helpful. Since this covers the cut at the endothelial side in the upper limbus area in the supine position and when the patient is upright, it prevents the outflow of aqueous humor until it is absorbed, gaining time for the first phase of wound healing.

In cataract surgery, it has proven effective to finally close the tissue in the area of the corneal accesses by intrastromal injection of BSS (hydrotamponade). If this does not succeed in exceptional cases, such as with too short incision length or in young patients, adaptation with a suture (Nylon 10-0) is also necessary.

21.1.5 What to do if the anterior chamber flattens?

If the anterior chamber flattens during the course of the operation, it should be checked whether there is excessive leakage from the incisions. This can be remedied by changing the instrument handling, which prevents gaping of the incisions. If necessary, excessively large, insufficient incisions are adapted with a suture. An increase in vitreous pressure (Vis a tergo) can also be considered as a cause. If there is simultaneous darkening of the red reflex, a spontaneous choroidal hemorrhage should be considered as the cause. In this case, the irrigation pressure of the machine (bottle height) should be increased. The instruments should be immediately removed from the eye through the incisions. After clarifying the situation (often the cause is the patient straining or an unconscious mispositioning of the instruments!), an attempt should be made to stabilize the depth of the anterior chamber by instilling a viscoelastic. If this succeeds, the procedure can be continued. If this is not possible, the procedure should be interrupted and, after further clarification of the general situation, continued promptly under general anesthesia by an experienced surgeon.

21.1.6 What should I do if the capsulorhexis slips into the periphery?

Anyone can face this problem, even after thousands of uncomplicated openings of the anterior lens capsule! There are findings, such as heavily fibrosed anterior capsules, aberrant zonular fibers inserting on the anterior lens surface, or partial zonulolyses, where it is unpredictable whether the rhexis can be completed intact. Therefore, the surgeon should be prepared and have a strategy for further action. In these situations, it has proven effective to inject viscoelastic again. This stabilizes the anterior chamber, and the procedure can be gently continued through the paracenteses. Using a tube-guided forceps and scissors (e.g., according to Koch, Chap. 5), the edge of the capsule opening running into the periphery is incised and grasped with the forceps so that the rhexis can be completed.

Depending on the overall situation of the capsular bag, the hardness of the lens nucleus, and the surgeon's experience, it will be decided how to complete the cataract surgery.

21.1.7 How should I proceed in the case of a posterior capsular defect?

The approach to a posterior capsule defect is crucially determined by the phase of the procedure in which it occurs or is detected. If it is clear after the capsule opening that the rhexis is not intact, it must be assumed that the tear running into the periphery can extend to the posterior capsule. Even in the further course—during phacoemulsification, cortex aspiration, and IOL implantation—the capsule can be injured.

In principle, when a capsule defect occurs, a particularly gentle approach must be taken. The irrigation pressure should be immediately reduced as soon as the capsule lesion is recognized. This is achieved, for example, by lowering the height of the infusion bottle (20 cm is recommended). Here too, the re-administration of viscoelastic can facilitate and make intraocular surgery safer. If the situation is very unclear, the nucleus can be prevented from dislocating into the vitreous cavity by placing the viscoelastic substance behind the nucleus, thereby possibly shifting it into the anterior chamber, to then gently deliver it through the extended tunnel as part of an extracapsular cataract extraction [3].

21.1.8 Which intraocular lens should be implanted?

In principle, beginners in ophthalmic surgery should only use implants that are routinely used in the training facility. This ensures that the mentor can instruct the young colleagues in the handling of the implants and take into account the peculiarities for the surgeon. This applies to the regular course of a cataract operation, i.e., phacoemulsification through a clear cornea approach with lens implantation in the capsular bag. The trainer also masters any complications that may arise. For beginners, multi-piece implants in the C-loop design (Chap. 10) made of hydrophobic material are recommended. These unfold more slowly and thus more controllably. They can also be fixed with the optics in the rhexis if necessary or, depending on the haptic diameter, also allow placement in the ciliary sulcus. Experience has shown that the selection of the implant and the implantation site must always be made depending on the current situation—possibly even immediately intraoperatively [6]!

21.1.9 What to do if the vitreous body prolapses?

A prolapse of the vitreous body is to be expected both in the case of a defect in the posterior capsule and in the case of extensive defects in the zonular fibers. The first measure in this case must always be: "Bottle down!" This means that the inflow from the irrigation must be reduced (see above). After that, the extent of the vitreous prolapse is assessed. If this is limited to a manageable area, the procedure can be continued. In this case, the placement of a viscoelastic can help to stabilize the prolapse or, if possible, to push it back. If this is not successful, an anterior vitrectomy is necessary, which should be performed bimanually through the paracenteses.

21.1.10 What should be considered in the presence of zonulolysis?

Defects in the lens support apparatus can occur, for example, in pseudoexfoliation syndrome, in Marfan syndrome, and after injuries. In this situation, a beginner in cataract surgery should hand over this procedure to an experienced surgeon or at least be assisted by them in individual steps! The extent of the zonulolysis is decisive for the further procedure [5]. In the case of defects that account for less than 3 clock hours, an experienced surgeon can often complete the procedure without complications. In the case of a larger extent of zonular insufficiency and already prolapsed vitreous body, the introduction of a tension ring can stabilize the capsular bag and the operation can be continued. The above-mentioned instructions should be taken into account. In cases where a zonular defect is more extensive and the capsular bag appears particularly mobile intraoperatively, conversion to an ECCE with removal of the entire capsular bag should be considered if necessary.

21.1.11 How do I proceed with the operation of a mature cataract?

This special situation requires careful planning and a special approach! Therefore, the procedure should be performed by an experienced surgeon or at least under the assistance of one. If it becomes apparent at the beginning of the operation that the red reflex (retroluminescence) is very weak, it is advisable to turn the patient's head to check if the eye can be positioned in such a way that a sufficient red reflex results in the pupil. Since the preservation of an intact capsulorhexis is crucial for the success of any cataract operation, the risk should be minimized by visualizing the anterior capsule using a dye in the absence of retroluminescence (Chap. 11). Subsequently, the procedure can usually be completed in the form of a planned phacoemulsification. Due to the initial situation, the likelihood of the previously discussed complications is significantly increased and may necessitate the approach according to the previously given instructions.

21.2 Incorporation of new tools into the surgical process

Thomas Hammer and Alexander Petzold

Even surgical beginners must orient themselves to the new technical possibilities. The principle here is: "Stagnation is regression." It has proven useful to learn new techniques in the context of congresses, courses, wet labs, and observerships (Sect. 21.3) and to apply them to patients only after thorough familiarization.

21.2.1 Intraoperative OCT

In recent years, optical coherence tomography has become established in ophthalmology for diagnostics in both two-dimensional and three-dimensional forms and has found many areas of application. The strengths of the OCT technique lie, depending on the wavelengths used, in a relatively high penetration depth (1 to 3 millimeters) with simultaneously high axial resolution (0.5 to 15 μm).

Since there are intraoperative situations in which the view into the anterior chamber of the eye is obstructed by corneal pathologies or, for example, in a DMEK surgery, the position and location of the Descemet membrane cannot be precisely identified with a conventional surgical microscope, the use of the OCT technique enables completely new possibilities. For instance, it is possible to obtain information about the position of the Descemet membrane using two-dimensional OCT technique, i.e., a section in the area of the x- and y-axis. This OCT technique has also been integrated into surgical microscopes in recent years. The OCT images are displayed either on a separate monitor or as an overlay in the operator's eyepiece. The focusing and control of the OCT imaging are done via the footpedal of the surgical microscope (Fig. 21.1). Often embedded in this are functions for capturing still images or video sequences. Besides its use in anterior segment surgery, the visualization of retinal structures with such OCT surgical microscopes is also possible (Table 21.1).

21.2.2 New Techniques in Phacoemulsification

The classic ultrasound technique operates via a vibrating piezo crystal, which transfers a vibration to the tip of the phaco handpiece. Since this crystal allows a back-and-forth vibration, the fragmentation of the nucleus occurs through constant repulsion and suction at the phaco tip. Due to the oscillations, heat is generated, which

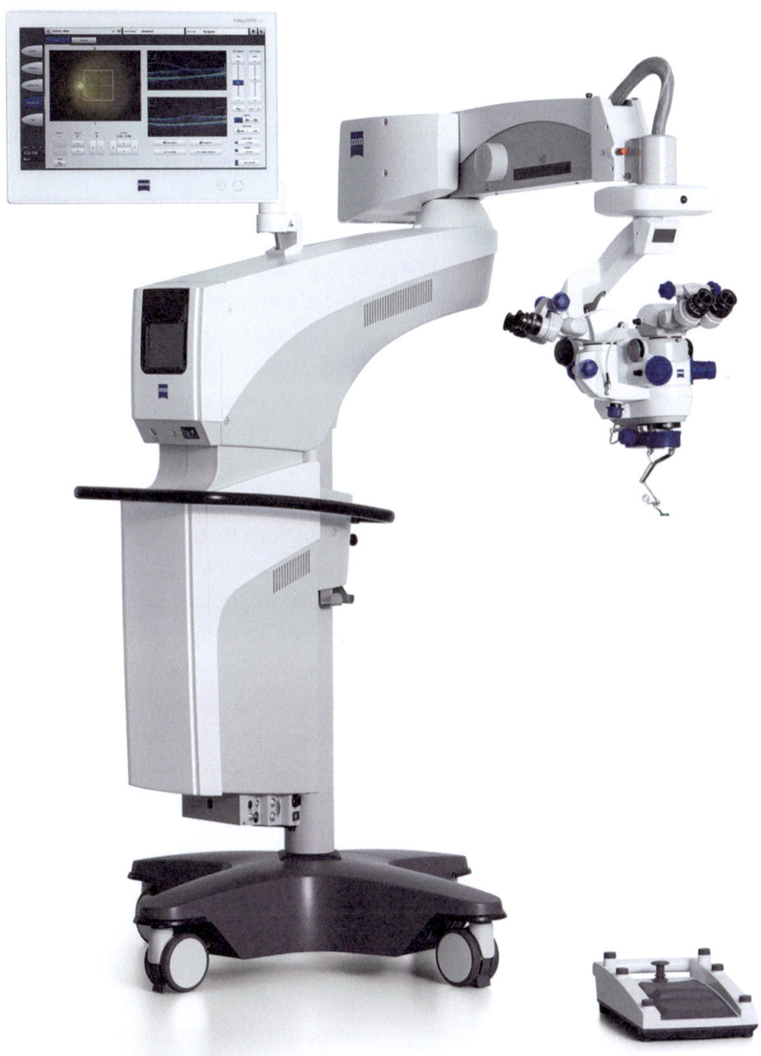

Fig. 21.1 Zeiss microscope with intraoperative OCT. (© Carl Zeiss Meditec AG)

Table 21.1 Currently available intraoperative OCT models

	Haag-Streit iOCT	Carl Zeiss Rescan 700	Leica EnFocus Ultra-HD
Scans/s	10,000	27,000	32,000
Depth (mm)	4.2	2	2.5
Resolution (μm)	10	5.5	4

in earlier years repeatedly caused damage in the corneal area, so-called "corneal burns," representing a thermal overload of the cornea, especially in the area of the phaco tunnel.

To reduce this, the pulsed technique was introduced. Depending on the manufacturer, this procedure is named differently. It works in such a way that the phaco tip oscillates briefly and then takes a short pause. This achieves, on the one hand, that the repelled nucleus fragment is re-aspirated to the phaco handpiece and further fragmented, and on the other hand, that cooling is generated by the fluid surrounding the tip. A further development of this pulsatile energy delivery is the torsional movement of the phaco tip. This is not a linear back-and-forth movement but a short rotational movement of the phaco tip. An oscillation of 5 to 10 degrees is achieved by the oscillation of the tip. This effect is particularly clinically relevant when the phaco tip used is angled and thus describes a kind of circular path. Through this technique, in combination with pulsed energy delivery, it is possible for the nucleus fragments to adhere to the phaco tip through suction and thus be fragmented. This results in fewer turbulences in the anterior chamber, and the lens parts to be fragmented float less. This technique overall leads to a reduction in thermal load while simultaneously improving lens fragmentation.

21.2.3 Femto-Phaco (Femtosecond Laser-Assisted Cataract Surgery [FLACS])

The operation of the clouded eye lens (cataract), with more than 20 million operations per year worldwide, is the most common procedure on humans. Due to the increasing life expectancy with rising population numbers and better medical care in developing countries, further increasing numbers of cataract surgeries are to be expected.

The lens operation, already performed in early antiquity, has experienced rapid innovation, especially in recent decades. This began with the implantation of the first artificial intraocular lens into a human eye by Sir Harold Ridley in 1949. Further milestones were the development of a continuous opening of the lens capsule by Neuhann and Gimbel and the introduction of ultrasound technology by Charles Kelman. With today's small incision technique, it is possible to insert foldable intraocular lenses through incisions of just under two millimeters at the corneal edge, which have also been available as multifocal optics since the mid-1990s.

With the application of femtosecond laser technology in the context of cataract surgery, another step towards an even safer and more precise operation is now being taken. Just as with Ridley and Kelman, there were initially intense discussions about the usefulness and benefits when this new technique was introduced by Nagy in 2008.

Meanwhile, however, there are many scientific publications that prove that the femtosecond laser makes new ways in cataract surgery possible.

Currently, there are five laser platforms from different manufacturers on the market. In all lasers, the device is coupled to the patient using a so-called patient interface. The fixation of the funnel-shaped suction ring to the patient's eye using a vacuum is similar to that of a Femto-LASIK (laser in situ keratomileusis).

After successful docking, either an OCT-based measurement is performed to create a treatment profile, or the necessary data is collected using Scheimpflug measurements. The planning software then allows various parameters, such as the location of the corneal incisions, the centering of the laser capsulotomy, the fragmentation pattern of the lens, as well as the length and depth of the keratotomies, to be varied according to the individual circumstances of the patient (Fig. 21.2).

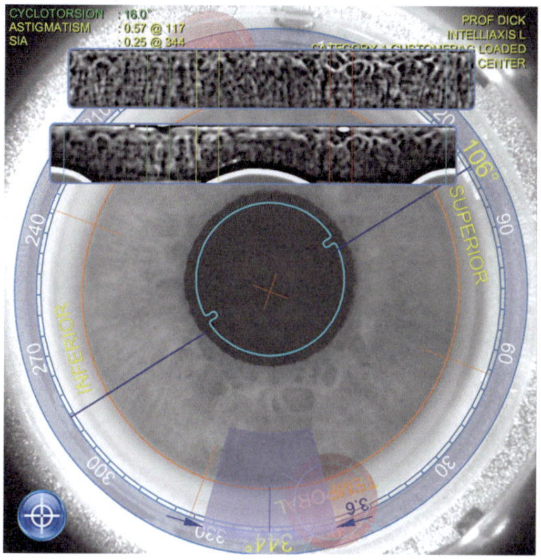

Fig. 21.2 Planning software LensAR. (With the kind permission of Ruhr University Bochum, Prof. Dr. med. Burghard Dick)

This technique enables a precision and reproducibility that was previously not achievable with the manual standard operation.

The use of femtosecond laser-assisted cataract surgery (FLACS) seems particularly sensible for eyes with an insufficient lens support apparatus, as the stress from manipulation on the loose zonular fibers is reduced. Hard nuclei also benefit from the use of the laser through the reduction of phaco energy. The predictability of the effective lens position can be improved by FLACS. This is made possible by the perfectly circular opening of the lens capsule with a uniformly overlapped optic edge and the centering of the laser capsulotomy on a desired target axis. This is especially important for premium lenses (multifocal lenses, toric intraocular lenses).

Novel lens designs are also made possible by the perfection of the laser and are already in use. With additional haptics at the edge of the optics, these lenses are suspended in the capsulotomy with the aim of reducing postoperative tilting, decentration, and rotation (Fig. 21.3).

With femtosecond laser-assisted astigmatic keratotomy (FSAK), it is also possible to safely treat astigmatism up to 1.5 diopters in the corneal area during cataract surgery.

The intraoperative alignment of toric intraocular lenses and the control of the postoperative position of the lens marking is made possible by a laser-created marking of the anterior capsule (Fig. 21.4).

With its accuracy and reproducibility, the femtosecond laser can contribute as part of modern cataract surgery to meeting the increased quality demands of patients, not only in terms of visual rehabilitation but also regarding safety, precision, and individuality.

21.3 Observerships

Erik Chankiewitz, Frank Wilhelm and Arne Viestenz

The word derived from the Latin word "hospitari" (to be a guest) has a very special significance for the training of ophthalmic surgeons. Unlike assistance (Latin "assistere", to support, to stand by), the observer has a purely passive role. The observer comes "as a guest" and receives "the gift of insight."

Why are observerships particularly important in ophthalmic surgery? Eye surgeries are mostly one-man operations, i.e., the surgeon is often the only one acting, making situational decisions and implementing them immediately. There is often no more experienced or/and learning assistant. Making decisions requires a lot of experience, which can be learned through observerships. Many techniques and tricks are not found in textbooks, and even in newer formats like surgical videos, often only the "ideal scenes" are edited together. During an observership, one learns about the real conditions and obstacles on the way to a perfect completion of the surgery. A surgeon can generally assume that he will take away new insights from every visit to another operating room. It is therefore advisable to take notes while watching the host operate and discuss them afterward. During the procedure, a discussion can only take place in exceptional cases—also considering the fact that most procedures in ophthalmology are performed under local anesthesia and a discussion with the surgeon could unsettle the patient.

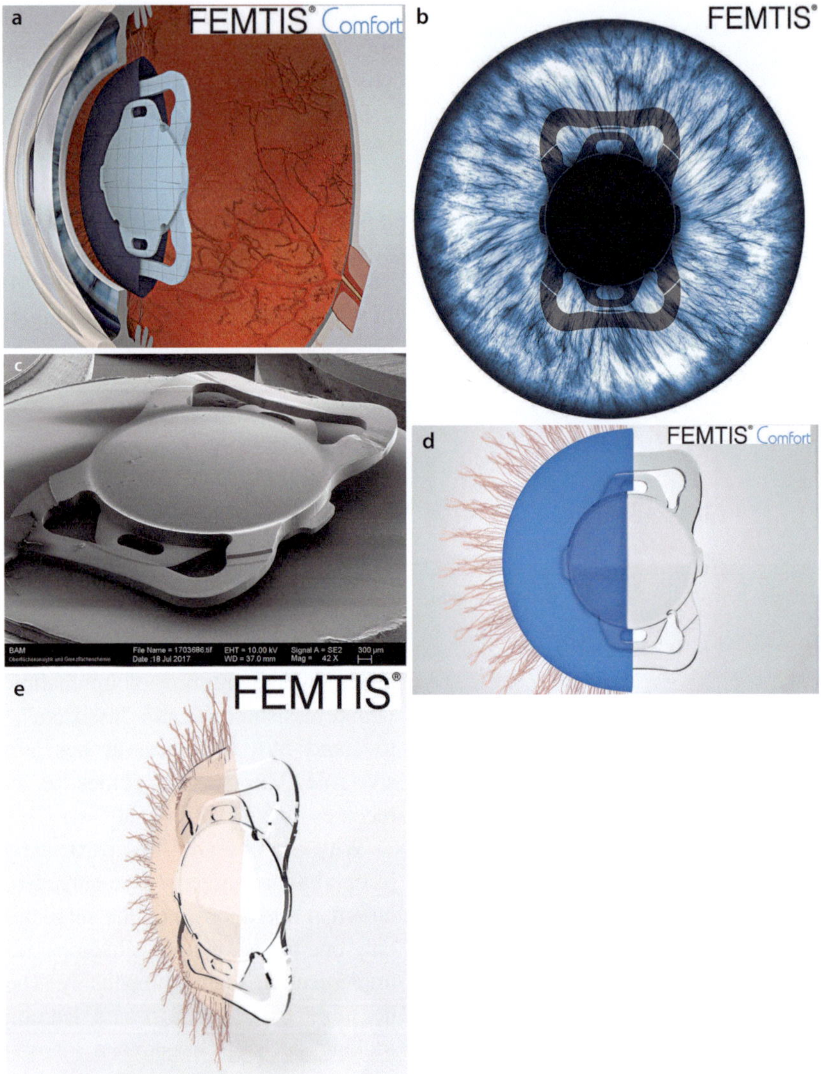

Fig. 21.3 (**a–g**) Femtis lens by Teleon

It has proven effective to learn a new surgical technique by watching an experienced colleague over the shoulder—through the co-observer. This also applies to the introduction of innovations (Section 21.2), such as intraocular lenses or devices. Here, representatives of the respective companies usually give recommendations and can arrange observerships with colleagues who have already established the new product.

Often, the less experienced individual is so impressed by a visit to another operating room that they want to change their entire concept. Here, the principle "less is more" applies, and if changes are made, they should be done gradually! This means that proven procedures should be maintained and then gradually changed in individual steps so that one can return to the established procedures without major problems if necessary.

The observership can take place at all levels and bring mutual insights to both experienced and inexperienced colleagues. Many observerships at the beginning of a training enable the young surgeon to better master difficult situations. One

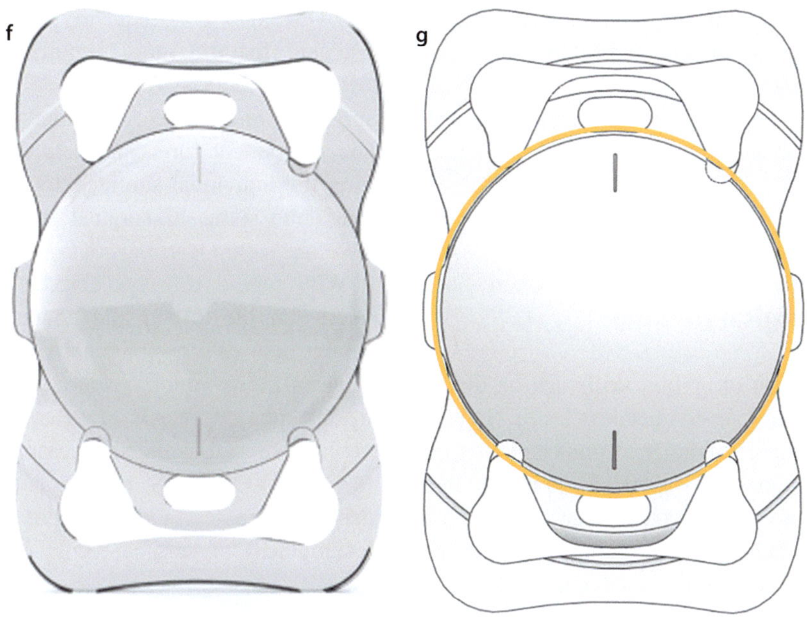

Fig. 21.3 (continued)

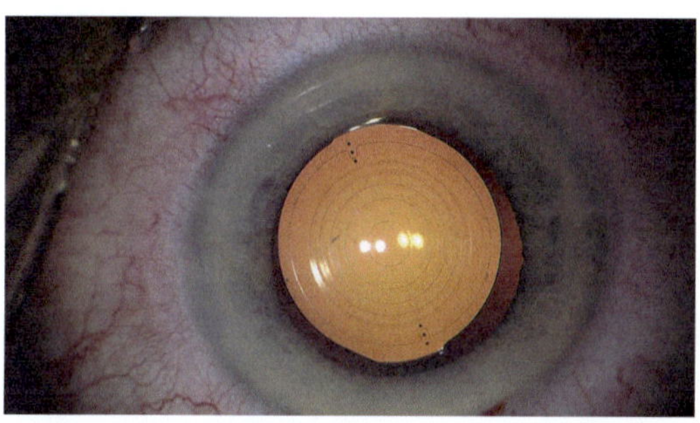

Fig. 21.4 Alignment of a toric intraocular lens with the capsule marking after measurement of the anterior segment of the eye

only pays attention to certain details after having performed some surgeries oneself.

Increasingly, observerships are contractually regulated to manage mutual claims. Usually, a request or even a small application letter precedes. Through the personnel department, the duration and location of the assignment and the liability insurance status are queried, and the observer is informed about confidentiality and behavior and must sign their consent.

Under German law, no tasks may be assigned to the observer, as this would then create a legal claim to a regular employment contract.

International observerships promote bidirectional knowledge transfer. During stays in less developed countries, simple techniques, solutions, and complication management are learned (Sect. 21.4). While observerships from developing societies provide an opportunity to establish modern techniques in the respective home countries.

21.4 Operating Abroad

Heiko Philippin, Karin Knoll, Martin Nentwich and Frank Wilhelm

Learning ophthalmic surgery involves alternating between theoretical training and practical steps. Both are shaped in form and content by cultural influences and national "habits." This is not limited to the surgical activity itself but is also evident, for example, in the composition of the surgical team, the handling of trainees, patients, and superiors or colleagues. Training and healthcare systems also differ in various countries. Therefore, a stay abroad can be very enriching. On the one hand, the characteristics of one's own training are more clearly perceived in a foreign environment, and on the other hand, the trainee can also learn from the strengths and weaknesses of other environments, not least other surgical techniques (Fig. 21.5).

21.4.1 Assessing the Status and Progress of One's Own Surgical Training

The acquisition of certain skills can be divided into five phases or competency levels (Dreyfus 1980): novice, beginner, competent, experienced surgeon, and expert. In practice, there are numerous variations of this classification, which are helpful for training planning and evaluation. For example, not only abroad, the ICO-OSCARS are frequently used, which are available for the most important ophthalmological procedures (OSCAR, "Ophthalmology Surgical Competence Assessment Rubric") [2]. The assessment forms are helpful for internalizing the individual surgical steps and can well assess the status of surgical training and also serve one's own learning control.

With regard to stays abroad, it should be noted that the timing and content of surgical training can differ significantly from those the trainee's home country, which is why specifying the training year is often not helpful. With the help of standardized assessment aids such as the ICO-OSCARS, trainers and mentors are also able to assess and document the status and development of surgical skills across national borders.

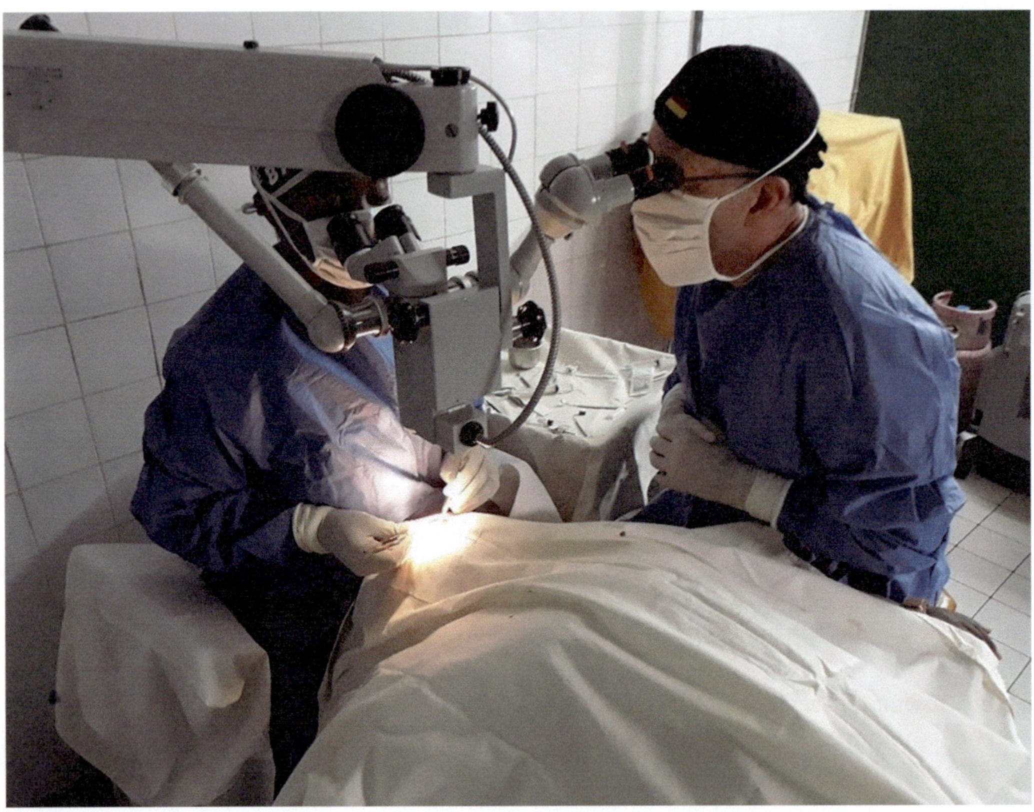

Fig. 21.5 Cameroon: Demonstration of regional surgical techniques during a mentor's visit. (Courtesy of Frank Wilhelm)

21.4.2 Planning a Stay Abroad

It is important to define fixed goals for planning and to allocate sufficient time for preparation.

Setting Goals for the Stay Abroad Planning begins with setting one's own expectations for a stay abroad within the framework of surgical training. Do you want to observe or be practically active? Learn a specific technique or broaden your general horizon? Depending on one's own training level, different goals are suitable (see also Table 21.2). Since learning ophthalmic surgery also significantly involves feedback from colleagues and observing experienced surgeons, both observations and practical training can be valuable. Especially after a certain basic level of surgical skills has been established, stays in a foreign environment become increasingly helpful, as the details of the operation are perceived more differentiatedly and tips can also be implemented more quickly and easily by the learner. Practical surgery usually requires a longer familiarization period and mutual acquaintance on site. An exception is short surgical courses offered for specific operations. These can vary greatly in price, quality, and adherence to ethical standards. It is usually worthwhile to first exchange ideas with colleagues who have recently completed such a course.

Planning Time for Preparation Performing surgery abroad usually requires a medical license, possibly additional professional liability insurance, and a work visa. The costs incurred must usually be borne by the intern. It is essential to inquire about the exact regulations on site and to allocate sufficient time for obtaining all documents. Often, about a year of lead time is required.

If possible, preparation with surgical videos in the respective local language is also recommended to learn the relevant technical terms in advance.

21.4.3 Operating Abroad

Once all the hurdles in preparation are overcome and one stands for the first time in the new operative environment, a very instructive and enriching time usually begins.

Every eye clinic has its own operating culture, and abroad, national regulations and customs additionally determine the atmosphere and procedures in the operating room. This starts with the size and task distribution of the operating team, the handling of patients, extends to the way feedback is given, and also includes specific surgical techniques. National professional societies also have a significant influence on the frequency and preference of various surgical techniques. It is always worthwhile to look beyond the national horizon, also to learn from the mistakes and successes of others.

A particularly favorable circumstance is when the mentor and the less experienced

Table 21.2 Different Stages of Surgical Training. There are mixed forms

Competence	Definition	Aspects
Novice	First steps learned, but still requires constant supervision	Short internships of a few weeks for general familiarization are useful. Practical training is most feasible in structured training programs and should be clearly agreed upon.
Beginner	Can independently perform the entire operation but still frequently needs support	Observing various surgeons in different clinics and countries is useful, as the surgical steps and their fine variations are already perceived. Practical training is rather difficult, usually requiring a long stay of 3–12 months.
Competent	Performs the operation independently and rarely needs support	Practical training is possible during a longer stay to deepen existing knowledge. Short observations are often sufficient to learn new techniques and subsequently apply them.
Expert	Operates independently with a lot of experience, teaches other surgeons	Benefits from observing other experienced colleagues. Acting as a trainer is possible, especially with regular assignments conducted over years.

colleague already know each other from mutual visits. Then the experienced mentor can better address the regional peculiarities during surgical training [8].

Examples of different variants of common surgical techniques are sutureless extracapsular cataract extraction ("sutureless ECCE") or releasable sutures in trabeculectomy. In these cases, adapted ICO-OSCARS can also be used for teaching and learning control.

21.4.4 Examples of Internationally Common Surgical Variants

The general course of a specific operation is usually fixed. However, regarding the small details, there are often many ways that can be taken. Since only relatively few of these individual steps are compared in randomized studies, much surgical practice is based on experience and traditional knowledge. This knowledge can be expanded through videos, but it is best learned by observing experienced surgeons or by independent operating under direct supervision.

Sutureless Extracapsular Cataract Extraction

Introduction

Sutureless extracapsular cataract extraction ("sutureless extracapsular cataract extraction", ECCE) is an advancement of the classic ECCE. It is widespread in many countries with a high number of patients with advanced cataracts. Additionally, the costs of the procedure can be kept low, as the purchase and maintenance as well as consumables of a phacoemulsification unit are eliminated, and PMMA intraocular lenses can be used. The surgical technique is a sensible option for any cataract surgeon in difficult situations, such as with a very hard lens nucleus.

Steps of Sutureless Extracapsular Cataract Surgery

1. Surgical preparation including peribulbar anesthesia and sterile draping
2. After inserting the lid speculum, a superior rectus muscle fixation suture may be placed, especially in deep-set eyes
3. Peritomy of the conjunctiva along the limbus over four clock hours and hemostasis
4. Scleral incision and preparation of a scleral corneal tunnel up to 1–1.5 mm into the clear cornea, without opening the anterior chamber yet
5. Paracentesis, filling the anterior chamber with viscoelastic
6. Completing the scleral corneal tunnel into the anterior chamber
7. Capsulotomy with the curved tip of a 26G needle, can-opener or envelope
8. Hydrodissection and dislocation of the lens nucleus into the anterior chamber
9. Extraction of the lens, e.g., with a lens loop or in fishhook technique
10. Removal of cortex and epinucleus remnants with the Simcoe irrigation/aspiration cannula
11. Implantation of the intraocular lens into the posterior chamber
12. Irrigation and aspiration
13. With correct tunnel construction, it self-seals in small incision techniques, so no suture is required. If the tunnel is not tight, a suture must be placed.

Trabeculectomy with Releasable Scleral Flap Sutures

The trabeculectomy is significantly less standardized than cataract surgery (Fig. 21.6). The application of Mitomycin C, scleral flap sutures, or conjunctival sutures of the filtering bleb are performed in various ways in different clinics and by different surgeons. A globally frequently

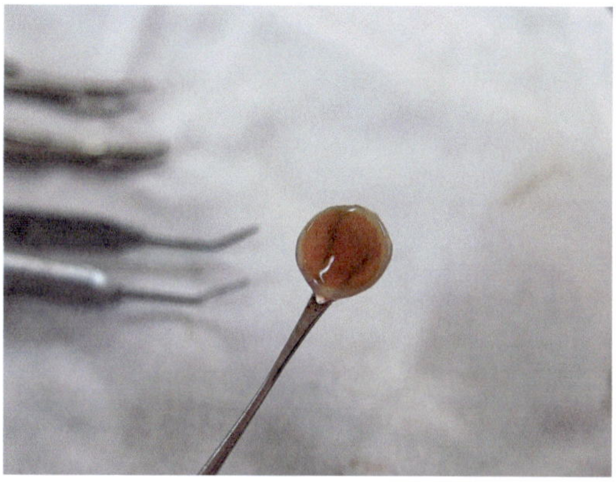

Fig. 21.6 Tanzania: A mature lens nucleus can be gently removed using sutureless extracapsular cataract extraction, here with a "lens loop". (Courtesy of Heiko Philippin)

used variant in the procedure of trabeculectomy (Fig. 21.7) is the use of releasable sutures instead of single knotted sutures to fix the scleral flap. In this case, a loop is knotted instead of a single thread. One end of this loop runs through the peripheral cornea. If the intraocular pressure is too high in the early postoperative phase within the first month, one or both threads can be easily pulled at the slit lamp with a needle and forceps, without the need for a laser and without leaving thread remnants in the tissue [10, 11].

Internet Resource For many surgeries performed worldwide, helpful resources can be found on the internet. Many surgeons offer videos that provide a good overview of surgical

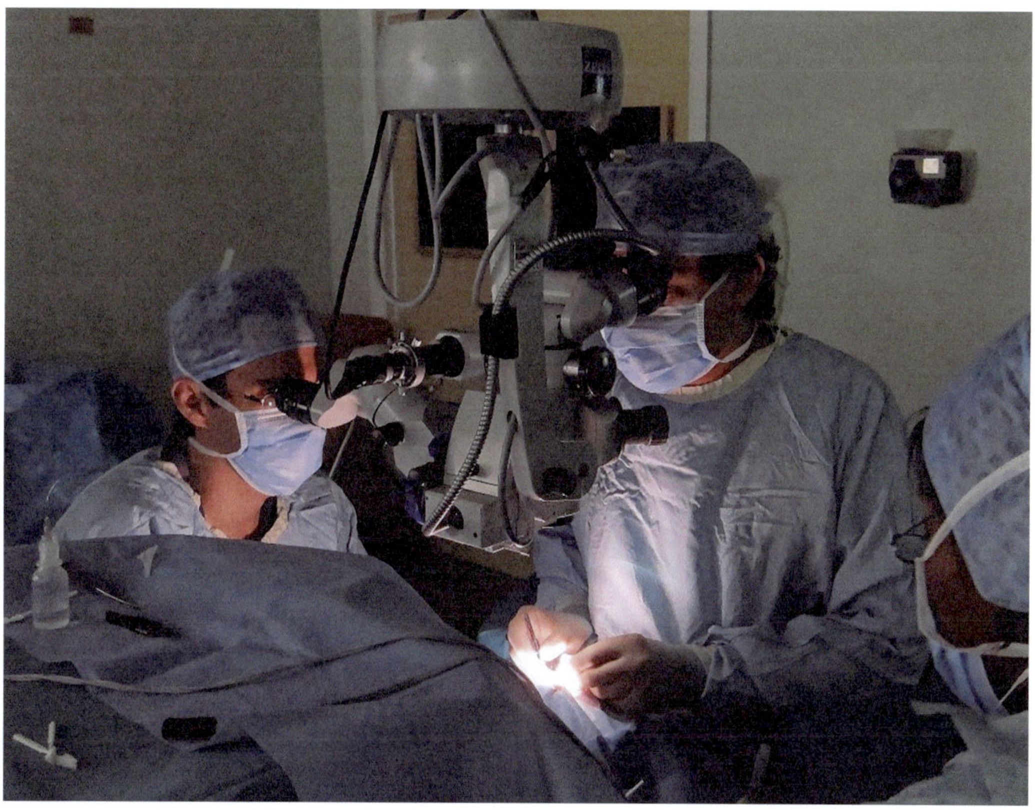

Fig. 21.7 United Kingdom: Observing a trabeculectomy with releasable scleral flap sutures during an international fellowship. (Courtesy of Heiko Philippin)

techniques and their differences. A free option for ophthalmological online training in general and specifically for global surgical techniques is "Cybersight" by Orbis (www.cybersight.org). The platform offers courses on, for example, phacoemulsification and sutureless ECCE ("sutureless ECCE").

References and Further Reading

1. Ahr WM (2021) Frühe Nachsorge nach unkomplizierter Kataraktoperation. Z prakt Augenheilkd 42:83–95; Dreyfus SE (2004) The five-stage model of adult skill acquisition. Bull Sci Technol Soc 24:177–181
2. Golnik KC, Beaver H, Gauba V, Lee AG, Mayorga E, Palis G et al (2011) Cataract surgical skill assessment. Ophthalmology 118:427.e1–427.e5
3. Holzwig DH (1997) Irisretraktor, ein Teilschritt in der Kataraktchirurgie bei engen Pupillen. In: 11. Kongress der Deutschsprachigen Gesellschaft für Intraokularlinsen-Implantation und refraktive Chirurgie. Springer, Berlin/Heidelberg, S 232–237
4. Kohnen S (2012) Kataraktchirurgie: Komplikationsmanagement bei Inzision und Kapseleröffnung. Ophthalmo Chir 24:147–154
5. Kohnen S (2016) Komplikationsmanagement in der Kataraktchirurgie: Linsensubluxation und Zonulolyse. Ophthalmo Chir 28:117–120
6. Pham DT (2016) Komplikationen bei der Intraokularlinsen-Implantation. Ophthalmo Chir 28:123–128
7. Pham DT (2017) Spätkomplikationen bei der Intraokularlinsen-Implantation. Z prakt Augenheilkd 38:64–68
8. Sachsenweger M (1990) Augenheilkunde in den Tropen. Gustav-Fischer, Stuttgart/New York, S 206s
9. Wirbelauer C, Schmidt S, Puk C (2018) Mechanische Pupillenerweiterung mit Ringen zur Kataraktoperation bei enger Pupille. Ophthalmologe 115:329–335
10. Zhou M, Wang W, Huang W, Zhang X (2014) Trabeculectomy with versus without releasable sutures for glaucoma: a meta-analysis of randomized controlled trials. BMC Ophthalmol 14:1–8
11. Khaw PT, Chiang M, Shah P, Sii F, Lockwood A, Khalili A. Enhanced Trabeculectomy – The Moorfields Safer Surgery System. Dev Ophthalmol. 2012;50:1–28.

MIX
Papier aus verantwortungsvollen Quellen
Paper from responsible sources
FSC® C105338

If you have any concerns about our products,
you can contact us on
ProductSafety@springernature.com

In case Publisher is established outside the EU,
the EU authorized representative is:
Springer Nature Customer Service Center GmbH
Europaplatz 3, 69115 Heidelberg, Germany

Printed by Libri Plureos GmbH
in Hamburg, Germany